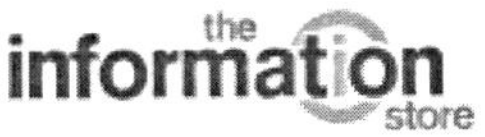
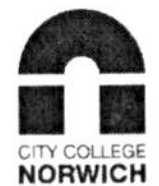

THIRD EDITION

THE **COMPLETE GUIDE** TO

FOOD FOR SPORTS PERFORMANCE

A GUIDE TO PEAK NUTRITION FOR **YOUR** SPORT

Dr LOUISE BURKE & GREG COX

ALLEN&UNWIN

First published in 2010

Allen & Unwin
83 Alexander Street
Crows Nest NSW 2065
Australia
Phone: (61 2) 8425 0100
Fax: (61 2) 9906 2218
Email: info@allenandunwin.com
Web: www.allenandunwin.com

Cataloguing-in-Publication details are available from the National Library of Australia
www.librariesaustralia.nla.gov.au

ISBN 978 1 74114 390 4

Text and cover design by Emily O'Neill
Illustrations by Ian Faulkner
Typeset in 11/14pt Granjon by Post Pre-press Group
Printed and bound in Australia by Griffin Press

10 9 8 7 6 5 4 3 2 1

For John and Jack,
(dreaming of the day that Jack kicks the winning goal
in the Saint's elusive premiership)

To Jen, Seb amd Izzy,
life will always be full and 'rockin' in our family

FOREWORD

by Nathan Deakes,
2007 World Champion in the 50km Road Walk

As an elite athlete, my eating habits are as important as each training session. After all, I wouldn't be able to complete my arduous workload without fueling my body correctly for both recovery and performance. Whilst dietary needs and demands are different for each sport and discipline, one constant does exist—the need to be vigilant and conscious of both food intake and quality on an individual basis.

Sports nutrition has developed greatly over the years. Stories of infamous pre-competition meals of steak and eggs are now replaced by carefully managed carbohydrate and amino acid intakes as witnessed in Tour de France cyclists. Today's high performing athletes are more aware of the benefits of carefully structuring their food and fluid intakes to enhance daily training, assist recovery and optimise competition performance. The field of sports nutrition is the most innovative and dynamic of all sport sciences. It makes perfect sense to be well informed in this very specialised field.

The Complete Guide to Food for Sports Performance provides an up-to-date, informative insight into various sports for athletes, coaches and administrators alike. Raising functional issues and providing practical advice, this book imparts sensible, no-nonsense guidance to help athletes gain that extra edge for peak performance.

Throughout my career, I have worked closely with both Louise and Greg as my sports dietitians, and I congratulate them on producing the third edition of *The Complete Guide to Food for Sports Performance*. I encourage every athlete, regardless of their level, to have a copy on their bookshelves.

CONTENTS

CHECKLISTS

CASE HISTORIES AND PROFILES

TABLES

FIGURES

ACKNOWLEDGEMENTS

This book is a product of our opportunities and environment at the Australian Institute of Sport. As Keith Lyons, our colourful friend and colleague, has pointed out, there is a collective experience of over 1000 years of work with athletes between the sports science and sports medicine professionals at the AIS. We couldn't have developed the expertise needed to write this book without the passion, motivation and generosity of our co-workers. Allan Hahn, Chris Gore, Kieran Fallon, Craig Purdam, Nick Brown, Bruce Mason, Damian Farrow and Julian Jones are the leaders of inspiring teams, and we thank them for driving the engine-room. We wish there was space to name all our daily collaborators from these areas. Let's just say that excellence and friendship comes in many guises—from the 'Eveready Bunny Genius' of Dave Martin to the 'Quiet Achiever' of David Pyne and the 'Closet Type A' of Peter Blanch. It's probably a good career move to single out our bosses—Peter Fricker is now the Fearless Leader of the Australian Institute of Sport, and Mark Peters was the Big Boss of the Australian Sports Commission while Dennis Hatcher was our first-line supporter while we updated this edition. We thank them for their moral and financial support for our work, and we look forward to working with our new bosses, Phil Borgeaud and Matt Miller.

Sports Nutrition at the AIS has been a thriving outfit since 1990, and we thank the members of our team, past (Benita Lalor, Gary Slater, Michelle Cort, Bethanie Allanson, Ruth Crawford, Michelle Minehan, Sofie Modulon, Nikki Cummings, Liz Williams, Mareeta Grundy, Prue Jackson, Ben Desbrow, Louise Bell, Lesley Irvine, Natasha Porter,

Kelly Meredith, Nick Petrunoff, Andrea Braakhuis, Claire Wood, Liv Warnes, Katherine Cook, Gail Cox, Maz Dickson, Kim Horne, Tracy Protas, Louise Baker, Emma Harriden, Vinni Dang, Mary Martin and Amanda Spratt) and present (Liz Broad, Nikki Jeacocke, Greg Shaw, Stephen Gurr, Christine Dziedzic, Jo Mirtschin and Lynne Mercer). Thanks for all you have done to make us look good.

Many colleagues from outside the AIS have directly and indirectly contributed to the information in this book. Again, there are too many to mention by name, but our colleagues from Sports Dietitians Australia and the newly formed PINES group make us confident that sports nutrition is in the right hands in Australia and around the world.

Finally, we are lucky that our coalface allows us to work with many of the most talented and hard-working coaches and athletes in Australia. Thanks for allowing us to share the highs and lows of your efforts to be the best that you can be.

Louise Burke and Greg Cox

INTRODUCTION

There have been exponential improvements in the science and practice of sports nutrition since the second edition of this book was released in 1995. Australia achieved its best results ever as host of the 2000 Olympic Games in Sydney, then defied tradition by reaching even greater heights at the 2004 Athens Olympics. Many factors contributed, but we like to think that the increasing role of sports dietitians in the preparation of our teams played a role. Certainly, recognition of sports nutrition's role has grown on our shores, through the work of groups such as Sports Dietitians Australia, and internationally through activities such as the launch of the International Olympic Committee Diploma of Sports Nutrition and the formation of Professionals in Exercise and Sports Nutrition (PINES). Of course, it is much easier to spread knowledge and practice guidelines via the Information Superhighway. It is hard to believe that the second edition of this book was written without the backdrop of the Internet, email, videoconferencing, and universal use of iPods, mobile phones, wireless and digital electronic connections . . . How did we ever operate back then?

What have been the major changes in sports nutrition over the past fifteen years? A number of expert groups have issued or reissued guidelines for the nutrition of athletes. These include the American College of Sports Medicine (Nutrition for athletes—2009; Creatine—2000; Fluid replacement—2007; Female athlete triad—2007); the International Olympic Committee (Nutrition for sport—2003); Fédération Internationale de Football Association (FIFA) (Nutrition for football—2005) and International Association of Athletics Federations (IAAF) (Nutrition for Athletics—2007). The major theme from the most recent scientific investigations and practice guidelines is a recognition of the individuality of each athlete's nutritional needs. No longer is it sufficient to promote a 'one size fits all' approach to sports nutrition. We now recognise that each sport has specific physiological, cultural and practical issues and that these create a backdrop of special nutritional needs for that sport. We also recognise that each athlete within a sport has his or her own special blend of nutritional needs and challenges, which change over a season and a career. This is true for both the elite competitor and the weekend warrior. Whichever end of the spectrum they come from, athletes will benefit from dietary strategies that allow them to train hard, adapt and recover quickly, stay healthy, achieve their ideal physique, then perform at their best in the competition arena. Today's sports nutrition climate promotes individual case management, based on finding practical ways to achieve guidelines that are underpinned by sound science.

The Complete Guide to Nutrition for Sports Performance was ahead of its time in taking a practical and individual approach to sports nutrition. This third edition continues that theme—transforming science into practice, then taking a real-life look at the special nutritional needs and lifestyles of various sports. We hope that past and new readers will use this very latest information to achieve their goals in sport.

Metric units are used throughout the book:

1 kilogram (kg)	= 2.2 pounds
100 grams (g)	= 3.5 oz.
250 g	= 8.8 oz.
1 litre (L)	= 35 fl. oz.
100 millilitres (ml)	= 3.5 fl. oz.
1 kilojoule (kJ)	= 0.24 kilocalories

While the metric unit for energy is the kilojoule, people are often still familiar with the old unit of the Calorie. Since energy is a basic issue in nutrition, it is useful to be able to understand the range of ways in which it may be described:

1000 kilojoules (kJ)	= 1 megajoule (MJ)
1 kilocalorie (kcal)	= 1 Calorie (Cal)
1 kilocalorie	= 4.2 kJ

Part I

PRINCIPLES OF SPORTS NUTRITION

1
Training nutrition: The principles of everyday eating

To many people, sports nutrition is about carbo-loading for a competition, or having the latest sports food or supplement. However, the 'big-ticket item' with the most potential to influence your sports performance is your training diet. On the basis of time alone, your training diet is the aspect of your total nutrition most likely to make an impact on your body. It also lays the groundwork that is critical to your long-term success. Everyday eating must keep you healthy and uninjured, and in top shape for your sport. And it must support you through all the training that is needed to get you to the starting line or opening bounce.

Daily training creates special nutritional needs for an athlete, particularly the elite athlete whose training commitment is almost a full-time job. But even recreational sport will create nutritional challenges. And whatever your level of involvement in sport, you must meet these challenges if you're to achieve the maximum return from training. Without sound eating, much of the purpose of your training might be lost. In the worst-case scenario, dietary problems and deficiencies may directly impair training performance. In other situations, you might improve, but at a rate that is below your potential or slower than your competitors. However, on the positive side, with the right everyday eating plan your commitment to training will be fully rewarded.

So what does a successful training diet look like? There is no perfect combination of foods or single eating plan that will meet the nutritional challenges of every athlete. When you read Part II of this book, you will find that nutritional needs and interests vary between sports. Imagine trying to find a single menu to encompass the food likes and dislikes, not to mention the lifestyles, of all athletes! While the focus and details will differ from one athlete to the next, there are certain goals that are common to all sports. Checklist 1.1 will help you to rate the success of your training diet. If you are achieving all these goals with your everyday eating plan, then congratulate yourself for having achieved peak training nutrition.

Obviously, peak training nutrition doesn't happen by chance. Before you can branch into the special and individual areas of sports nutrition, you must start with some general principles, based on the common ground shared by all athletes. Once you have a structure in place, you can fine-tune your eating plan to respond to your particular nutritional needs and dietary goals. At each level, knowing more about what is in food and how to select and prepare it will give you more control over what you eat. You can choose to meet your dietary challenges in ways that are both enjoyable to you and complementary to your busy schedule. So let's start with the basic principles.

1.1 Enjoy a variety of food

Most countries have a set of dietary guidelines, and most begin with a recommendation to 'eat a variety of foods every day'. Some qualify this, saying, 'eat a variety of nutrient-dense foods every day'. Others have even quantified this information—the old Japanese guidelines recommended that we 'eat at least thirty different foods each day'. But what does variety really mean, and why does it come up over and over as the No. 1 nutrition recommendation?

We tend to take an overly simplistic view of the food we eat, focusing on one or two nutrients, such as iron, cholesterol or sugar. One side-effect of this habit is that we pin labels on food—for example, we might believe that yoghurt is 'good' for us while chocolate is 'bad'. In fact, it's the way we use food that determines whether it's a good or bad choice in assisting us to meet our specific nutrition goals. This depends on what we are trying to achieve and what else we eat over the course of the day. For instance, a banana mega-smoothie might be a great afternoon snack for a hungry basketball player with high energy (kilojoule) needs. But it would blow the kilojoule budget of a tiny gymnast, and wouldn't be well tolerated by a runner at the 30-km mark of a marathon. The real value of a food needs to be judged in context. This is a key theme that we will return to many times in this book.

One of the problems with the simplistic branding of foods as 'good' and 'bad' is that it can lead to narrow and rigid eating. Some people try to follow a 'good diet' by giving up all the foods they consider 'bad'. Athletes are particularly skilled at this because they are motivated (often obsessively so) and good at self-discipline. It takes mental toughness to stare at a black line on the bottom of a pool for hours on end, or to run kilometre after kilometre in the zone—and this focus can easily be extended to breakfast, lunch and dinner. Of course, other factors such as fussy eating, real or perceived food intolerances, poor domestic skills and a tight budget can all lead to a narrow, unvarying diet.

To understand what is at stake, we need to appreciate how marvellously complex our food really is. Nutrients and food chemicals do not exist in isolation and are not consumed that way. There is more to an orange than vitamin C, and more to meat than protein. What's more, each food is greater than the sum of its components, because the chemicals in a food interact with each other and with the chemicals in other foods eaten at the same time. Although some popular diet books have spread the myth that certain foods shouldn't be eaten in combination, the truth is that the nutritional quality of a meal is often improved by mixing and matching foods. For example, the iron in cereal foods is better absorbed in the presence of vitamin C, making a glass of orange juice a clever accompaniment to your breakfast cereal.

An emerging theme in nutrition is the recognition that we have barely begun to learn about the full range of chemical and physical properties of food. To paraphrase the former US Secretary of Defense, Donald Rumsfeld, our food is full of 'known unknowns' and 'unknown unknowns' as well as all the things we do know about. We often discover that a certain group of people enjoys unusually good health or a low risk of developing the diseases of ageing—for example, cancer, diabetes, high blood pressure and cardiovascular diseases. This is often attributed to their dietary patterns—for example, the fact that they eat lots of fruits and vegetables or certain types of oils. We next jump to the conclusion that the health benefit comes from a well-known nutrient found in these singled-out foods, and that we could share this benefit by taking the nutrient in pill or powdered form. After all, it's much simpler to pop a pill to stay healthy than to make radical changes to your eating. The problem with this logic is that joining the dots so crudely skates over the complexity of all those unknowns in the original food supply.

Newspapers and scientific journals continue to report on our identification of ranges of antioxidants and active ingredients in plant foods—often termed 'phytochemicals' or 'phytonutrients'. Table 1.1 provides a list of just some of these chemicals—within each category, there may be hundreds of individual compounds. While supplements and functional foods (foods to which some special ingredients are added) can contribute to nutritional goals, at this stage they lag well behind the genius of Mother Nature. In the future, with improved knowledge, we may be able to unravel some of her mysteries to make firm recommendations about these phytonutrients. For the moment, enjoying a wide variety of nutrient-dense foods, both in your general diet and at each meal, provides the best way to sample a little of everything food has to offer.

Seen from another angle, consuming a varied diet is 'eating in moderation'. Harmful substances can occur naturally in foods (e.g. the poison solanine, which occurs in green sprouting potatoes) as well as being overrepresented in manufactured foods (e.g. the unhealthy 'trans' fatty acids which arise when vegetable oils are processed). Since the nutritional problems in countries such as Australia and the United States are linked mostly to overconsumption of dietary compounds, eating a wide variety of foods is a good way to keep your intake of all food components within healthy bounds. The nutrition education campaigns in most countries still feature a pictorial model of a healthy diet—such as a pyramid or triangle or food plate—in which different types of foods can be arranged with the priority on 'most of what you need' topped off by 'a little of what you fancy'.

Last, but by no means least, a varied diet offers greater opportunities for flexibility, enjoyment and adventure with food. Newer dietary guidelines in many countries make a definite point of promoting the experience of eating. For example, the new Japanese guidelines urge people to 'have delicious and healthy meals that are good for your mind and body; enjoy communication at the table with your family and other people, and participate in the preparation of meals'. It might seem strange that government departments feel the need to formally promote these ideas. However, in many countries, it is a sad reality that each succeeding generation has less exposure to family mealtimes, learning to cook, understanding food composition or appreciating the food culture of the preceding generation. Use Checklist 1.2 to ensure that you are maximising the benefits of variety.

1.2 Eat the right type and amount of fats and oils

In the old days we simply said 'eat less fats and oils', based on the observation that the typical Australian diet contains more fat than is necessary or healthy. The direct benefits of cutting back on fats include promoting healthy weight or weight loss and reducing the risk of some lifestyle diseases. Indirect benefits include making room in the energy budget for some more valuable foods and nutrients. Nutrition guidelines recommend that total average fat intake be reduced by a quarter, to less than 30 per cent of total energy. For people needing to reduce body fat, a further reduction to 20–25 per cent of intake may help to reduce total energy intake. But guidelines for a lower average fat intake were never meant to promote a 'no-fat' intake. After all, fats and oils are widely distributed in foods and have many benefits. They provide a concentrated source of energy, and they make meals tasty, satisfying and rich in texture. They also supply essential fatty acids and fat-soluble vitamins, which are important to health. We need a minimum of 20–40 g (1–2 tablespoons) of the right fats each day to get enough of these nutrients.

Newer nutrition guidelines target not just the total *amount* of fat in our diets, but also the *types* of fats and oils we eat. Depending on their chemical structure, different fats have different effects on your weight, on how well your body responds to insulin, and on blood fat and cholesterol levels. Unfortunately, most of us overeat the 'unhealthy' fats and undereat the 'healthy' ones. The fats we overconsume are the saturated types and trans fatty acids. Saturated fats come mostly from animal sources such as meat and dairy foods, but they are also found in coconut and palm oils. Because these oils are perfect for many aspects of food manufacture, they end up in deep-fried foods, pastry items, confectionery, biscuits and snack foods. Many of us fail to recognise the high fat content of such foods, or we mistake it as being healthy because the oil is labelled as a vegetable one. Trans fats occur naturally in small amounts in meat and dairy foods, but they are also artificially created when polyunsaturated and monounsaturated fats undergo processing (hydrogenation) during food manufacture. As a result, these fats are overrepresented in diets high in processed foods. Both saturated and trans fats increase the unhealthy type of blood cholesterol known as LDL (low density lipoprotein) cholesterol while trans fats also decrease the healthy cholesterol known as HDL. Our efforts to reduce our intake of fats and oils should focus on the unsaturated types.

The preferred fats are polyunsaturated and monounsaturated. Monounsaturated fats are found in many vegetable oils and animal fats, but the richest sources are olives/olive oil, peanuts/peanut oil, other nuts, canola oils and avocadoes. These fats have a small lowering effect on LDL cholesterol levels and do not appear to be as 'fattening' as their advertised kilojoule content. Polyunsaturated fats come in various forms and have favourable effects on blood fat levels. One family, known as the omega-3s, is found in a small number of vegetable oils, such as canola and linseed, and in larger amounts in oily fish. Some functional foods with added omega-3s are also appearing on our supermarket shelves. Omega-3 fats appear to offer a range of health benefits—lowering blood fat levels and blood pressure, reducing the build-up of fatty deposits in blood vessels and blood clots, and preventing irregular heart rhythms. They may also have beneficial effects on immune and inflammatory diseases such as asthma, eczema, psoriasis, rheumatoid arthritis and inflammatory bowel disease. There is also encouraging news linking omega-3s to improved insulin sensitivity and lowered risk of diabetes, along with better brain functioning and maintenance.

Another group of polyunsaturated fats is the omega-6 series, found in the majority of vegetable oils (safflower, sunflower), as well as wholegrain cereals and nuts. Although they have a positive effect on blood fat levels, they are structural competitors to the omega-3 series and may counteract their effects—for example, by increasing inflammation. Unfortunately, we now consume a diet heavily skewed to omega-6 fatty acids rather than the omega-3 family, so nutritional guidelines promote a better balance by increasing intake of the first and reducing intake of the second. Checklist 1.3 provides strategies to achieve all the guidelines related to fats and oils.

While athletes need to think about eating for their future health (life does go on after the Olympic Games!), they are understandably more interested in the here and now, specifically, the role of dietary fat in sports performance. The traditional view on this front is that although dietary fats and oils are the most concentrated source of food energy, they do not provide the major source of fuel for exercising muscles. Instead, body carbohydrate stores provide the critical energy source for strenuous activity. These, however, are limited in size. Body fat stores, on the other hand, are in plentiful supply even in the leanest of athletes, and could provide fatty acids for hours and days of exercise. From time to time, interest is rekindled in making endurance and ultra-endurance athletes more effective at burning body fat as a muscle fuel by adapting them to high-fat diets. This strategy will be discussed in more detail in the next chapter, but at this stage it doesn't appear to have much to offer the majority of athletes. In fact, a high fat intake could be of disservice to an athlete if it displaces carbohydrates whose kilojoules were needed to meet muscle fuel needs.

Fat intake can have an indirect effect on sports performance. Fats and oils have twice the energy density of protein and carbohydrate—that is, more than twice the kilojoules per mouthful. This means that it is easy to overshoot your daily energy requirements with a diet based on fatty foods, especially in a food culture that encourages large servings and frequent eating. What's more, there is some evidence that diets high in saturated and trans fats are especially efficient at increasing body-fat stores. On the other hand, a switch to lower-fat eating can help to reduce body-fat levels or protect you from gaining body fat, since you have to eat more mouthfuls to meet your energy needs. Of course, as we will see in the next section, this principle doesn't work if you simply replace fat with other energy-dense foods or unnecessarily large portions of low-fat foods.

1.3 Eat the right amount of nutrient-dense carbohydrate foods

If the messages regarding fats and oils needed fine-tuning, then it's fair to say that the carbohydrate message has required an overhaul. When the original guidelines that promoted a higher carbohydrate intake were released, nutrition experts had in mind that people would eat more wholesome, fibre- and nutrient-rich foods such as wholegrain breads and cereals, fruits and vegetables to replace their reduced intake of foods high in saturated fats. We expected benefits in terms of better fuel intake for active people, lower food-energy density to assist with weight control, and overall improvements in nutrient density (more vitamins and minerals per mouthful). We didn't anticipate that the food industry would respond with a huge array of low-fat carbohydrate-rich foods, or that consumers would respond by eating them in such huge amounts. Some of these foods (e.g. low-fat versions of yoghurt and flavoured milk) might offer good nutrient value, but they weren't always lower in kilojoule content, since extra sugar kilojoules often replaced most of the lost fat ones. In other cases, a low-fat label gave people an excuse to eat carbohydrate-rich foods with limited nutritional value in extra-large portions. Think buckets of 97 per cent fat-free ice-cream, jumbo low-fat muffins, family-size packets of 'natural' no-fat confectionery. No wonder the proposed health benefits of high-carbohydrate eating didn't eventuate. No wonder we got fatter. No wonder the next phase was a return in popularity of low-carbohydrate and moderate-carbohydrate diets.

But even if the high-carb eating of the 1990s didn't benefit everyone, surely athletes were better off? After all, the critical source of fuel for exercising muscles comes from your body's carbohydrate stores—blood glucose (a small amount), and glycogen stored in the liver and muscles (larger stores, but sufficient only for up to 90 minutes of moderate to high-intensity exercise). Against this background, you would think that athletes would benefit from carbohydrate loading 24/7. Think again. The problem with this idea is that it treats all athletes as having the same high fuel requirements and a large energy budget. This isn't the case. In the second section of this book we will find plenty of examples of athletes with low to moderate fuel needs and a focus on weight control.

Our latest guidelines still recommend that Australians should allow nutrient-rich carbohydrate foods to make up around half of their total energy intake. However, there is now greater recognition that carbohydrates shouldn't be considered a bottomless well, and that the quality of carbohydrate-rich food choices is important. Even in sports nutrition, many dietitians avoid using the term 'high-carbohydrate diet' because of the way it has been misinterpreted by athletes and coaches. 'Targeted' carbohydrate eating is probably a better term since it implies matching intake to daily fuel needs. In fact, some Australians, including some athletes, do need to cut back on their intake of certain carbohydrate-rich foods.

Does this mean that lower-carb eating plans are here to stay? Those of us who've been in nutrition for a long time know that ideas are constantly recycled and the present fashions will probably disappear, only to be reinvented further down the track. There are good lessons in some of the diets based on moderate-carbohydrate eating (e.g. the CSIRO diet), although many athletes will need to adjust such plans to increase their intake of fuel foods. On the other hand, the Atkins diet and other strict low-carb diets will not cure the world's nutrition problems or provide a long-term solution to obesity and overweight. In fact, they suffer from some of the same problems that 'sunk' the high-carb movement—people take them to extremes, use them to justify eating food with low nutrient content, and fail to understand what sensible portion sizes really are. More information on this will be provided in a case history in the second part of this book.

Whatever our carbohydrate target is, we need to think carefully about the types of foods and drinks we use to reach it. We used to think about carbohydrates based on structure—'simple' carbohydrates (or sugars) of one or two molecules, or 'complex' carbohydrates (or starches) made up of thousands of sugar molecules joined together. The sugars were allegedly the bad guys, causing tooth decay, shooting blood-sugar levels up and down, and failing to provide vitamins and minerals. The complex carbohydrates were the good guys, reversing all these problems. Thankfully, we have moved on from this to a less black-and-white view. There are many features of carbohydrate-rich foods that could be considered, but for the purposes of sports nutrition we will focus on three: total nutritional value, effect on blood glucose and practical issues. Many 'ready reckoners' of carbohydrate-rich foods, like the one in Chapter 2, show the total amount of carbohydrate provided by various foods and drinks, but in any given situation certain foods may confer an advantage because of one or all three of these features. Different situations have different demands—it's all about 'horses for courses' rather than 'good' and 'bad' carbohydrate-rich foods.

Total nutritional value

Most of the time, athletes should aim to get maximum nutritional value from the kilojoules they eat. While a system describing the nutritional value of foods will always be arbitrary, we can try to simplify carbohydrate-rich foods into categories of 'wholesome/nutrient-dense' and 'refined'. 'Wholesome' or 'nutrient-dense' carbohydrate-rich foods can also be described as those providing valuable amounts of vitamins, minerals, protein or fibre for a moderate kilojoule intake. By contrast, 'refined' carbohydrate-rich sources are foods or drinks that have been processed to remove much of their original nutritional value, or foods in which fat and sugar add lots of kilojoules to dilute the total nutrient–energy ratio. Table 1.2 provides examples of carbohydrate-rich foods that might fall into the 'wholesome' and 'refined' categories, and shows how poorly 'simple' and 'complex' labels track nutritional value. For example, just as some simple carbohydrate-rich foods provide valuable fibre and vitamins (for example, fruit), other 'complex carbohydrate'-rich foods are a negligible source of fibre, vitamins or minerals (for example, a Danish pastry). There are also carbohydrate-rich foods that contain significant amounts of both 'complex' and 'simple' carbohydrates (for example, a breakfast cereal combining grains and dried fruit). And of course, the total nutritional value of a meal or snack is based on the company that the carbohydrate-rich food keeps. Pasta coated with a buttery sauce is a different choice from pasta tossed with lean meat and vegetables; white bread and jam should be judged differently from a multigrain sandwich with chicken and salad.

Fibre is one component of most wholesome carbohydrate-rich foods. Actually, fibre is a family of compounds whose members include soluble fibre, insoluble fibre and the more newly recognised 'resistant starch'. Different types of fibre have different effects on the digestion and metabolism of food. These include aiding digestion, regulating blood glucose and blood cholesterol levels, and perhaps reducing the risk of some cancers. Fibre is also useful in making food and meals filling—an invaluable aid when you're cutting back on kilojoules to lose body fat.

Fibre is found in fruit and vegetable foods—or, more precisely, fibre occurs naturally in these foods. Quite often the processing of food removes much of the fibre—not just in the food factory, but in the restaurant or in your kitchen. It's not uncommon for people to eat processed food minus its fibre, then buy a fibre supplement in the belief that this is 'healthy'. The best guideline is to eat fibre as it naturally occurs in the variety of foods that you eat. This will ensure that you get a mixture of the fibre types, and that the quantity of fibre varies with your energy and nutrient intake.

Like anything else, too much fibre has its disadvantages. Adding bulkiness and volume to foods is useful for those with low energy requirements, but it can make life difficult for athletes with higher energy needs. For them, high-fibre foods may exceed their stomach's comfort limit. Too much fibre intake, or a sudden increase in fibre intake, can also lead to flatulence and diarrhoea. Fibre-rich foods may not be the best choice just before training or competition. So be guided by a sensible amount and variety of fibre intake. Most times you will be pleased to enjoy the fibre that naturally occurs in your carbohydrate-rich foods. However, know the limits and the times for limiting!

Although replacing wholesome carbohydrates with sugary foods might be seen as forgoing some health benefits, it is worth considering the common charge that sugar is directly harmful to health. Most of the time when we use the term sugar, we mean sucrose, the most commonly occurring simple carbohydrate in the Western diet. Of all carbohydrate-rich foods, it is the most refined, being extracted from sugar cane and purified to remove all other compounds—including nutrients. In some parts of the world, high-fructose syrups refined from corn are replacing sucrose as a cheaper form of sweet kilojoules. Whatever the form—sucrose, high-fructose corn syrups, honey or glucose—it's all 'empty' kilojoules.

Several health problems have been linked to *excessive* intake of these refined sugars and their association with other unhealthy eating habits. The current intake of sugar in Australia is almost a kilogram a week, or about 20 per cent of total energy intake. This is way more than most people need, which explains why one of the dietary guidelines for Australians is 'consume only moderate amounts of sugars and foods containing added sugars'. Sugar is a compact and delicious high-kilojoule food that is easily overeaten. And it often keeps bad company—think of sugar-coated saturated fats such as chocolate, cakes and ice-cream. A combination of high kilojoules and fat, and in many cases the relative absence of fibre, vitamins and minerals, is where the potential for overuse and detriment to health lies. Sugar intake is also strongly linked to tooth decay. Of course, it is a bit more complicated than this. Tooth decay occurs when the bacteria in plaque turn carbohydrates into an acid that erodes tooth enamel. So any sticky carbohydrate that is left on the teeth will cause problems. Dental health is not only a matter of making good food choices, but also of ensuring that teeth have minimal contact with foods by brushing after eating and recognising the risks associated with constant grazing.

Effect on blood glucose

We've already mentioned the old theory that simple sugars cause rapid surges and plunges in blood sugar levels, and that complex carbohydrate foods maintain more even levels. However, research has shown that this is a myth; in fact, each carbohydrate-rich food has a unique effect on blood glucose concentrations and metabolic processes, and this effect is quite unconnected to its structure. Blood glucose changes are related to the speed with which the food is digested and absorbed. Many factors influence this—including the type and amount of fibre in a food, the way in which complex carbohydrate molecules are joined, and even the physical form of the food (whether it is thick and sticky, in whole pieces or mashed up, and even hot versus cold). You can't predict how a food will affect blood glucose levels—you can only measure the results.

The Glycemic Index (GI) is a ranking system created to compare carbohydrate-rich foods according to the blood glucose responses produced in a standard test. Test subjects eat the food first thing in the morning in a serve that provides 50 g of carbohydrate. The resulting blood-glucose curve is compared to the response achieved when 50 g of carbohydrate is consumed from standard food known to produce a high glucose response (by convention, either pure glucose powder or white bread). The foods are then classed as 'high GI'—those that produce more than 70 per cent of the blood-glucose response to the standard—and 'low GI'—those that produce less than 55 per cent of the standard response. Table 1.3 provides a list of the published GI values for some common carbohydrate-rich foods. In Australia, the GI Symbol Program allows food manufacturers to have their products officially tested and carry information about their measured GI on labels and promotional material (*www.gisymbol.com.au*). Although there are differences between specific products, some foods play against the stereotypes of carbohydrate foods. For example, bread and potatoes typically have a higher GI than sugar. It's just more evidence of the need to throw out our previous ideas about the value of simple or complex carbohydrates.

In some areas of nutrition, particularly in the prevention and treatment of diabetes and high blood-fat levels, the Glycemic Index has been used to design eating patterns that manipulate blood-glucose levels into the favourable zone. Lower-GI meals or diets have sometimes also been associated with better 'satiety' (the feeling of fullness or satisfaction that we feel after eating). Several popular diet books promote reduced-GI eating as a way to prevent or treat overweight, since kilojoule intake will be reduced if people feel less inclined to overeat or snack unnecessarily. Some people propose that certain areas of sports nutrition might be improved by the ability to control or produce a predictable blood-glucose response. It is often suggested that high-GI carbohydrate-rich foods are most appropriate for replenishing muscle glycogen stores after strenuous exercise, while low-GI carbohydrate-rich meals are best for a pre-competition meal. Although these ideas aren't universally true, some athletes in some situations may benefit from choosing foods in a certain GI class. Remember, though, this is just one more piece of the food puzzle, not a universal tick of approval for a particular type of food.

Practical issues

It doesn't matter how good a food looks on paper. Food doesn't become 'nutrition' until a person has actually eaten it. Unfortunately, athletes often find it a challenge to eat the amount of carbohydrate they need at crucial times. For a start, an athlete may simply not like a food. What if Brussels sprouts were found to contain a magic ingredient for sports performance? Other challenges include appetite, availability of food, and stomach 'fullness'. These challenges most often appear at the crucial times before, during and after exercise.

The key to sports nutrition is finding practical ways to consume the carbohydrate you need to meet the fuel needs for your particular situation. At times you may need to find a carbohydrate-rich food that's easy to eat when you're on the move, for example, or when gut issues are important—one that's not too fibrous or filling. On other occasions, you may need a portable and non-perishable food that can travel with you to training or a competition venue. In these situations, logistics may take priority over perfect nutritional qualities—and a sports dietitian may actually prescribe a sugary food over a high-fibre food that's full of vitamins! This is all part of dietary balance.

Checklist 1.4 provides some hints for getting the general balance of carbohydrates right—neither overemphasising them nor shunning them in fear—and for putting your focus on the wholesome choices. In the next chapter, we will find strategies for fine-tuning the carbohydrate intakes of athletes to meet their fuel needs during both exercise and recovery. Finally, the case histories in Part II provide examples of how athletes can choose carbohydrate-rich foods to suit the practical challenges of their sport. They also illustrate how special sports foods such as sports drinks, gels, bars and liquid meal supplements are tailor-made to help you reach nutritional goals for sport more easily.

1.4 Replace your daily fluid losses

Water is our most important nutrient. Dehydration is quickly felt and not only affects performance but at times can put life itself at risk. The nutrition guidelines in most countries encourage us to 'drink plenty of water'. There are two angles to this advice, and two sides to the water story. The first issue is the size of the fluid losses that we need to replace each day—losses that occur through urine production, bowel movements, sweat and even our breath. On average, these losses total around 2.5 litres per day, which might be the source of the generic advice that we should drink 'at least eight glasses of water each day'. But these losses can increase under different scenarios:

- if the weather or our personal environment (e.g. heating in the house) is hotter
- if the air we breathe is drier (e.g. due to air-conditioning or being at altitude, including in a pressurised plane cabin)
- if we exercise at high intensities or for prolonged periods
- during episodes of diarrhoea or vomiting.

Most of us manage to replace most of our daily fluid losses most of the time. Our fluid intakes are driven by a complex interaction of thirst (which tells us when we need to drink) and social customs or habits (for example, drinking with meals, or our rituals of 'breaks' during the workday or school day). Many people don't realise, however, that half of our fluid intake typically comes from food. Some foods have a high fluid content—for example, milk, fruits and vegetables, as well as jelly, yoghurt, ice-cream, soups and sauces. But even quite 'solid' foods like bread contribute fluid.

When our fluid losses stay constant, we probably 'luck' into a pattern that looks after our fluid needs. Some groups, such as children and the elderly, and some individuals aren't as good at getting this right—perhaps they don't read their thirst signals as well, perhaps it is more difficult for them to get access to fluids and high-fluid foods, or perhaps they aren't as good at drinking the volumes they need. Other high-risk scenarios involve a sudden change in fluid losses, fluid availability or drinking customs—for example, the onset of hot weather, an abrupt increase in sweat losses during exercise, or travel and new patterns of eating and drinking. Even if these changes lead to increased thirst or an increased awareness of the need to drink, there is often a lag of several days before we boost our fluid intake sufficiently to meet our new needs.

Reduced urine output can be a signal of inadequate fluid intake; it may show up in the form of less frequent visits to the toilet, or a change from clear, plentiful urine to small amounts of dark and concentrated urine. The first sample of the morning is the best indicator of urine volume and characteristics. Some athletes use special machines or 'urine sticks' to obtain information about the concentration of their urine. When this exceeds certain cut-off values, they know that their drinking patterns are not keeping up with their daily fluid needs and must be adjusted. Part of the Big Picture is to look after acute fluid needs during and after exercise. These will be covered in more detail in Chapter 2 (Fine tuning) and Chapter 4 (Competition nutrition). But it is also important for athletes to get their everyday hydration patterns right so they can avoid starting a training session or competition event already dehydrated. Obviously, this would compound the challenge of managing during- and after-exercise fluid intake, and create a vicious cycle of poor hydration.

The second issue that we need to consider is what we are using to replace our fluid losses. Does the advice to drink 'at least eight glasses of water' mean that we should drink only water or that we should consume this volume on top of all the other fluids and fluid-containing foods in our diet? If you Google this advice, you will find that some sources do advise people to drink at least this amount of actual water each day. Others even say that tea, coffee and caffeine-containing soft drinks not only can't be counted in our daily fluid intake, but will add to our water requirement because of the dehydration they cause. But if you read further you will find that neither the source nor the scientific evidence behind 'eight glasses' is provided. In fact, many nutrition experts consider this 'rule' to be an urban myth. As outlined above, each individual should drink enough fluids to replace their specific fluid losses each day, and adjust this intake as the losses and fluid needs change. This fluid intake comprises all drinks and the fluids found in foods. Caffeine does have a small, though usually insignificant, diuretic effect (increasing urine loss). But the overall effect of drinking tea, coffee and cola drinks on our hydration is positive—they add to our total fluid intake.

Deciding what we should drink needs to be done with our overall nutrition goals in mind. Some fluids may contribute towards other nutrition goals—for example, milk will help us to meet protein and calcium goals, and juice may be a quick and easy way for an athlete with high energy needs to 'eat' a fruit/vegetable serve. Many athletes forget that drinks are a quickly consumed source of kilojoules and nutrients—and that this can be both a boon and a danger. 'Drinking' food is useful when we don't want to have to chew our way through large amounts of fuel—if we're a growing basketball player who needs an afternoon snack that won't blunt our appetite for the evening meal, say, or a runner who needs a source of carbohydrate to consume at an aid station during a marathon. But it's a disadvantage if we have reduced energy needs; in that case we'd be better off savouring the slower and more filling experience of eating.

Anyone who is over thirty should be able to remember the time when a tap was the source of most of their daily drinks. Today, for many people tap water has been replaced by soft drinks, grande lattes, frappes, juices and even bottled water! What's more, cups and bottles have upsized considerably, so that in some places it is possible to buy a bucket of drink as a single serve, or to receive 'bottomless' cups and endless refills. Expense and wastage of resources are some of the downsides of this cultural shift. The nutritional consequences include our increasing inability to judge appropriate portion sizes or respond appropriately to thirst. In addition, the intake of unnecessary amounts of sugar in sweetened beverages such as soft drinks, flavoured mineral water and even sports drinks is blamed for contributing to obesity rates. Even juices, with their antioxidants, are considered by nutritionists a second-class alternative to eating the real thing.

At the beginning of this section, we warned that there were two sides to the message of 'drink plenty of water'. The new side is an emerging story with sad consequences. As is often the case in nutrition, it is possible to misinterpret good advice so that it becomes dangerous. Many health-conscious people seem to have become 'welded' to a drink bottle, continually swigging down fluids during work, study and other activities. This might be a good practice for athletes with very heavy training programs in hot weather who need to replace litres of fluid each day. But what about moderately active people who spend most of the day in air-conditioned comfort? We used to think that the worst consequence of drinking too much fluid was a frequent need for toilet breaks. But it seems we now need to publicise the fact that drinking too much fluid can be life-threatening.

When fluid is consumed at a rate that outstrips the capacity of your kidneys to produce urine, blood constituents, including sodium, can be diluted. At extreme levels, this condition (called hyponatraemia) can lead to confusion, irritability, coma and death. It used to occur, rarely, in people who had psychological problems that caused them to drink large volumes of fluid. More recently it has shown up as a result of 'odd' behaviour, such as participating in a radio competition to see who can drink the most fluid before they have to wee. Worryingly, it has been reported in marathons and Ironman triathlons among well-meaning recreational competitors who thought they were doing the right thing by drinking large amounts in the days leading up to the race, and making further excessive use of the aid stations during their event. Such exaggerated behaviour and its potentially fatal outcomes are still relatively rare, but they are completely preventable. The guidelines in Checklist 1.5 should help you to find a healthy balance with your daily fluid intake. More information about drinking during and after exercise sessions is found in Chapters 2, 4 and 5.

1.5 Look after your electrolytes ('salts')

Sodium is the most important electrolyte found outside the body's cells, while potassium is its 'counterweight' inside the cells. The sodium concentration helps to regulate blood pressure and volume, and assists in balancing the distribution of fluid and nutrients between the inside and outside of cells. When the sodium concentration falls outside its normal range, the delicate balance is disturbed and body function is impaired. (In the previous section we heard that low blood sodium levels, arising from excessive fluid intake and the resulting dilution of all blood contents, can be fatal.)

Fortunately, your body has a fairly complex system involving your kidneys and thirst to regulate how much sodium and water are taken in and how much of these and other electrolytes (potassium, chloride, etc.) are excreted in urine. Electrolytes, particularly sodium, are also lost in other body fluids, particularly sweat. Massive losses of sweat can potentially deplete the body's electrolyte stores. But with training and acclimatisation, it can adapt to a hot environment by diluting sweat and thus conserving electrolytes. It then 'expects' you to replace net losses through your diet. In this way, within a broad range of challenges the body can manage its electrolyte levels quite well. However, the life of an athlete isn't always a series of gentle challenges, and you may at times throw your body into some extreme situations. Either heavy loss of electrolytes or excessive intake of them can threaten your vital electrolyte balance.

The more common problem is one of overconsumption, and the usual suspect is sodium. In fact, eating patterns in Australia and other Western countries make excessive salt intake almost unavoidable. Sodium, like the other electrolytes, is found naturally in many foods. However, our dietary patterns have distorted our sodium intake through the addition of large amounts of salt (sodium chloride) to our foods and our meals. Other sodium compounds include MSG (monosodium glutamate), sodium bicarbonate, and some vitamin C tablets (sodium ascorbate). Our kidneys generally manage our excess intake of sodium by excreting it in urine. However, one in five people will develop high blood pressure. Overdosing on salt also interferes with calcium balance and can thus contribute to lowered bone density in those at risk. Since we don't always know who is at risk for these problems until it is too late, nutrition guidelines encourage all Australians to moderate their salt consumption.

Athletes who sweat a lot are one of the few groups of people who may need to deliberately consume salt. Particular athletes may be at risk of salt depletion if they experience very large sweat losses in hot weather, particularly if they are 'salty sweaters' (people whose sweat contains a high concentration of sodium). These athletes may need to use electrolyte-containing drinks during and after exercise, as well as adding a little extra salt to their post-exercise meals. This is mentioned in Checklist 1.6 and covered in more depth in Chapter 4 (Competition nutrition) and Chapter 5 (Promoting recovery).

1.6 Using alcohol sensibly

Alcohol can be an enjoyable part of most lifestyles, including that of an athlete. It is hard to think of a celebration without champagne—and hopefully you will have many sports successes to celebrate! The issue with alcohol is how well you use it, and unfortunately, in some sports alcohol is used very badly. Despite many campaigns and 'player conduct codes', the newspapers still print plenty of stories about the antics of football players, cricketers and other athletes who get drunk after competition, in the off-season, or on the post-season trip. These binges may result in trips to jail, brawls and domestic violence, car accidents, and, on unfortunate occasions, death. Even if it doesn't hurt your body, drinking to excess could hurt your reputation and 'market value' to sponsors and others.

A nutrition textbook will warn you about the health and social consequences of alcohol abuse, including its contribution to the annual road toll. For most athletes, however, cautionary tales about liver cirrhosis seem of little relevance. But drinking doesn't have to reach the level of serious abuse or alcoholism before it affects sports performance. With this in mind, we shall consider alcohol's effects solely from the viewpoint of exercise.

The immediate effects of drinking alcohol include dilation of blood vessels (vasodilation) and depression of the central nervous system. As a result, you will feel a little flushed (losing more heat through your skin) and your sensitivity will be dulled. So while you may think you are giving a great performance, be it in the disco or on the playing field, in fact your judgement, coordination and vision will be impaired. The severity of these effects will depend on how much alcohol you drink and on your individual tolerance (note that females tend to have poorer tolerance). However, most people will experience the initial effect after consuming 20–30 g of alcohol. Figure 1.1 illustrates the alcohol content of various drinks.

Alcohol does not help with fluid replacement—in fact, it acts as a diuretic and may reduce the rate at which you are rehydrating. And despite what you may have heard about carbo-loading with beer, alcoholic drinks will not top up your muscle glycogen stores. Most of the kilojoules in alcoholic drinks come from alcohol, not carbohydrate. Furthermore, alcohol is high in kilojoules—29 kJ, or 7 Calories, per gram (see Chapter 2)—and can quickly cause an energy surplus. It seems to promote the deposition of body fat, especially around the abdomen.

The bottom line is that alcohol should not be consumed just before or during exercise. The penalties for heavy intake at such times include poor hydration, lowered fuel stores, impaired skills, poor sleep and a greater risk of hypothermia in a cold environment (heat loss through the skin will interfere with normal temperature regulation). After exercise, alcohol intake should not compromise your recovery goals. You should follow your nutrition plans for rehydration, repair and refueling before you consider drinking alcohol. You should also weigh up the effect of alcohol on recovery from injuries. The standard treatment for soft-tissue injuries and bruising is to ice and elevate the affected area to constrict blood flow to it. The injured athlete who consumes alcohol immediately after the event may cause extra swelling and bleeding, delaying recovery and in some cases even exacerbating the damage. The most sensible choice for an injured athlete is to avoid any alcohol in the 24–48 hours post exercise.

So should you worry about occasional alcohol binges—or perhaps the weekly post-match 'wind-down'? The answer is that even a single episode of excessive intake will cause some damage. In particular, it will delay recovery and injury repair after exercise. Slow recovery could be crucial if your next competition is a day or even a week away and catches you at less than your best. Even if competition is some time away, you should consider whether your next training sessions will be disrupted and whether you can afford this.

The real problem with alcohol occurs when drinking binges are repeated, as often occurs after weekly matches in team sports. Repeated bingeing will slowly but surely erode your skills, your fitness and your sports career. That is a fact—even if everyone on the team does it and it appears to be normal (or desirable) behaviour. Another thing to remember is that alcohol is high in kilojoules and low in nutritional value. Heavy consumption and bingeing will lead to weight gain. Have you noticed how much heavier you are on your return from the end-of-season trip?

Alcohol is not 'sweated out' or 'exercised off'—these are just more of the locker-room tales that help to sustain alcohol misuse in sports. It is a drug that, at high levels, causes damage to many organs and tissues in your body. The only way to prevent this from happening is not to drink to excess. That said, alcohol can be a small part of a healthy diet. A drink after a hard day's training can help you relax, and a few drinks can add sparkle to social occasions. If you choose to drink, make it work for you, rather than letting it lower your sports potential to the level of those who would have you believe that 'team bonding' (getting drunk together) is all that sport is about. Checklist 1.7 provides hints on how to drink sensibly for sport.

CHECKLIST 1.1
Are you achieving your peak training diet?

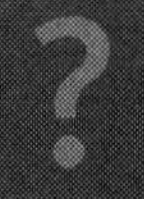

- Do you meet the energy and fuel requirements needed to support your training program?
- Can you achieve and maintain body weight and fat levels that are good for your long-term health and performance in your sport?
- Do you refuel and rehydrate appropriately during key training sessions to perform optimally at each session?
- Do you promote recovery between training sessions with practices that will rapidly replace fluid and fuel stores and all the nutrients that enable the body to adapt to the training load?
- Do you provide your body with all its nutrient needs, remembering that requirements for some nutrients will be increased by a strenuous training program?
- Do you reduce your risk of getting ill or injured by consuming the energy and nutrients that maintain good health?
- Do you create opportunities in training to try out your competition eating practices (such as the pre-event meal, or eating and drinking during an event)? Practice makes perfect and can help you identify many of the things that could go wrong on the big day.
- Do you make well-considered decisions about the use of supplements and specialised sport foods that have been shown to enhance training performance or meet training nutrition needs?
- Do you think about the future? Do you take into account the nutrition guidelines for long-term good health? (Not only will this affect the quantity and quality of your own life, but others who admire your sporting achievements may follow suit.)
- Does food provide pleasure in your day? Are you able to enjoy social eating opportunities with your family and friends?

TABLE 1.1
Phytonutrients (plant compounds) with potential health benefits

Phytochemicals are compounds found in plant food which appear to have a variety of activities, including

- Acting as antioxidants
- Altering the effect of the hormone oestrogen
- Helping to fight cancer-causing agents
- Limiting inflammation
- Limiting blood clotting
- Helping to reduce blood cholesterol levels
- Enhancing immune function

Family and examples	Examples of good food sources	Examples of believed actions
Carotenoids • Beta-carotene	• Yellow-orange and dark-green fruit and vegetables	• Antioxidant activity • Cancer protection • Immune system function
• Lycopenes	• Red-pink vegetables • Dark-green vegetables	• Protection against prostate cancer
• Lutein and zeaxanthine	• Green and yellow-orange fruits and vegetables	• Protection against macular degeneration (eye disease)
Flavonols • Quercetin	• Tea, onions, berries, grapes, apples	• Strong antioxidant activity • Anti-inflammatory activity • Anti-cancer properties
• Resveratrol	• Grapes, wine, peanuts	• Reduction of damage to arteries caused by certain blood fats
Catechins	• Green tea, black tea	• Strong antioxidant activity • Prevention of formation of cancer-causing agents

Family and examples	Examples of good food sources	Examples of believed actions
Anthocyanins	• Blue-purple fruits and vegetables	• Strong antioxidant activity • Mild antibacterial agent
Isoflavones • Genistein	 • Soybeans and soy products (e.g. soy milk, tofu), other beans and legumes	Phytoestrogens • Sharing activities of the hormone oestrogen such as reducing symptoms of menopause and assisting bone health • May also interfere with oestrogen synthesis and reduce risk of breast cancer
Lignins	• Flax-seeds, pumpkin seeds, sesame seeds, bran and wholegrains, beans	• Phytoestrogens (as above)
Phenolic acids • Capsaicin • Ellagic acid • Curcumin	 • Hot peppers/chillies • Raspberries, strawberries, red grapes and kiwifruit • Mustard, tumeric	 • Regulates blood clotting • Increases enzymes that get rid of cancer-causing agents • Anti-inflammatory properties • Blocks cancer-causing agents
Terpenes	• Citrus fruit (especially skins)	• Neutralises cancer-causing agents • Reduces growth of cancers

Family and examples	Examples of good food sources	Examples of believed actions
Saponins	• Soybeans, legumes, some herbal compounds	• May reduce blood cholesterol levels • May reduce growth of cancers
Phytates	• Wholegrains and bran, nuts, oats, soybeans, and seeds	• Binds to minerals to prevent free-radical production—may have anti-cancer outcomes
Indoles and Isothiocyanates	• Cruciferous vegetables (cabbage, broccoli, cauliflower, Brussels sprouts)	• Increases enzymes that get rid of cancer-causing agents • Reduces the growth of cancers
Allicin	• Onion, garlic, leeks, chives	• Antibacterial and antiviral activity • Blood-thinning activity
Phytosterols	• Soybeans and other plants—now added to a range of 'functional foods' such as margarines	• Has cholesterol-like activity, reducing the absorption of food cholesterol and lowering blood cholesterol

CHECKLIST 1.2
Maximising food variety

- Colour your eating with a rainbow of fruits and vegetables every day—aim for a daily goal of at least five serves of veggies and two serves of fruit to find this colour diversity:

- Pink-red (e.g. tomatoes, watermelon, ruby and pink grapefruit, cherries and red berries, rhubarb)
- Yellow-orange (e.g. carrots, pumpkin, sweet potatoes, peaches, apricots, papaya, cantaloupe, mango)
- Green (e.g. broccoli, beans, dark lettuce, silverbeet, spinach, peas, avocadoes, green capsicums, green apples)
- Blue-purple (e.g. purple grapes, raisins, blueberries, blackberries, raspberries, plums, eggplant)
- White (e.g. mushrooms, bananas, onions, cauliflowers, potatoes)

- Be prepared to try new foods.
- Make the most of foods in season.
- Visit markets to see the new produce on offer.
- Google new recipes or information on preparing unfamiliar foods.
- Explore all the varieties of a food—for example, try breads and cereals made from grains other than wheat (rye, multigrain, fruit breads, etc.).
- Mix and match foods at your meals.
- Avoid meals made up of just one food type, such as a fruit-only lunch or toast-only breakfast.
- Make the most of buffet eating—but instead of simply eating more food, mix and match more *types* of foods to make up the quantity you need.
- Enjoy recipes or meal ideas that use layers or combinations of foods—for example, combination stir-fries, fruit or vegetable salads, sandwiches with multi-layer fillings, mixed vegetable soups, raw vegetable platters with dips.
- If you are cooking for one, make the most of fresh or frozen vegetable medleys to add diversity to your meals, or make up a larger recipe with multiple ingredients and save/freeze portions for later meals.
- Add fresh herbs for extra flavour and for the plant nutrients they provide.

- Think carefully before you banish a food or food group from your diet, even if it contains a problematic ingredient. Consider what other value the food may have—in particular, which extra nutrients it could supply. Consider ways to reduce or modify your intake of the food rather than discarding it entirely.

CHECKLIST 1.3 The good oil on fats

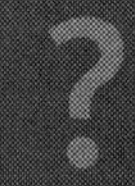

Reduce intake of total fats and saturated fats

- Choose lean cuts of meat, chicken, fish and seafood. Eat a portion size that is right for your overall energy and protein needs rather than letting these foods dominate the plate.
- Avoid high-fat sausage and luncheon meat products. Look for processed meats with a relatively low fat content (95 per cent or more fat-free).
- Make use of low-fat or non-fat dairy products such as skim and low-fat milks, ricotta and cottage cheese, and low-fat yoghurt.
- Be aware that even reduced-fat hard cheeses are quite high in fat (around 25 per cent fat by weight compared with 30–40 per cent for 'normal' cheese). Use these in preference, but limit the serving size—e.g. have just a slice in a sandwich or a sprinkle on a pizza. Some hard cheeses and cheese slices contain only 7–10 per cent fat by weight. While these are the best choice in terms of fat content, you may prefer to use small amounts of richer tasting cheeses in some situations.
- Become a whiz at low-fat cooking. Grill, bake on a rack or in foil, barbecue, microwave, steam, or 'dry fry' with a non-stick frypan smeared with a little oil.
- Use phyllo (filo) pastry as a low-fat alternative in pies, strudels and other pastry-goods. Spray or brush a little oil on the top sheet and between sheets.

- Avoid creamy dressings and cream-based sauces. Use an oil-free dressing or make your own dressings with a little olive oil and vinegar.
- Replace butter and margarines on bread with salsa, mustards or other tasty fat-free spreads.
- Cook with reduced-fat ingredients. Find an alternative for high-fat ingredients—e.g. plain yoghurt or evaporated skim milk instead of cream; skim milk instead of full-cream milk; evaporated skim milk with coconut essence instead of coconut milk.
- Enjoy low-fat versions of yoghurt, Frûche or custard, or a low-fat ice-cream (96 per cent or more fat-free) as quick and nutritious desserts or as toppings for fruit-based desserts.
- Beware of labels that say 'lite' or 'light'. This does not necessarily mean light in fat or kilojoules. In fact, it may simply mean light in salt, colour or flavour. 'Low cholesterol' is another misleading term, since foods can still be high in oils and kilojoules without containing cholesterol. Learn to read labels!
- Enjoy chocolate, biscuits, pastries and rich cakes as a treat. If you go for quality in the foods that are special to you, you won't mind a smaller quantity.
- Keep away from the bowl when snack foods such as chips, corn chips and roasted nuts are on offer. These are high in fat as well as being very 'more-ish'. Many brands of pretzels, air-popped corn and toasted pita-bread strips provide a low-fat alternative, and vegetable sticks are a better vehicle for dips.
- Take special care with take-away foods—especially if they're fried, battered or in pastry. Hopefully, they do not make up a big part of your diet. When you do eat them, choose the lower-fat types or order a small serve only (add other nutritious foods to make up the rest of the meal).

Increase omega-3 fats and keep these in balance with omega-6 fats

- Eat oily fish at least twice a week—salmon, tuna, trout, mackerel or sardines. Plan evening meals around fish or have canned fish in your lunch-time sandwich.
- Invest in a good non-stick frypan and/or wok. Brush or spray with a small amount of canola or flax-seed oil for omega-3s. Alternatively, use a monounsaturated oil such as olive, rather than safflower or another omega-6-based oil.
- Use canola spreads for bread and toast rather than other polyunsaturated margarines or butter.
- Replace roast vegetables and chips with 'dry-baked' items: Cut potatoes (or pumpkin, carrot etc.) into chips or chunks. Spray or brush the tray with enough oil to stop sticking, then brush the chips with a little canola oil and some herbs. Bake in a hot oven.
- Consider using linseed (flax-seed) and soy breads, or functional foods with added omega-3s.
- Enjoy leafy green veggies—they are also a small source of omega-3s.
- Add walnuts to main-meal salads or eat them as a snack with dried fruit.

Eat a little monounsaturated fat

- Replace butter with a spread of avocado or olive-oil-based margarine.
- Oven bake or stir-fry using a little olive oil.
- Replace salad dressings with a little olive oil and vinegar and herbs.
- Add dry-roasted or raw nuts to salads and stir-fries.

TABLE 1.2
Wholesome and refined carbohydrate-rich choices

Wholesome/nutrient-dense carbohydrate-rich choices	Refined/nutrient-poor carbohydrate-rich choices
SIMPLE CARBOHYDRATES	
• Fresh fruit • Canned and stewed fruit • Dried fruit • Juice (in small quantities) • Flavoured milks, especially low-fat brands • Yoghurts, especially low-fat brands • Custard, especially low-fat brands • Frûche/*fromage frais*, especially low-fat brands • Fruit smoothies • Liquid meal supplements (e.g. PowerBar Proteinplus, Sustagen Sport) • Some low-fat and fruit-based desserts and cakes (e.g. crumbles, fruit muffins) • Light-style muesli cereals with grains and dried fruits	• Sugar • Jam, honey • Nutella • Syrups, toppings • Soft drinks, cordial, flavoured mineral water • Sports drinks • Sports gels • Lollies, chocolates • High-fat cakes, pastries, biscuits and desserts
COMPLEX CARBOHYDRATES	
• Breads, muffins, bagels etc, especially wholegrain types • Breakfast cereals, especially wholegrain types • Pasta and noodles • Pizza bases on healthy pizzas • Rice and other grains • Starchy vegetables (potatoes, sweet potatoes, corn, etc.) • Lentils, baked beans and other legumes • Rice cakes, rice crackers and low-fat dry biscuits/snacks (e.g. pretzels) • Some low-fat and fruit-based desserts and cakes (e.g. crumbles, fruit muffins)	• French fries • Pastry • Crisps, Twisties etc • High-fat cakes, pastries, biscuits and desserts

Note that some foods contain a mix of carbohydrate sources and that the nutritional value of a carbohydrate-rich source is affected by the company it keeps.

CHECKLIST 1.4
Balancing carbohydrate with fuel needs

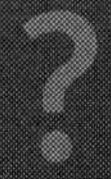

Know your needs

- Anchor your total carbohydrate intake around your exercise patterns. Plan to eat more when you are training more or at higher intensity than usual, or when you are fuelling up for an endurance event. Scale back when you are more sedentary.
- When you are training hard or competing in endurance events, use some of your extra carbohydrate intake for fuelling before, during and after sessions. This will help to give you energy when it is needed most and to aid recovery between sessions.
- If you are not sure of your fuel needs or you're trying to train hard on a low energy budget, consult a sports dietitian for an individualised nutrition plan.

Focus your carbohydrate budget on nutrient-dense carbohydrate-rich foods

- In general, when fuel needs are high, make a carbohydrate-rich food the focus of each meal and build the rest of the meal around it. When carbohydrate needs are more modest, look for recipe ideas and food choices that include carbs but don't make them the centrepiece. Specific examples are given below.
- Choose breakfast cereals from the low-to-moderate sugar, high-fibre range. Be wary of toasted mueslis—they are high in fat and energy-dense. Instead, choose the lighter blends of cereal flakes with dried fruits and other ingredients or use the toasted variety as a sprinkle on top of unsweetened cereal.
- Explore breads—pita, bagels, rolls, crumpets, damper and fruit bread, to name but a few. When carbohydrate needs are high, choose thick-sliced loaves, foccacias or rolls to increase the bread part of the sandwich. When needs are more modest, enjoy thin-sliced breads, open sandwiches, pita-bread 'pizza's, and wraps.

- Become versatile with pastas, rice, couscous and noodles in all their shapes and sizes. When fuel needs are high, consider recipes where they are the core (e.g. rice in risottos or paella, pasta with sauce, special fried rice). When carbohydrate needs are more modest, choose recipes in which they play a secondary role (e.g. noodles in a laksa, pasta sheets in lasagne). Alternatively, enjoy them as a side dish (e.g. rice or couscous with a stir-fry). Side dishes offer the best flexibility to scale your serving up or down.
- Try legumes (kidney beans, lentils, chickpeas, baked beans etc.) in pasta sauces and casseroles to replace some or all of the meat, fish or chicken. Make a meal out of a hearty soup or bean salad.
- Make the most of starchy vegetables—potatoes, sweet potatoes and corn. Baked potatoes and corn on the cob can pep up a meal, and stuffed potatoes make a delicious main course.
- Note that other vegetables, particularly salad vegetables, are good sources of fibre as well as some vitamins and minerals. However, they do not provide a large carbohydrate serve, so depending on your fuel needs you may have to add higher-carb foods to the meal. A bread basket is a quick way to make up for a lack of fuel foods at a meal.
- Enjoy the sweetness and variety of fruit at meals and as snacks. Fresh is usually the most nutritious form—but make good use of juices and dried, canned and stewed fruits.
- Cook cakes, muffins and puddings with fruit and other low-fat ingredients—for example, fruit crumbles, baked fruit, pancakes with a fruit coulis, fruit strudels made with low-fat filo pastry.
- Enjoy sweetened dairy foods as a dessert or snack—non-fat fruit yoghurts, light Frûche, and low-fat ice-cream and low-fat custards. These may be eaten with fruit or to complement a fruit-based dessert.

Hints for increasing your fibre intake

- Generally, choose foods with the fibre content left intact by:
  - selecting wholegrain breads and breakfast cereals, wholemeal pastas and brown rice.
  - enjoying some of your fruits and vegetables raw—for example, fresh fruit, salads, crunchy vegetable sticks, fruit salad, whole fruits blended into smoothies. Eat the skins and seeds where appropriate.
  - cooking fruit and vegetables lightly, leaving them a little crisp rather than overcooked. Again, leave the skins on where appropriate.
- Cook with wholemeal flour. Many recipes involving flour can be made with it or with a mixture of half white and half wholemeal.
- Experiment with vegetarian recipes. Try legumes and other types of wholegrains and cereals.

Hints for using sugar well

- Learn to read labels in order to recognise sugar by its other names (sucrose, fructose, corn syrup, glucose, etc.).
- Look at the total amount of sugar that you eat. Let sugar be part of your carbohydrate intake rather than dominating it.
- When weight loss is desired, be extra vigilant: reduce sugar intake and save the kilojoules for more nutritious carbohydrate foods.
- Enjoy sugar-coated-fat foods as a treat. Think of chocolate, ice-cream, and rich cakes as fun foods rather than energy foods, and give them a special, rather than a regular place in your eating plan. Quality over quantity is the best guideline.
- Except when a carbohydrate drink is specifically required for your sports performance, stick to water, plain mineral water and low-joule drinks.
- Gradually cut down the sugar you add to your coffee or sprinkle on your breakfast cereal.

- Look for 'unsweetened' and 'no-added-sugar' labels.
- Experiment with reducing the sugar in your baking and dessert recipes.

Hints for caring for your teeth

- Limit the number of times you expose your teeth to sugary or sticky carbohydrate foods or drinks each day.
- Try to brush after meals or snacks. Sugar-free gum may be an alternative between meals to promote salivation or dislodge particles stuck to teeth.
- Repeated sipping of sugary drinks over a prolonged session of exercise is good for performance, but not great for teeth. Blame the drinking pattern as much as the product—sports drinks, soft drink, cordial and juice all have the potential to erode tooth enamel. Limit such sipping to situations where it actually fuels your sports performance, rather than when you are sitting on the couch watching a movie.
- Use a sports bottle or drinking straw that squirts the water to the back of your mouth, or clean off your teeth by following up with a swig or swallow of water.

TABLE 1.3
Glycemic Index of some common carbohydrate-rich foods

	Food	GI
High GI (>70)		
	Glucose powder	100
	Cornflakes	77
	Coco Pops	77
	White rice, boiled	88
	Instant mashed potato	86
	Boiled Pontiac potato	88
	Baguette bread	95

	Food	GI
	Bagel	72
	Gatorade	78
	Jelly beans	78
Moderate GI (55–70)		
	Sucrose	61
	Honey	58
	White bread	70
	Wholemeal bread	69
	Vita Brits	70
	Basmati or Doongara rice	58
	Watermelon	72
	Sultanas	56
	Soft drink	68
	Cordial	66
	Orange juice	52
Low Glycemic Index (<55)		
	Coca-Cola	53
	Mixed-grain breads	49
	Porridge	49
	All-Bran	30
	White pasta, boiled	38
	Wholemeal pasta, boiled	37
	Baked beans	48
	Kidney beans	27
	Milk	31
	Banana	52
	Apple	38
	Apple juice	39
	Chocolate	42
	Fruit-flavoured yoghurt	33
	Fructose	19

Note: These published GI values of selected Australian foods have been derived from studies using glucose as the standard food. These examples were chosen to show that the GI of a carbohydrate-rich food is not readily predictable. A more complete list of foods is available from www.Glycemicindex.com

CHECKLIST 1.5
Looking after daily fluid needs

- Be aware of the factors that drive your daily fluid losses—weather, surrounding temperature, training and competition exercise (intensity, duration and condition of exercise). At times you might want to measure your fluid/sweat losses under these conditions (see Figure 2.3). Otherwise, be aware of changes in these factors and be prepared to increase or decrease your fluid intake as required.
- Track how well hydrated you are on a daily basis and adjust your fluid intake according to these clues:
  - How many times do you need a wee break during the day? Is this more or less than other people? Does this cause problems in your daily activities?
  - What are the characteristics of your first urine of the morning? What is the volume? Is it light and pale, or dark and concentrated? If you are able to measure USG (urine specific gravity), is it less than 1.020?
  - Do you have to get up in the night for a wee? Is this interfering with your sleep and recovery?
  - Do you become thirsty over the day? Rate the intensity of your thirst.
  - If you weigh yourself first thing in the morning, is your morning waking weight stable, or does it yo-yo from one day to the next?
- Be aware of your daily fluid intake patterns and how well these meet your fluid needs. Do you need to change the volume and timing of your drinking?
  - Do you drink anything when you first get up in the morning?
  - What do you drink at your meals?
  - Do you take specific breaks during the day? What do you drink during these breaks?

- ○ Do you have a drink with you during your daily activities?
- ○ Do you drink before you go to bed?
- ○ Do you drink fluids overnight?
- ○ Do you have a special drinking plan for before, during and after your exercise sessions?

- Be aware of the sources of your daily fluid intake, and of any change to your routine or environment that might affect these. Plan ahead for times when you may have less access.
- Are you choosing a fluid that is right for your needs?
- Are you always able to get access to fluids when you need them?

CHECKLIST 1.6
Salt—friend or foe?

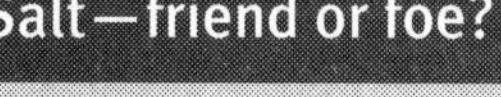

Most of the time, go easy with salt

- In general, there is little need to add salt to your food, either in cooking or at the table. Learn to enjoy the natural taste of your cooking.
- Experiment with herbs, spices, lemon juice and other salt-free flavourings to make your meals tasty.
- Go easy also with salty sauces and flavourings (for example soy sauce, stock and Vegemite).
- Prefer fresh to packaged or canned foods.
- Read labels to check the salt content of processed foods such as soups, spreads, sauces, cheeses and some cereals. Look for new varieties that are labelled salt-reduced, no-added-salt or low-sodium.
- Reduce your intake of salty snack foods (crisps, salted nuts, corn chips, etc.), processed foods and take-aways. These foods

are also often high in fat and relatively low in nutrients. As well as adding salt to your diet, they help to perpetuate your taste for salt.

- Make this campaign a gradual process. Your taste buds will gradually adapt (and even thank you!).
- If you have high blood pressure or a family history of it, take extra care with salt.

You may need extra salt if you have large sweat losses or are a 'salty sweater' (your sweat dries with white crystals on your skin and clothes)

- If you have lost large amounts of sweat in a single session of exercise, include a salt-added drink such as a sports drink or oral rehydration solution (e.g. Gastrolyte) in your recovery routine. Alternatively or in addition, include salt-added foods such as bread, pretzels or breakfast cereal in your recovery snacks/meal, or add a little salt to your next meal.
- If you suddenly increase your training loads or travel to a hot climate, you may need to add a little salt at your meals until you adapt to the conditions.
- If you are undertaking a prolonged event in extreme conditions (such as an Ironman triathlon in a hot environment), consult a sports dietitian to develop an appropriate plan for fluid and electrolyte replacement during training and the race.
- If you are a salty sweater or suffer from cramps that may be due to extreme electrolyte losses, consult a sports dietitian who can carry out 'sweat testing'. Estimating your sweat sodium levels and sweat sodium losses will help the dietitian formulate a plan for sodium intake.

CHECKLIST 1.7
Safe and sensible ways with alcohol

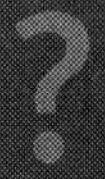

- If you choose to drink alcohol, learn to enjoy a couple of glasses per occasion. It is much better to have a couple of drinks throughout the week than save up for a binge on Saturday night (or after your competition).
- Generally, avoid alcohol in the 24 hours before competition.
- Avoid any alcohol for 24 hours post-exercise if any soft-tissue injury or bruising has occurred.
- Enjoy alcohol after competition in ways that limit the damage to yourself, your recovery and your performance:
    - Rehydrate, refuel and repair with carbohydrates, protein and other important nutrients before you start with alcoholic drinks.
    - Once you are ready to consume alcohol, set yourself a limit of a certain number of drinks and stay on top of how much you have consumed (see Figure 1.1 for a guide to the alcohol content of drinks).
- Don't get caught up in group drinking situations:
    - Avoid being in a 'shout' or round.
    - If you are caught in a shout, use your turn to buy a non-alcoholic drink.
    - Look after your friends or team-mates. Develop a buddy system and learn to recognise the signs of excessive alcohol intake.
- Use tricks to pace yourself or 'make the alcohol go further'. These strategies will allow you to keep to your drink limit:
    - Keep busy and alternate alcoholic drinks and non-alcoholic drinks.
    - Drink low-alcohol beers.
    - Mix your wine or spirit coolers with mineral water, order half-nips of spirits in mixed drinks, or alternatively order a small measure of spirits in a large glass of a non-alcoholic mixer.

   - Make plenty of non-alcoholic drinks available, both as thirst quenchers and as an enjoyable alternative to alcohol. These could include fruit juices, plain mineral water and soft drinks, as well as special non-alcoholic cocktails.
- Use the advice that accompanies drink-driving laws in your state as a useful guide to sensible drinking:
   - Make yourself a designated driver for social activities. This will allow you to look after your goals as well as take care of your friends' transport needs.
- If you need to restrict your energy intake, treat alcohol as a luxury item. There are more nutritious ways to consume kilojoules.

FIGURE 1.1

What is a 'drink' of alcohol? We talk of a 'standard drink' as the serve that contains about 10 g of alcohol. However, as shown in the figure on the right, what many people consider a single 'drink' may be equal to more than one standard alcohol serve.

Number of Standard Drinks

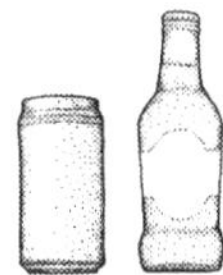

1.5 375 ml Full Strength Beer
4.9% Alc./Vol
1 375 ml Mid Strength Beer
3.5% Alc./Vol
0.8 375 ml Light Beer
2.7% Alc./Vol

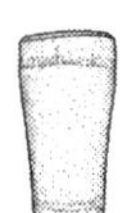

1.1 285 ml Middy/Pot Full Strength Beer
4.9% Alc./Vol
0.8 285 ml Middy/Pot Mid Strength Beer
3.5% Alc./Vol
0.6 285 ml Middy/Pot Light Beer
2.7% Alc./Vol

1.5 375 ml Pre-mix Spirits
5% Alc./Vol

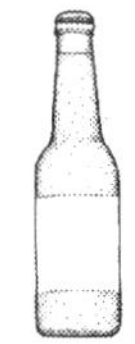

1.5 340 ml Alcopops
5.5% Alc./Vol

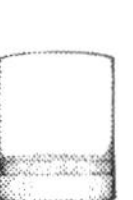

1 30 ml Spirit Nip
40% Alc./Vol

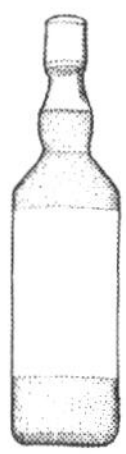

22 750 ml Bottle of Spirits
40% Alc./Vol

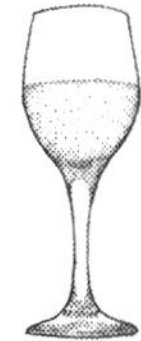

1 100 ml Standard Serve of Wine
40% Alc./Vol

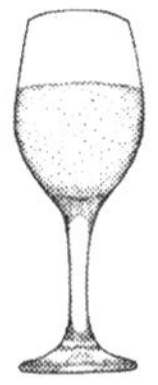

1.8 180 ml Average Restaurant Serve of Wine
12% Alc./Vol

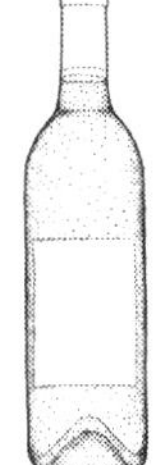

7 750 ml Bottle of Wine
12% Alc./Vol

2
Fine tuning: How much and when?

Now that the basic principles are in place, we can start accounting for your individual characteristics and planning for your specific needs. The task is to estimate your requirements for various nutrients, and then arrange these within your energy budget. Of course, you will need to consider how best to arrange your food intake over your busy day—to gain nutritional advantages as well as meet your schedule of commitments.

2.1 Energy

The first feature of food is the energy (kilojoules, or if you're old fashioned, calories) it provides. How many kilojoules should I eat each day? Athletes frequently throw this question at sports dietitians with the expectation of an immediate answer with accuracy to three decimal places. Such precision is impossible, because your body is a unique energy system with its own tally of energy needs. In a nutshell, you need enough energy to be you!

There are a number of components that make up your total energy requirements:

1. *Basal metabolic rate*

Your Basal Metabolic Rate (BMR) is the energy required just to keep your body functioning. This varies according to a number of factors:

- Your age—it decreases as you get older
- Your body mass—it increases with a larger body mass

- Your body composition—it increases with greater muscle mass and decreases with greater fat stores
- Your gender—it is higher in men than women
- Other factors, including body hormones.

Typically, basal metabolic rate accounts for 60–70 per cent of total energy requirements. However, it can vary greatly between people—which can be a great source of frustration and discouragement to those who 'drew the short stick'.

2. *Activity*

Activity typically accounts for 15–30 per cent of total energy requirements, but the intensive training or competition programs of some athletes may increase this contribution to 50 per cent or even more. Scientists divide our activity into two components. First, there is voluntary physical activity. This includes not only planned exercise but the movements undertaken in our household chores, employment or daily activities—things that our modern lifestyles have managed to make minimally energy-consuming. This is unfortunate, because these things could play a significant role in helping with weight control for many people. Planned exercise—usually training—is the major form of physical activity for most athletes. The energy cost of this varies greatly with the type, intensity and duration of the exercise.

Currently, there is a lot of interest in another component of our physical activity. This is given various names, such as spontaneous physical activity or 'fidgeting', but it basically refers to the movements we make without purpose or intention—swinging legs, tapping fingers, moving around in our chairs, pacing . . . You probably know some people who simply can't keep still, and others who can assume the stance of a statue (especially when watching TV or staring at a computer screen!). Scientists have observed this behaviour carefully and have found that the energy cost of fidgeting can be significant. What's more, it can differentiate people who are likely to gain weight from those who less likely to. In fact, prolonged sitting is a separate risk factor for the development of the 'metabolic syndrome' of obesity, diabetes and cardiovascular disease. Even a regular exercise program may not be enough to make up for long periods of uninterrupted sitting.

3. *Thermic effect of food*

Whenever we eat, our metabolic rate increases while we do the work of digesting it and processing the nutrients in it. This accounts for less than 10 per cent of our total energy budget, but will obviously differ among people according to how often and how much they eat.

4. *Growth, including pregnancy and breast-feeding*

Children and adolescents may need plenty of additional kilojoules to provide for new bone and body tissues as they grow.

Knowing a bit about these factors helps to predict which athletes will have large energy budgets and which ones will have smaller energy needs. Growth, a big body size (especially large muscle mass), and lengthy high-intensity training sessions all predict high energy needs. This explains why adolescent basketballers, heavyweight rowers, marathon runners and triathletes are generally high energy consumers. Females typically have smaller energy requirements than their male counterparts, and a small body size and a skill-based training program also predict lower energy needs. Female gymnasts and ballet dancers are good examples of athletes with relatively small energy budgets. Of course, these generalisations are by no means hard and fast—in fact, energy requirements are individual and specific to each athlete.

So how can you tell what your energy budget should be? There are specialised techniques for measuring energy expenditure, including monitoring metabolism for a period in a special room called a metabolic chamber. Alternatively, you can swallow a special type of water (called doubly labelled water) and track what happens to the hydrogen units and the oxygen units separately. Unfortunately, these techniques are expensive and require high-tech equipment and scientific support. At present, they are really only used as a research tool. You can also measure the energy cost of various activities—from lying down to exercising—by capturing all the air you breathe in and out in a special bag and calculating the volumes of oxygen and carbon dioxide in the expired air. If done with the right expertise, this technique can measure some of the components of your total energy expenditure. While it won't be able to sum up all your energy needs for a day, it may be useful to see if key components are as expected. Again, however, this technique isn't widely accessible.

A sports dietitian has the expertise to make an *estimation* of the main components of your energy requirements—your BMR, activity costs, and growth if appropriate. You can use some of the information in this book to do some rough calculations of your own energy needs, based on the *average* energy costs of various activities for people of different sizes, ages and genders (see Figure 2.1). Remember, however, that the actual requirements of individuals vary to a remarkable degree around these predicted values, and that the purpose of doing such a calculation is simply to find a ball-park figure for your expected energy requirements.

Most of the time, we are in energy balance, meaning that we match our energy expenditure to our energy intake. However, your body has a buffer for this equation. The body's fat stores provide an energy reserve to store extra kilojoules when you consume more than you expend, or to make up the deficit when the reverse occurs. This is how you gain or lose weight through body fat. Even when you are in energy balance (neither gaining nor losing body fat), you will not necessarily have to eat exactly the same number of kilojoules as you expend for that day. In the short term—say over a couple of days—there may be little correlation between your energy input and output. However, over a period of a week or more, this balance is usually maintained with considerable precision.

You should not be surprised if your predicted energy requirements are quite different from those of other athletes—even athletes in the same sport as you. The most important thing is that they are right for you. Once you have an idea of your daily kilojoule budget, your next task is to learn how to 'spend' it wisely, on the nutrients that are important for your health and performance. These nutrients will now be covered in more detail.

2.2 Carbohydrate

Your carbohydrate requirements are based on how much fuel your muscles need—to replace the fuel that you burn up in daily exercise and to restore muscle glycogen levels. This will depend on the amount of training (or competition) that you undertake each day, and the size of your muscles. This is why it is a good idea to provide guidelines based on body size (weight), which can be scaled up and down according to daily activity levels. A general estimation of the daily carbohydrate needs of athletes in various sports and situations is presented in Table 2.1.

TABLE 2.1
Estimated carbohydrate needs of athletes

	Situation	Carbohydrate targets per kg of the athlete's body weight**
Daily needs for fuel and recovery*		
Minimal	Light training program (low intensity or skill-based exercise)	3–5 g per kg each day
Moderate	Moderate exercise program (i.e. ~1 hr per day)	5–7 g per kg each day
High	Endurance program (i.e., 1–3 hr per day of moderate- to high-intensity exercise)	6–10 g per kg each day
Very high	Extreme exercise (i.e., >4–5 hr per day of moderate- to high-intensity exercise, such as Tour de France)	10–12 g per kg each day
* Note that large athletes and athletes undertaking a weight loss program may be better suited to reduce their fuel intake to the needs of the previous category		
Special situations requiring fuel		
Maximal daily refuelling	Post-event recovery or carbohydrate loading before an event	7–12 g per kg for each 24 h
Speedy refuelling	Less than 8 h recovery between two demanding workouts	1–1.2 g per kg immediately after first session Repeated each hour until the normal meal schedule is resumed.

	Situation	Carbohydrate targets per kg of the athlete's body weight**
Pre-event fuelling	Before an endurance event	1–4 g per kg eaten 1–4 hr before exercise
During exercise	Moderate-intensity or intermittent exercise of >1 hr Ultra-endurance events (e.g. Ironman, Tour de France)	30–60 g/hr Perhaps up to 1.5 g per min (e.g. 60–90 g per h)

So a female basketballer (60 kg) whose daily training involved 60–90 minutes of actual exercise would need about 300 g of carbohydrate a day. A 65-kg male triathlete fuelling up for a long race might aim for about 650 g of carbohydrate to stock up 1–2 days before the event. A light breakfast providing about 120 g of carbohydrate would fit the guidelines for his pre-race meal. Look at Table 2.8 for a ready reckoner of the carbohydrate content of various foods. Using this guide and its 50-g fuel portions, our triathlete would need to eat around 13 'large serves' of carbohydrate foods on these days—for example, two large bowls of cereal (2 serves), six slices of bread (2), two English muffins (1), three tablespoons of jam (1), four pieces of fruit (2), two glasses of juice (1), 500 ml of soft drink (1), one sports bar (1) and three cups of cooked pasta (2)! And the pre-race breakfast might include up to 6 'medium' serves of carbohydrate—two slices of raisin toast (2), a glass of orange juice (1) and a powerbar (about 3).

Do you need to count up all your carbohydrates each day? For most athletes, this is probably an unnecessary task. Generally, the priority is to establish a baseline amount of carbohydrate required for a rest day or light training day. On heavy training days, additional carbohydrate can be incorporated before, during or after exercise to support performance and facilitate recovery. The food hints summarised in Checklist 1.4 should help you form habits that will adjust your carbohydrate intake to reflect your daily exercise patterns. Athletes who need to consume large amounts of carbohydrate and kilojoules or those who need to monitor their body weight may be helped by periodically calculating the amount of carbohydrate foods needed, since their appetite and/or typical meal patterns may not reflect their daily requirements. In special situations such as carbo-loading, when you need to maximise glycogen storage, carbohydrate counting will ensure that you achieve your daily target of 7–12 g of carbohydrate per kilogram of your weight.

2.3 Protein

The protein needs of athletes have been hotly debated for many years. In the past, strength athletes have argued that more was better for growing muscles, whereas endurance athletes almost ignored protein, focusing mainly on carbohydrate to fuel exercise. More recently, the publicity surrounding high-protein diets to aid weight loss has struck a chord with weight-sensitive endurance athletes, with some now eating protein at the expense of carbohydrate. So is all the hype deserved?

It is clear that protein requirements are increased by exercise—first, to account for the small contribution of protein to muscle fuel, and second, to account for any extra muscle that is laid down to increase muscle size and strength or repair damaged tissue. Some scientists have estimated the likely increase in protein requirements for athletes in heavy training who might max out these extra protein demands. The suggested maximum needs for daily protein are found in Table 2.2.

This summary shows that the total protein needs of many athletes will still be met by the general recommendation of 1g of protein per kilogram of body weight—e.g. 60 g for a 60 kg athlete. But athletes whose daily training sessions are lengthy and intense (burning up a significant total of protein fuel), or who are in a muscle-gain stage of their programs, will require an increase in their protein allowance. Athletes who are growing will need to cover these physiological requirements as well. However, don't go rushing for a protein powder yet—although protein requirements increase in absolute terms (you may need more total grams of protein), the extra kilojoules in your diet to fuel exercise should automatically allow you to eat more protein without having to consciously emphasise protein foods.

Protein foods should be chosen with a range of nutritional goals in mind—that is, you should choose those which have a good fat profile and are also good sources of other nutrients. Table 2.9 provides a ready

TABLE 2.2
Estimated protein needs for athletes

	Example of athlete or situation	
Daily needs		Protein needs per kg of the athlete's body weight
Australian RDI	Sedentary adult male Sedentary adult female	0.84 g 0.75 g
Suggested target	Recreational level sports activity	~1 g
Suggested targets	Strength-training athletes —maintenance or steady-state phase —muscle gain or increased training phase	1.2 g– 1.6 g
Suggested targets	Endurance training athletes —moderate volume/ intensity program —prolonged strenuous training/competition	1.2 g– 1.7 g
Suggested targets	Team athletes —moderate training —hard training or match program	1.2 – 1.7 g
Suggested target	Adolescent + growing athletes	2.0 g
Suggested target	Female athletes	15% less than males
Australian RDI	Pregnant athletes	Extra 14 g per day in 2nd and 3rd trimester
Australian RDI	Breast-feeding athletes	Extra 20 g per day

	Special situations	Total protein needs
	After resistance workout to promote maximal muscle gain	20 g
	Recovery after strenuous endurance or intermittent/ team training session	20 g

Source of Australian RDIs: NHMRC, Australian Government, 2006

reckoner of the protein content of some valuable foods. Lean animal protein foods are able to supply all the body's essential amino acids, as well as calcium (dairy foods) and iron (meats and shellfish). They may also be good sources of omega-3 fats—especially fish. If you look at the vegetable protein foods, you will see that some of these appear as good carbohydrate sources also. The ready reckoner should convince you that it doesn't take half a cow to make up your daily protein needs—cereal with skim milk for breakfast, a chicken sandwich for lunch and a small steak for dinner will provide over 60 g of protein for a 60-kg squash player. Studies typically show that most athletes eat well above these protein targets. In fact, the only athletes really at risk of failing to meet these guidelines are those who eat very restricted diets—low in energy, low in variety, or low in both.

Is it bad to eat a high-protein diet? This question has different answers, depending on what you mean by 'high protein'. Some athletes can eat protein in quantities far greater than the suggested targets simply because they have high energy needs. In these cases, their total energy budget will allow them to meet all their other nutritional goals as well. The disadvantage of eating lots of protein may simply be that protein-rich foods tend to be the most expensive items in a shopping trolley, especially when they are specialised protein supplements or sports foods. However, other athletes may choose protein foods at the expense of their other real needs and create a disadvantage for themselves. There are some hypothetical problems with a very high protein intake—such as an extra load on your kidneys, extra water needs and a negative effect on calcium balance. But these problems appear to be more of a possibility than a reality in otherwise healthy people. Some athletes have freely chosen protein intakes of 3–4 times their body weight for lengthy periods without apparent problems. So the worst feature of an unnecessary intake of protein may simply be that it is unnecessary. In fact, one of the consequences of a high protein intake is that your body increases the amount of protein it simply burns for fuel rather than making it available for the manufacture of new body proteins. This is wasteful.

A new reason for athletes to be less concerned about the total *amount* of protein they eat is the growing evidence that the *timing* of one's protein intake is a critical factor in optimising the results of training or achieving recovery goals. When protein is eaten in the hour or so after a resistance/weights workout, there is a substantial increase in protein synthesis in the muscle. Eating protein in the immediate recovery period after strenuous endurance exercise also achieves this effect. Of course, the stimulus of endurance exercise serves to create proteins to repair damaged muscle or to create new enzymes that will make the athlete better at his exercise tasks. Meanwhile, the stimulus of resistance training serves to create new muscle to make the athlete bigger and stronger. The exciting news from recent studies is that gains made by this strategic timing of protein intake around training sessions are real and stand out even from the results of eating protein over the rest of the day. There are lots of questions to ask. How much protein do you need to optimise the effect? Or, in the case of athletes with low energy budgets, how little protein can you eat and still get a worthwhile outcome? What about the ideal timing—before, straight after the exercise, or after a delay? In one single snack or meal, or as a series of nibbles? Does the type of protein matter? Animal or vegetable? Whey? Amino acids? Does it matter or help if other nutrients such as carbohydrate are eaten at the same time? It may take until the fourth or fifth edition of this book before all the answers to these questions are found. For the moment, we have put the results of our present knowledge into the recommendations in Chapter 5 (Promoting recovery).

To close this section, we will make some comments about vegetable proteins. Protein is made from various combinations of small chemical building blocks called amino acids. Some of these amino acids can be manufactured in the body by rearranging the structure of other compounds, while the other amino acids (called the essential amino acids) can be obtained only by eating food. Animal protein foods contain a good variety of amino acids, including all the essential ones. On the other hand, plant foods tend to have one or more of the essential amino acids in short supply. This could be a problem if plant foods make up most or all of your diet—for example, if you are a vegetarian.

Fortunately, however, while one vegetable protein food will contain a good supply of some essential amino acids but be lacking in one or two others, another vegetable protein food will have the reverse problem. By cleverly mixing and matching these foods throughout the day, you can put together a full house of amino acids. This is known as complementing vegetable proteins, and can also be done by mixing a vegetable protein, with a small amount of animal protein, such as a dairy food. Figure 2.2 shows you which protein foods can complement each other, and some typical examples of how it can be done at the same meal. The recent thinking is that it is OK to achieve this mixing and matching over three or four meals rather than having to do it at the same meal. But is still good to have a feel for foods that 'go together'.

2.4 Vitamins

Helped along by some clever advertising from vitamin-supplement makers, most people think of vitamins as the most important nutrients in their diet and the ones most likely to run into short supply. One of the advertising promises associated with vitamin supplements is 'having more energy', and it targets time-poor, overstressed people who don't get enough sleep, skip meals and make poor food and lifestyle choices.

The truth is somewhat different. While an adequate vitamin intake is essential to good health and optimal training nutrition, vitamins are not the first nutrients that are likely to go missing in a poor diet. And as pointed out in Chapter 1, foods contain a lot more than vitamins, so replacing a variety of nutritious foods with a vitamin supplement misses out some of the important food components we now know about.

In the correct sense of the term, vitamins do not provide energy—that is, they do not contribute any kilojoules to the body. But various vitamins are involved in the production of energy from fuel stores by acting as catalysts for metabolic reactions. Vitamins are involved in many other reactions, too—including the production of red blood cells, the action of antioxidants, the repair of tissues, and the synthesis of protein. When vitamin levels drop below a certain mark, these body processes will be impaired, and sports performance has been shown to suffer. However, if your vitamin supply is continually maintained, metabolism will continue unimpeded.

Nutrition experts have set a recommended intake for most of the vitamins (known as the Recommended Dietary Intake, or RDI). The RDIs for vitamins are set as a general target, and most people's diets provide intakes well above these levels. A diet that provides less than the RDI for a vitamin is not necessarily deficient in that vitamin, because quite a large safety margin has been set. However, if your usual diet consistently supplies you with less than about two-thirds of the RDIs, some expert dietary advice and remodelling is suggested. In some cases there is insufficient evidence to set an RDI, and another estimate is made of an Adequate Intake (AI) level.

If you have nutritional shortfalls, your best line of attack will be not to take a vitamin supplement but rather to change your diet. After all, because nutrients exist together in food, it is likely that any diet that is low in one or more vitamins is also failing to meet other goals of peak training nutrition. Taking a vitamin supplement might be a short-term solution to prevent or reverse your low vitamin intake, but how will it help your high fat intake or your low carbohydrate supply? And how will you find a source of all the antioxidants and phytochemicals that food has to offer?

After looking at the population RDIs for vitamins, athletes usually ask two questions:

- Does heavy exercise increase the requirements for vitamins?
- Will extra vitamins, especially in large doses, improve performance by speeding up metabolism?

The second question really belongs to the area of dietary supplements and nutritional ergogenic aids (performance boosters), and will be covered in Chapter 6. On the trail of extra vitamin needs, research has not been able to show that the vitamin requirements of athletes are raised above the RDI. Table 2.10 summarises food sources of each vitamin, with the RDIs from the new Nutrient Reference Values for Australia and New Zealand published in 2005. In terms of vitamin intake, the two biggest assets that an athlete's diet can have are a high energy intake (more food should mean more nutrients) and a wide variety of foods (as you learnt earlier, variety increases your opportunities to get a little of everything you need). The athletes who are most likely to run into problems with vitamin intake are those on very restricted diets (e.g. fad diets, strict vegetarian diets, fussy eaters) and those with low energy intakes (low energy consumers and people on weight-loss diets). In these situations, a sports dietitian can help you to maximise your dietary intake, and may also suggest a low-dose vitamin supplement to help fill any remaining gaps.

2.5 Iron

Iron is an important nutrient in sports performance, since it is a component of the oxygen carriers in the blood (haemoglobin) and in the muscles (myoglobin). In addition, iron is involved with some of the enzymes that promote exercise metabolism. An iron deficiency will reduce the oxygen supply to muscles as well as slow down some of these metabolic reactions. Obviously, this is not compatible with optimal performance.

If the situation worsens and blood haemoglobin levels become lowered (in the condition called anaemia) the symptoms become more drastic—severe fatigue, cramps, headaches and often shortness of breath. It is at the anaemia stage that we know for sure performance is impeded. It has been harder to find clear proof that low iron stores in the absence of anaemia actually lower the quality of performance. There may be some impairment of the ability to adapt to training, and athletes certainly complain of extra fatigue and failure to recover between sessions. Nevertheless, even if low iron stores do not directly cause changes to performance, this condition should be treated to stop the progression to anaemia.

Iron requirements for athletes provide a few challenges. First, females need to eat more iron than their male counterparts to account for the blood losses of menstruation. The tricky part is that females usually need to eat fewer kilojoules than males and must therefore find more iron per mouthful in their diet. Second, heavy exercise increases iron requirements by increasing iron losses from the body. Iron can be lost through sweat and gastrointestinal bleeding—particularly if you take a lot of anti-inflammatory drugs for injuries. Red blood cells are destroyed by continual jarring and impact, whether in contact sports or from pounding the pavements while running. A guide to iron requirements for sedentary individuals is provided in Table 2.3 below. The upper ranges suggested for endurance athletes, while not real RDIs, represent a guess at the worst-case scenario where an athlete is experiencing iron drain from all exercise-related sources.

TABLE 2.3
Iron needs for athletes

Population	Daily iron needs (RDIs)
Adolescent boys (growth)	11 mg
Adolescent girls (pre onset of periods)	8 mg
Adolescent girls (growth + periods)	15 mg
Adult males	8 mg
Endurance training males—heavy training	8–17.5 mg
Adult females (menstruating years)	18 mg
Endurance training females—not menstruating	8–17 mg
Endurance training females—menstruating years	18–23 mg
Adult females (post-menstrual)	8 mg/d
Pregnant females	27 mg/d

Source for RDIs for iron: NHMRC, Nutrient Reference Values for Australia and New Zealand. Australian Government 2006.

The final complication in the iron story is that the kinds of people who need iron most often steer away from the most iron-rich foods. Dietary iron is found in two forms—a special form called 'heme' iron that occurs in some animal foods, and a simpler form known as 'non-heme' iron, found in plant foods. Table 2.11 shows the iron content of some common serves of food.

The importance of this classification is twofold—foods with heme iron generally have more iron overall, and the heme iron is well absorbed. By contrast, the non-heme iron is poorly absorbed and can be further tied up by other factors in food such as tannin (in tea), phytates (in wheat bran and wholemeal cereals) and oxalates (in spinach). Athletes whose diets are based heavily, or solely, on plant iron foods—such as vegetarians or endurance athletes who are overly focused on carbohydrates—may find that the iron they consume is inadequate and metabolically unavailable.

Some special tactics are needed to put an iron boost into the optimal training diet. This will include clever mixing and matching of foods to make use of low-fat heme foods, and to take advantage of dietary factors that actually enhance the absorption of non-heme iron—the presence of vitamin C and meat/fish/poultry. Checklist 2.1 provides a summary of useful strategies to provide an iron boost.

2.6 Calcium

The best-known function of calcium in the body is its role in bone, since 99 per cent of the body's calcium is in the skeleton. A growing awareness of bone health in athletes has put the spotlight on calcium in recent years. Osteoporosis, or severe loss of the mineral content of bones, is typically a process of ageing. Bones that have lost mineral content are thinner and more fragile. Remember how your grandmother shrank in height as she got older and her spine compressed, and how she broke her hip after a fall? Osteopaenia is the term used to describe a reduction in bone density that is part-way along the spectrum to osteoporosis. These conditions result from of a loss of bone mineral content, the failure to gain a healthy peak bone mass in the first place, or a combination of both.

Risk factors for osteopaenia include:

- Age
- Gender (being female)
- Race—Asian and Caucasian women are at greater risk, especially those who are small-boned
- Family history
- Inactivity and lack of weight-bearing exercise
- Conditions involving reduced levels of the female hormone oestrogen. Oestrogen levels fall after menopause in women, causing a rapid decline in bone mass over the next few years.

- Lifestyle issues, including a low intake of calcium, lack of vitamin D due to inadequate sunlight exposure, inadequate energy intake, smoking and excessive alcohol intake
- Some medical conditions and some medications.

The special circumstances of impaired bone health in athletes will be discussed in more detail in Chapter 3. For now, we will concentrate on helping you to achieve a healthy intake of calcium, said to play a facilitating role in bone health. Think of it as contributing to superannuation for your bones—the more bone mass you can store now, the better protected you will be when bone loss occurs in later life. And you may be helping to reduce the risk of stress fractures in your present athletic career. Of course, stress fractures, as we shall see later in a case history, also reflect the volume of training you are doing, the surfaces and shoes involved, and how good your biomechanics are. Too much repeated pounding or a hard fall will eventually crack any bone—but soft bones increase the risk in any situation.

Targets for calcium intake are presented in Table 2.4 based on the RDIs for sedentary people. The greatest calcium requirements occur when you are growing or have low oestrogen levels.

TABLE 2.4
Calcium needs for athletes

Population	Daily calcium needs (RDIs)
Young boys and girls	1000 mg
Adolescent boys and girls (growth)	1300 mg
Adult males	1000 mg
Adult females (during menstruating years)	1000 mg
Adult females (non-menstruating and post-menopausal)	1300 mg
Pregnant females	1000 mg
Breast-feeding females	1000 mg

Source: NHMRC, Nutrient Reference Values for Australian and New Zealand. Australian Government 2006.

Checklist 2.2 provides hints for achieving a calcium-rich diet—with emphasis on foods that also fit with other sports nutrition goals. This is important information, since studies show that more than half of all women fail to meet the recommended dietary intake of calcium. Risk factors include inadequate kilojoule intake, which limits the intake of all nutrients, and failure to consume calcium-rich dairy foods.

You can see from Table 2.12 that dairy foods are a rich source of calcium—in fact they provide 60–75 per cent of the calcium in a typical Western diet. It is unfortunate that they've suffered from bad publicity in recent years. Like red meat, dairy foods were caught up in the cholesterol concerns of the 1970s, being labelled as 'fattening' and full of saturated fat. They have also been accused by many 'alternative health' followers of causing all manner of allergies, 'mucus' formation and other health problems. Among younger populations, milk has lost its status as the preferred drink. School milk programs no longer run, and many teenagers reach into the fridge for a fizzy drink or fruit juice rather than the milk carton each time they are thirsty. This is a double whammy for bones. Not only is a good calcium source removed from the diet, but the cola drink that is often chosen as a replacement is high in phosphorus, which has an impact on calcium balance. In fact, some studies have shown a relationship between bone fractures in active young people and their consumption of fizzy drinks or cola drinks.

Most of the health prejudices against milk can be dismissed for lack of supporting evidence. For example, no relationship between milk intake and mucus production has been found. And although some babies suffer from cow's-milk intolerance during their first months of life, most outgrow this in early childhood. Low-fat and reduced-fat dairy products have grown almost exponentially in both quality and range over the past five years, and now offer athletes many ways to enjoy valuable protein and calcium for a lower kilojoule cost.

Lactose intolerance is a problem for only a small percentage of Caucasians, but larger proportions of other racial groups, such as Asians and Australian Aborigines. It is not an allergy to milk; rather, those who are lactose intolerant lack adequate amounts of the enzyme lactase, which aids the digestion of lactose, the principle carbohydrate in milk. Inadequate digestion of lactose can lead to gastric discomfort, flatulence and diarrhoea. However, this problem does not prevent those affected from consuming dairy foods. For a start, products such as yoghurt and cheese do not contain large amounts of lactose, and it is now possible to buy special tablets which can be added to milk to 'predigest' the lactose. Even so, lactose intolerance is rarely absolute: most people can tolerate small amounts of lactose-containing products, especially when they are consumed with other foods as part of a meal.

All in all, dairy products can form a valuable part of the athlete's peak training diet. If you haven't drunk a glass of milk since you were in school, there are many other ways to enjoy low-fat dairy foods—Checklist 2.2 shows many high-calcium meal and snack ideas that also incorporate carbohydrate-rich and low-fat foods. Three or more choices such as these each day will help you to meet your calcium goals. For those who can't or won't eat dairy products, calcium-enriched soy products are an alternative. Note that soy milk contains a similar amount of fat to whole milk, so you should choose a low-fat brand. Soy versions of yoghurt, cheese and other dairy products are also often available. Other foods can make a calcium contribution—for example, fish that is eaten bones and all, green leafy vegetables and tofu—but most of us will not eat these foods regularly enough to make them our most important calcium source. Some athletes will not be able to meet their calcium goals from diet alone and may be prescribed a calcium supplement. This should be done on the advice of a sports dietitian or doctor after making sure that dietary potential has been reached.

2.7 Other minerals

Although we have picked out calcium and iron for special comment, many other minerals and trace elements are needed for health and performance. Food variety and adequate energy are the keys to meeting needs for compounds such as zinc, magnesium, copper and phosphorus. Table 2.10 provides an overview of dietary sources of the minerals for which RDIs have been set.

2.8 Fluid

It is hard to believe how the simplest and most important of our nutrients has become such a controversial area in sports nutrition. In Chapter 1 we covered the principles for meeting daily fluid requirements—neither over-drinking nor under-drinking, and making good fluid choices. Fluid needs around exercise are a bit more complicated, because sweat losses can be variable and the opportunities to drink can be governed by the rules or challenges of the sporting activity. In the chapters on preparing (Chapter 4), competing (Chapter 4) and recovering (Chapter 5) from a sporting event, we will outline strategies for addressing fluid needs before, during and after an event. On each occasion we will try to make sense of the present discussions about fluid intake for sport. This does not mean that these arguments aren't relevant to training. Rather, training sessions provide the key opportunities to learn about fluid needs and to develop a plan for meeting them. Good fluid management in training will help you to get the best out of each workout and fine-tune a race or competition plan.

A simple way to assess fluid losses during exercise is to monitor weight changes over the session. Essentially, each kilogram of weight loss is equivalent to a litre of sweat. There are some ways in which this is an oversimplification. For example, we burn up some fuel during exercise that contributes to a smallish weight loss. And there are ways in which errors can creep into the calculations. Sweat can be caught up in hair and clothes so that it's included in a weight measurement when it is really no longer part of the body's fluid stores. Figure 2.3 provides some guidelines on how to get a general idea of fluid-balance issues resulting from exercise. It is valuable for athletes to make such assessments from time to time to get a feel for the fluid-management issues in a range of exercise challenges and situations. This will help to formulate and evaluate good drinking plans.

2.9 Timing of meals

Being an athlete often means having a hectic lifestyle. Your daily schedule may include work or school, training (or competition), perhaps some physiotherapy or a massage, adequate sleep—and who knows what other commitments. Somewhere among all these activities, food has to be squeezed in, and unfortunately it often becomes an afterthought.

For best results, your training diet needs to be planned rather than haphazard. That way you will be sure that you are achieving all your nutrition goals. The timing of food—eating when your body most appreciates it—is also important.

Your daily timetable and your commitments are unique. A good start to organising your nutrition needs is to plot your total commitments for a week into a grid, and then use coloured pens to fill in each day's nutrition needs and opportunities. See Checklist 2.3 for some hints on drawing up a daily food and fluid schedule. Note that careful timing of eating and drinking before, during or after training sessions (and competitive events) will play an important role in optimising your performance and recovery.

2.10 Periodising your nutrition program

In most sports, athletes periodise their training. There may be a base phase after the off-season in which high volumes of training are used to regain conditioning or to gain muscle mass. This may be followed by a transition phase and competition preparation, then competition, recovery and the start of a new cycle. Within these macro cycles, there are micro cycles with sessions of different duration, intensity and purpose—hard day, easy day, etc. Clearly, as your exercise needs change, your nutrition needs do too. In the previous section, we promoted the idea of setting up some baseline eating routines and scaling up or down with extras and training-based snacks according to your workouts and their goals. Energy needs will go down during periods of inactivity, while protein and carbohydrate needs will increase as you train more. This is the simplest way of periodising your nutrition.

However other approaches are being tried. One involves trying to adapt endurance athletes to high-fat diets to make them better at 'fat-burning'. Even the leanest of athletes carries several kilograms of body fat that can be used by the muscles as a fuel for exercise. The training undertaken by these athletes helps them to use this fuel instead of muscle glycogen. This is an advantage since it allows the limited glycogen stores to last longer before they are depleted and the athlete gets fatigued.

We have been involved in studies that showed that training alone doesn't max out the fat-burning capacity of muscles, even in elite athletes. In fact, if these athletes switch to a diet that is high in fat (65 per cent of energy) and restricted in carbohydrate (less than 20 per cent of training) over five days of hard training, they can 'retool' their muscles to be more efficient at using fat at the same exercise intensity. By itself, this change doesn't appear to benefit sports performance. After all, it is just switching from one fuel source to another. However, the experiment became interesting when we found that the muscle retains this fat-burning memory at least for a day or so after the high-fat diet is removed. This provided a blueprint for a new way to 'load up' for an endurance or ultra-endurance event. Five days of 'fat adaptation', followed by a day of carbohydrate loading, produced an athlete with full glycogen stores and an enhanced capacity to use them slowly. Even when carbohydrate was eaten before and during exercise, the body still used fat as a fuel source in preference to glycogen.

On paper, this looks like the best of both fuel worlds. However, a whole series of studies has failed to find any evidence that this approach made an athlete go faster in a time trial. What's the problem? Are we unable to measure performance well enough to detect a useful change? Do some athletes respond better than others, making the results of a group study unclear? These explanations are still plausible. However, new evidence emerged that the fat adaptation doesn't just slow down the use of glycogen fuel during exercise, it can actually impair the muscles' ability to use it. This isn't such a problem for low- to moderate-intensity exercise, where fat burning can keep up with the required rate of power production. However, your 'top gear' absolutely demands the rapid power production that of which only carbohydrate is capable. Without it, an athlete can't be part of a breakaway, surge up a hill or sprint to the line. These are the event-defining moments in most sports. So there is a risk of losing out on an important part of performance, as well as the discomfort of undertaking fat loading. (It isn't pleasant forcing yourself to train hard on a low-carbohydrate, high-fat diet.) As a result, we can't recommend this once-promising strategy.

'Train low, compete high' is the other dietary periodisation protocol that has captured the interest of athletes, coaches and sports scientists. This refers to strategies in which the athlete deliberately trains with low glycogen levels over a longer period, then switches to full fuel stores for the competition phase. The idea is based on studies which show that the training stimulus provided by a given exercise session is increased when muscle runs low on glycogen. It seems that low glycogen levels trigger a greater response from some of the important proteins involved in adapting to training. In other words, the athlete can 'train smarter'—get a better return for the same stimulus.

Again, this strategy sounds appealing and has reinvigorated interest in low-carbohydrate diets. However, before you rush for an Atkins cookbook, it needs to be pointed out that the current studies on this topic have manipulated glycogen levels by changing training patterns rather than by restricting carbohydrate. Instead of training for one session each day, subjects in 'train low' studies do two training sessions every second day and have a rest day in between. And they eat a carbohydrate-focused diet that is able to restore glycogen from day to day—around 8 g per kilogram of body weight per day! So the real story is that the first training session of a Big Day is done with high fuel stores, while the second one is done in a depleted state. (The protocol should really be called 'training 50 per cent low' or 'training 50/50'). This is a far cry from following a low-carbohydrate diet for prolonged periods. For a start, chronic fuel depletion is likely to interfere with training itself. And there are possible risks of illness, injury and staleness or overtraining when muscles, brain and the immune system are chronically fuel-depleted.

So is training smarter better than training harder? There are some issues with this cool-sounding idea. The study that started all the interest in this program involved untrained people who did the same training session every day. This is, again, a very different scenario from one where highly conditioned athletes do a lot of training, with the flexibility to train harder in volume or intensity depending how they feel or improve. In fact, two separate studies have now implemented a three-week 'train 50 per cent low' scheme with endurance athletes. Half of each group alternated between a 100-minute moderate-intensity training session on one day and a high-intensity interval-training session (8 × 5 minutes of all-out effort) on the next. The other half completed the same sessions but arranged them one after another on a single day, with a rest day in between.

Both studies found that the athletes who did their interval training 'low' had greater improvements in muscle markers of training enzymes and signalling proteins. But these athletes also suffered when doing these workouts. They were forced to do each rep at a lower power output than the fully recovering 'high' training group. They may have suffered less as the weeks progressed, but overall they ended up doing less work in these key training sessions. In case you're thinking that they made greater gains for less 'cost', consider that both groups spent the same number of minutes in training and trained as hard as they were able to (in fact, the 'low' training group felt terrible and needed to be bribed to get the best out of their legs). The 'low' trainers just couldn't produce the same power. Nevertheless, at the end of the training block, both groups improved equally (~10 per cent) on a one-hour performance ride. So, the 'train low' program produced neither detectable benefits nor drawbacks to a 'competition' performance. A scientist might argue that the performance ride just couldn't pick up the advantages that were present in the muscle, and that under different conditions 'training low' might achieve benefits. However, a coach might argue that high-calibre athletes need to train at high intensities and produce high power outputs—and that over a longer time or with a more sensitive performance test, the 'low' training group might suffer in competition.

So where does that leave us with training high or training low? In real life, athletes who train hard do a mixture of both. Whether by design or accident, some sessions are done with low fuel availability—for example, it's more practical to do early-morning sessions before breakfast, it may not be convenient to have a sports drink available throughout long training sessions, and the timetabling of some workouts won't allow for full recovery between sessions. Other sessions are done with longer recovery time or at times of the day when it is easier to fuel up. It is perhaps the right blend of training low on some occasions and training high for key performance sessions that prepares the athlete properly. That is why coaching—and sports nutrition—should be considered an art as well as a science.

FIG 2.1
How to predict your daily energy requirements

Step 1.	Find an estimate for your Basal Metabolic Rate from Table 2.5. Find a value that is closest to your weight and age
Step 2.	Rate your daily activity level. Either multiply your whole day by a single factor (Table 2.6) or rate the activity level of your non-sporting life and add the exercise as a separate calculation. Note that most athletes are quite sedentary outside their specific sporting activities, so it may be appropriate to choose the Sedentary or Light Activity factors.
Step 3.	Multiply your BMR by your activity factor
Step 4.	Add up the cost of your sporting activities for the week (use Table 2.7). Divide the weekly activity level by 7 to gain an approximation of the daily cost of your exercise and add it to the figure from Step 3. Note that these figures are meant to provide only a ballpark approximation
Example:	Molly is a 22-year-old runner who weighs 60 kg. She runs 4 days a week @ 5 min per km pace with each session lasting about 50 min. She does one interval-training session lasting about an hour. Her total mileage is 50 km. She walks around the university campus and considers her overall activity level to be light
Calculations:	Step 1 BMR = ~ 5.8 MJ (Table 2.5) Step 2 Activity level of non-exercise = 1.5 (Table 2.6) Step 3 BMR × activity level = 5.8 × 1.5 = 8.7 MJ Step 4 Weekly training cost = 50 min × 52 kJ/min × 4 (running) + 60 min × 55 kJ/min (intervals averaging at 4.5 min/km) = 13700 kJ or 1.37 MJ Daily training cost = 1.37/7 = 1.96 MJ Total = 10.66 MJ (2540 kilocalories)

TABLE 2.5
Basal Metabolic Rate for reference adults

Daily energy (MJ/day)				
	Age			
Body weight	15–18 yrs	19–30 yrs	31–50 yrs	51–70 yrs
Men				
50 kg	6.6			
56 kg	7.0	6.4	6.4	5.8
64 kg	7.6	6.9	6.7	6.1
71 kg		7.4	7.1	6.5
79 kg		7.9	7.5	6.9
88 kg		8.4	7.9	7.3
Women				
50 kg	5.7	5.2	5.2	4.9
56 kg	6.0	5.6	5.5	5.2
64 kg		6.0	5.7	5.4
71 kg		6.5	6.0	5.7
79 kg		7.0	6.2	6.0
88 kg				

Note: Kilocalories can be calculated by dividing by 0.0042
Source: Nutrient Reference Values for Australia and New Zealand, NHMRC, 2005

TABLE 2.6
Average activity levels expressed as multiples of BMR

Activity level	Males	Females
Bed rest	1.2	1.2
Very sedentary	1.3	1.3
Sedentary/maintenance	1.4	1.4

Activity level	Males	Females
Light	1.5	1.5
Light–moderate	1.7	1.6
Moderate	1.8	1.7
Heavy	2.1	1.8
Very heavy	2.3	2.0

Source: Recommended Nutrient Intakes, NHMRC, Australia, 1990

TABLE 2.7
Estimated energy cost of activity (kilojoules/minute)

Activity	Body weight				
	50 kg	60 kg	70 kg	80 kg	90 kg
Aerobics					
—beginners	22	26	30	34	39
—advanced	28	33	40	45	51
Badminton	20	24	28	33	37
Ballroom dancing	11	13	15	17	19
Basketball	29	35	40	46	52
Boxing					
—sparring	46	56	65	74	84
—in ring	29	35	40	46	52
Canoeing					
—leisure	9	11	13	15	17
—racing	22	26	30	34	39
Circuit training	22	26	30	34	40
Cricket					
—batting	17	21	24	28	32

	50 kg	60 kg	70 kg	80 kg	90 kg
—bowling	19	22	26	30	34
Cycling					
—9 km/hr	13	16	18	21	24
—15 km/hr	21	24	28	33	38
—racing	35	42	49	56	63
Football	28	33	39	44	50
Golf	18	21	25	28	32
Gymnastics	14	16	19	22	25
Hockey	18	20	24	29	33
Judo	41	49	57	65	73
Running					
—5.5 min per km	40	49	57	65	73
—5 min per km	44	52	61	70	78
—4.5 min per km	48	55	65	75	85
—4 min per km	54	65	76	87	98
Skiing					
—cross-country	35	42	49	56	63
—downhill (easy)	18	21	25	29	33
—downhill (hard)	29	35	40	49	55
Squash	44	53	62	71	79
Swimming					
—freestyle	33	40	46	52	59
—backstroke	36	43	49	56	63
—breast stroke	34	41	47	54	61
Table tennis	14	17	19	23	26

	50 kg	60 kg	70 kg	80 kg	90 kg
Tennis					
—social	15	17	20	23	26
—competitive	37	44	50	58	65
Volleyball	10	12	15	17	19
Walking					
—10 min per km	21	26	30	35	39
—8 min per km	25	30	35	40	45
—5 min per km	44	52	61	70	78

Notes: All figures are approximate values only.
Kilocalories can be calculated by dividing kilojoule values by 4.2
Source: Adapted from Katch, F.I., and McArdle, W.D., *Nutrition, Weight Control and Exercise*, Lea and Febiger; Philadelphia, 1988

TABLE 2.8
Ready reckoner of carbohydrate-rich foods

Carbohydrate food	Amount for 50 g ('large serve') carbohydrate	Amount for 15 g ('medium serve') carbohydrate
Bread and cereals		
Wheat biscuit cereal (e.g. Weetbix)	60 g (5 biscuits)	22.5 g (1½ biscuits)
Flake/bubble breakfast cereal (e.g. Cornflakes, Weeties, Rice Bubbles, CocoPops)	60 g (2 cups)	20 g (¾ cup)
Flake + fruit breakfast cereal (e.g. Sustain™)	75 g (1¼ cups)	20 g (⅓ cup)
Toasted muesli (e.g. Komplete)	70 g (⅔ cup)	20 g (2 tbsp)

Carbohydrate food	Amount for 50 g ('large serve') carbohydrate	Amount for 15 g ('medium serve') carbohydrate
Porridge made with milk	350 g (1 ⅓ cups)	110 g (~½ cup)
Porridge made with water	590 g (2¼ cups)	200 g (¾ cup)
Rolled oats	85 g (~1 cup)	30 g (~⅓ cup)
Bread	120 g (~4 slices regular or 3 thick slices)	30 g (~1 slice regular)
Bread rolls	90 g (1½ 10 cm diameter)	30 g (~½ 10 cm diameter)
Pita and Lebanese bread	100 g (2 small or 1 large pita)	30 g (⅓ large pita)
Chapati	140 g (4)	35 g (1)
English muffin	130 g (2 full muffins)	30 g (½ full muffin)
Crumpet	125 g (2½ crumpets)	40 g (¾ crumpet)
Bars, biscuits and cakes		
Cereal bar	2 × 40 g bars	25 g (⅔ × 40 g bar)
Muesli bar	90 g (3 × 30 g bars)	30 g (1 × 30 g bar)
Rice cakes	6 thick or 10 thin	2 thick or 3 thin
Crispbreads and dry biscuits	6 large or 15 small	2 large or 5 small
Fruit-filled biscuits	5	1½
Plain sweet biscuits	8–10	2–3
Cream-filled/ chocolate biscuits	~ 4–5	~ 1–2
Cake-style muffin—commercial	1½ medium or ¾ large	½ medium

Carbohydrate food	Amount for 50 g ('large serve') carbohydrate	Amount for 15 g ('medium serve') carbohydrate
Pancakes	170 g (3 medium)	55 g (1 medium)
Scones	105 g (3 small or 1 ½ commercial large)	35 g (1 small or ½ commercial large
Iced fruit bun	~100 g (¾ commercial medium)	~30 g (¼ commercial medium)
Croissant	130 g (1½ commercial medium)	~35 g (⅓ commercial medium)
Pasta, rice and noodles		
Rice, boiled	170 g (1 cup)	55 g (⅓ cup)
Pasta or noodles, boiled	220 g (1½ cups)	75 g (½ cup)
Canned spaghetti	440 g (large can)	130 g (½ cup)
Rice-cream or creamed rice	330 g (1⅓ cups)	120 g (½ cup)
Fruit		
Fruit crumble	½ cup (commercial)	2 tbsp (commercial)
Fruit packed in heavy syrup	270 g (1 cup)	80 g (⅓ cup)
Fruit stewed/canned in natural juice	450 g (1¾ cups)	130 g (½ cup)
Fresh fruit salad	515 g (2½ cups)	155 g (¾ cup)
Bananas	2 medium	1 medium
Mangoes, pears, and other large fruit	2 large or 3 medium	½ mango, 1 × medium pear
Oranges, apples and other medium-size fruit	2 large or 3 medium	1 medium
Grapes	340 g (2 cups)	100 g (⅔ cup)

Carbohydrate food	Amount for 50 g ('large serve') carbohydrate	Amount for 15 g ('medium serve') carbohydrate
Sultanas and raisins	70 g (5 tbsp)	20 g (1½ tbsp)
Dried apricots	115 g (22 halves)	35 g (7 halves)
Strawberries	7 × 250-g punnet	2 × 250-g punnet
Melon	6 cups (diced)	2 cups (diced)
Grapefruit	3 × large	1 large
Vegetables* and legumes (note that most vegetables have a low carbohydrate content)		
Potatoes (raw)	370 g (2 × large or 3 medium)	120 g (1 medium)
Sweet potato (raw)	280 g (2 cups)	105 g (¾ cup)
Corn	325 g (1¼ cups creamed or 2 large cobs)	80 g (⅓ cup or 1 medium cob)
Baked beans	440 g (1 large can)	140 g (1 cup)
Lentils (cooked and drained)	530 g (2½ cups)	220 g (1 cup)
Soy beans and kidney beans (cooked and drained)	400 g (2 cups)	130 g (⅔ cup)
Dairy products		
Milk	1 litre	300 ml
Flavoured milk	600 ml	150 ml
Custard	330 g (1¼ cups)	90 g (⅓ cup)
'Diet' yogurt and natural yogurt	5 × 200-g individual cartons	1½ × 200-g individual cartons
Flavoured non-fat yogurt	1½ × 200-g individual cartons	½ × 200-g individual carton

Carbohydrate food	Amount for 50 g ('large serve') carbohydrate	Amount for 15 g ('medium serve') carbohydrate
Ice-cream	250 g (~5 scoops or 1½ cups)	75 g (~½ cup)
Sugars and confectionery		
Sugar	50 g (3 tbsp)	15 g (1 tbsp)
Jam	80 g (3 tbsp)	25 g (1 tbsp)
Syrups	70 g (2½ tbsp)	20 g (¾ tbsp)
Honey	60 g (2 tbsp)	20 g (¾ tbsp)
Chocolate	80 g	25 g
Filled chocolate bars (e.g. Mars Bar)	70 g	20 g (e.g. Fun Size Mars Bar)
Jubes/jelly confectionery	80 g	25 g
Drinks		
Fruit juice unsweetened	600 ml	200 ml
Fruit juice sweetened	500 ml	150 ml
Cordial (25 per cent prep)	600 ml	200 ml
Soft drinks and flavoured mineral water	400 ml	125 ml
Fruit smoothie	300–400 ml	~100 ml
Sports foods		
Sports drink (e.g. Gatorade)	800 ml	200 ml
Liquid meal (Sustagen Sport/PowerBar Proteinplus)	250 ml made from milk or 80 g powder with water	¼ cup made with milk or 20 g powder with water

Carbohydrate food	Amount for 50 g ('large serve') carbohydrate	Amount for 15 g ('medium serve') carbohydrate
Sports bar (e.g. 65 g PowerBar Performance Bar)	1¼ bars	~ ⅓ gel
Sports gel (e.g. 40 g PowerBar Powergel)	2 gels	~ ½ gel

Source: The carbohydrate composition data were estimated using FoodWorks Professional Edition, Version 3.02, © 1998–2005 (Xyris Software, Brisbane, Australia). Food composition data were compiled from Nuttab 95; AusFoods; Australian AusNut and nutritional information from food manufacturers entered into the standardised Australian Institute of Sport Recipe database.

TABLE 2.9
Ready reckoner of protein-rich foods

Type of protein source	Amount of product needed to provide 10 g protein
Animal foods	• 2 small eggs • 250 ml reduced-fat or low-fat milk • 40 g (2 slices) of reduced-fat cheese • 70 g cottage cheese • 200 g carton low-fat fruit yoghurt • 250 ml low-fat custard • 35 g lean beef, lamb or pork (cooked weight) • 40 g lean chicken (cooked weight) • 50 g grilled fish • 50 g canned tuna or salmon
Vegetable foods	• 4 slices (120 g) wholemeal bread • 2 cups (120 g) wholegrain cereal (e.g. Sustain™) • 2 cups (300 g) cooked pasta • 2 cups (380 g) cooked rice • 1 cup (220 g) lentils or kidney beans • 210 g (1½ cups) baked beans • 100 g tofu or soy meat • 300 ml soy milk • 50 g nuts or seeds

Type of protein source	Amount of product needed to provide 10 g protein
Supplements and sports foods	• 10 000 mg free-form amino acids • 15–20 g high protein powder or protein hydrolysate • ~100 ml liquid meal supplement (e.g. Sustagen Sport or PowerBar Proteinplus) • 60 g sports bar (e.g. PowerBar Performance Bar) • 20–30 g high protein sports bar (e.g. PowerBar Proteinplus Bar)
Less expensive alternatives to sports foods and supplements	• 25 g (~3 tbsp) skim milk powder • 250 ml homemade fruit smoothie (Recipe for 600 ml = 250 ml low-fat milk, 200 g fruit yoghurt, 1 banana or cup berries) • 150 ml fortified milk shake (Recipe for 600 ml = 500 ml low-fat flavoured milk + 4 tablespoons ice-cream + ¼ cup skim milk powder)

Source: The protein composition data were estimated using FoodWorks Professional Edition, Version 3.02, © 1998–2005 (Xyris Software, Brisbane, Australia). Food composition data were compiled from Nuttab 95; AusFoods; Australian AusNut and nutritional information from food manufacturers entered into the standardised Australian Institute of Sport Recipe database.

TABLE 2.10
Vitamins and minerals: where to find your RDI

Vitamin	Functions	RDI (daily target)	Good food sources
Vitamin A	• Protects eyesight against night blindness • Essential for normal bone development • Healthy skin and mucous membranes • Antioxidant activities—assists with cancer protection • Immune system function—resistance to infection	(As retinol equivalents) Males 900 µg Females 700 µg	Occurs as retinol (fat soluble) • Oily fish • Egg (yolk) • Full-fat dairy products • Fortified margarine Occurs also as beta-carotene, which is converted to retinol (plant foods) • Yellow, orange and green fruits and vegetables

Vitamin	Functions	RDI (daily target)	Good food sources
Vitamin B1 (thiamine)	• Energy metabolism from food • Carbohydrate metabolism • Function of heart and nervous system	Males 1.2 mg Females 1.1 mg	• Fortified and wholegrain breads and cereals • Yeast extract (e.g. Vegemite, Marmite) • Legumes • Poultry • Soy Milk • Fish • Potatoes and watermelon • Organ meats (liver/pâté) • Pork
Vitamin B2 (riboflavin)	• Energy metabolism from food • Carbohydrate, fat, protein metabolism • Growth	Males 1.3 mg Females 1.1 mg	• Milk and dairy foods • Yeast extract (e.g. Vegemite, Marmite) • Green leafy vegetables • Fortified and wholegrain breads and cereals • Organ meats (liver/pâté)
Vitamin B3 (niacin)	• Energy metabolism from food • Carbohydrate, fat, protein metabolism • Cholesterol metabolism	Males 16 mg Females 14 mg	All protein sources, namely • Fish, liver • Meat, cheese, poultry • Grains, eggs • Fortified cereals • Potatoes • Nuts and legumes
Vitamin B12	• Red blood cell formation • Manufacture of DNA and nerve cells • Carbohydrate and fat metabolism	Males 2.4 µg Females 2.4 µg	• Animal foods—liver, lean meat, oily fish, seafood, eggs, milk and dairy • Plant foods—fortified soy milk

Vitamin	Functions	RDI (daily target)	Good food sources
Folate	• Red blood cell formation • DNA metabolism • Prevention of neural tube defects *in utero* • Reduction of homocysteine (risk factor for heart disease)	Males 400 μg Females 400 μg	• Wholegrain breads and cereals • Eggs, lean beef • Legumes and nuts • Green leafy vegetables • Broccoli • Organ meats (liver/ pâté)
Pantothenic acid	• Carbohydrate, fat, protein metabolism	*Males 6.0 mg *Females 4.0 mg	Made by bacteria in gut. • Present in all plant and animal foods. Best sources: • Eggs • Organ meats (liver/ pâté) • Fish and lean meat • Yeast extract (e.g. Vegemite, Marmite) • Wholegrain breads and cereals
Biotin	• Fat and protein metabolism • Growth • Nerve cell function	*Males 30 μg *Females 25 μg	Made by bacteria in gut. • Most vegetables • Banana, watermelon, grapefruit, tomatoes, strawberries • Peanuts • Milk • Egg (yolk) • Liver/pâté • Wholegrain breads and cereals

Vitamin	Functions	RDI (daily target)	Good food sources
Vitamin C	• Wound healing • Antioxidant activity • Formation of collagen in bones, teeth and blood vessels • Resistance to infection • Absorption of non-heme iron	Males 45 mg Females 45 mg	• Citrus fruits and juices • Tropical fruits and juices • Berries • Green leafy vegetables • Tomatoes, capsicums, broccoli, brussel sprouts, potatotes
Vitamin D	• Absorption of calcium and phosphorus • Bone and teeth health	*Males 5–15 μg *Females 5–15 μg	Most Vitamin D is formed from sunlight acting on skin • Dietary sources: • Oily fish • Butter and margarine
Vitamin E	• Antioxidant activity • Prevention of cancer and heart disease • Cell membrane	(as alpha-tocopherol equiva-lents) *Males 10 mg *Females 7 mg	• Wheatgerm and wholegrain cereals • Vegetable oils • Nuts and seeds • Eggs (yolk) • Offal
Vitamin K	• Blood clotting	*Males 70 μg *Females 60 μg	• Made by bacteria in gut. • Dietary sources: • Liver • Soybean and other vegetable oils • Green leafy vegetables • Wheat bran • Milk

Mineral	Functions	RDI	Good food sources
Phosphorus	• Partner to calcium in bone and teeth formation • Protein and nucleic-acid formation	Males 1000 mg Females 1000 mg	Widely distributed in foods
Zinc	• Wound healing • Enzyme component • Sexual maturation and function • Taste, smell and sight	Males 14 mg Females 8 mg	• Lean meat • Offal • Oysters, shellfish • Wholegrain bread and cereals • Eggs, poultry • Legumes and nuts
Magnesium	• Bone structure • Muscle contraction and nerve function • Enzyme systems	Males 400–420 mg Females 310–320 mg	• Widely distributed with richest food sources: • Wholegrain breads and cereals • Green leafy vegetables • Lean meat • Legumes and nuts • Tofu, milk, yoghurt
Iodine	• Brain function • Prevents goitre	Males 150 µg Females 150 µg	• Iodised table salt • Fish and shellfish • Seaweed
Selenium	• Antioxidant activity • Can protect against heavy-metal poisoning	Males 70 µg Females 60 µg	Content of grains and vegetables depends on selenium content of the cell in which they are grown • Lean meat • Fish, oysters • Offal, chicken
Molybdenum	• Iron metabolism	Males 45 µg Females 45 µg	Widely distributed in cereals and vegetables according to the molybdenum content of the soil

Mineral	Functions	RDI	Good food sources
Copper	• Co-factor in enzyme activity • Red blood cell formation • Formation of melanin in skin • Nervous-system function	*Males 1.7 mg *Females 1.2 mg	• Shellfish • Liver/pâté, kidney • Legumes, nuts and seeds • Dried Fruit • Tofu • Wholegrain breads and cereals
Chromium	• Growth • Part of glucose tolerance factor—a complex that enhances insulin action	*Males 35 μg *Females 25 μg	• Yeast extract (Vegemite, Marmite) • Wholegrain bread and cereals • Liver/pâté • Oysters, seafood • Lean meat • Eggs (yolk)
Manganese	• Enzyme function and activation	*Males 5.5 mg *Females 5.0 mg	Widely distributed in foods
Fluoride	• Healthy bones and teeth • Possibly prevents osteoporosis	*Males 4.0 mg *Females 3.0 mg	• Fluoridated drinking water
Potassium	• Major electrolyte inside the cell—balances with sodium outside the cell • Nerve impulse transmission • Counteracts effects of sodium on blood pressure • Enzyme function	*Males 3800 mg *Females 2800 mg	Widely distributed • Fruits and vegetables • Meat and fish

* There are no RDIs for this nutrient. However a level of Adequate Intake has been set.

Source: NHMRC, Nutrient Reference Values for Australia and New Zealand. Australian Government, 2006.

TABLE 2.11
Ready reckoner of iron-rich foods for the optimal training diet

Heme iron foods		
Food	**Serve**	**mg iron**
Liver	100 g (cooked weight)	9.3
Liver pâté	40 g (2 tbsp)	4.0
Lean steak	100 g (cooked weight)	~3.0
Chicken (dark meat)	100 g (cooked weight)	1.1
Fish	100 g (cooked weight)	0.3–1.9
Oysters	100 g (raw)	3.9
Salmon	100 g (small tin)	0.9
Non-heme iron foods		
Food	**Serve**	**mg iron**
Eggs	100 g (2)	1.6
Fortified breakfast cereal	30 g (½–1 cup)	2.5–5.00
Wholemeal bread	60 g (2 sl)	1.4
Spinach (cooked)	145 g (1 cup)	4.4
Lentils (canned and drained)	220 g (1 cup)	3.1
Kidney beans (canned and drained)	190 g (1 cup)	4.0
Textured vegetable protein	100 g dry	10.4
Tofu	100 g cooked	1.2
Sultanas	50 g	0.9
Dried apricots	50 g	1.6
Almonds	50 g	1.8

Source: The iron composition data were estimated using FoodWorks Professional Edition, Version 3.02, © 1998–2005 (Xyris Software, Brisbane, Australia). Food composition data were compiled from Nuttab 95; AusFoods; Australian AusNut and nutritional information from food manufacturers entered into the standardised Australian Institute of Sport Recipe database.

CHECKLIST 2.1
Hints for an iron boost

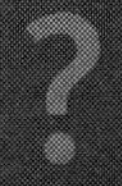

- Include heme iron from animal food sources regularly at meals. It provides a source of well-absorbed iron and, via the presence of a 'meat factor', enhances the absorption of non-heme iron from these and other foods consumed at the same meal. The frequency of eating heme iron sources may be more important than the total quantity of meat eaten:
    - Include small amounts of lean red meats in meals at least 3–4 times each week.
    - Consider shellfish or liver (e.g., pâté) as an alternative to red meat.
    - Add chicken and pork meats and dark cuts of fish at other meals to provide a reasonable source of iron and to enhance iron absorption at the meal.
- Choose ways to integrate high-iron eating with your other nutritional goals, such as adding meats to a high-carbohydrate meal:
    - Examples: sandwich with roast beef, pasta with Bolognese sauce, lamb kebabs with rice, beef stir-fry with vegetables and noodles.
- Include foods that are good sources of non-heme iron at most meals, especially meals at which heme sources are not eaten. Note that many of these foods also assist the athlete to meet carbohydrate targets:
    - Use cereal foods that are iron fortified (e.g., many commercial breakfast cereals).
    - Include iron-rich foods such as wholegrain cereals, dried fruit, legumes, eggs, nuts and seeds, and green leafy vegetables in meals and recipes.
- Mix and match foods at meals so that factors that enhance iron absorption are present where non-heme iron provides the major

source of iron or where factors that inhibit iron absorption are also present:

  - Vitamin C—example, omelette with tomatoes, orange juice with breakfast cereal
  - Meat factor—examples are provided above

- Reduce the impact of food factors that inhibit iron absorption from sources eaten at the same meal. Either separate these factors from heme-iron containing meals, or add a factor to enhance iron absorption:
  - Phytates (wholegrain cereal)—example, don't add wheat bran to your meals. You probably don't need it, and it will impair your absorption of iron from the meal
  - Tannin (tea, coffee)—drink tea and coffee between meals rather than with them
  - Calcium
  - Peptides from soy products
- If you are a vegetarian and reliant on non-heme iron:
  - Work extra hard on the non-heme mixes and matches
  - Think about cooking in cast-iron pots.
- See a sports dietitian if you are unable to follow such food patterns or suspect you are not consuming enough iron. An iron supplement may be part of the plan, but it should not be a substitute for dietary changes.

TABLE 2.12
Calcium-rich foods for the optimal training diet

Food	Serving	mg Calcium
Skim milk	200 ml (glass)	255
Low-fat calcium-enriched milk	200 ml (glass)	285
Soy milk	200 ml (glass)	27

Food	Serving	mg Calcium
Fortified soy milks	200 ml (glass)	230
Reduced-fat cheese	20 g (1 slice)	163
Cottage cheese	115 g (½ cup)	94
Low-fat fruit yoghurt	200 g (carton)	358
Light *fromage frais*	130 g (carton)	96
Low-fat ice-cream	20 g (2 tbsp)	30
Salmon (with bones, drained)	100 g (small tin)	310
Sardines (drained)	100 g	380
Oysters (raw)	100 g	135
Almonds (raw)	50 g	117
Tahini	20 g (tbsp)	66
Spinach (cooked)	145 g (1 cup)	90
Tofu (cooked)	100 g	330

Source: The calcium composition data were estimated using FoodWorks Professional Edition, Version 3.02, © 1998–2005 (Xyris Software, Brisbane, Australia). Food composition data were compiled from Nuttab 95; AusFoods; Australian AusNut and nutritional information from food manufacturers entered into the standardised Australian Institute of Sport Recipe database.

CHECKLIST 2.2
Hints for a calcium boost

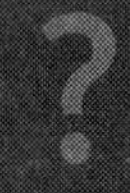

- Adopt food patterns that include regular servings of dairy foods. One serving is equivalent to 1 cup of milk, 40 g or 2 slices of cheese, or a 200 g carton of yoghurt:
    - Adults: 3 servings a day
    - Children and adolescent athletes: 4 servings a day
    - Note that athletes with menstrual disturbances may need 5 servings a day
- If you are unable or unwilling to consume dairy foods, opt for a calcium-fortified soy alternative.
- Be aware of other foods that can increase total calcium intake, including fish eaten with bones, green leafy vegetables, and some nuts and legumes.
- Be aware that in some countries, everyday foods such as orange juice can be fortified with calcium to provide a substantial and regular source of calcium. Some low-fat dairy foods are also calcium-enriched.
- Organise your calcium-rich eating to meet other goals such as restricting energy intake or meeting fuel targets. The following meals and snacks are calcium-rich, carbohydrate-rich and low in fat:
    - Cereal and low-fat milk
    - Fruit and low-fat fruit yoghurt/low-fat custard/creamed rice
    - Wholemeal sandwich with salmon and salad (eat the bones!)
    - Homemade pizza topped with low-fat cheese slices or a sprinkle of reduced-fat mozzarella cheese
    - Banana smoothie made with low-fat milk, banana and low-fat ice-cream/yoghurt
    - 'Skinny' hot chocolate or cappuccino plus toast or English muffin
    - Liquid meal supplement (e.g. PowerBar Proteinplus, Sustagen Sport)

- If you can't fit enough calcium-rich foods into your diet, see a sports dietitian to devise a suitable meal plan. When dietary intake of calcium is insufficient, calcium supplements may be prescribed.

CHECKLIST 2.3
It's all in the timing!

- Write down your schedule of training and other daily commitments for the week ahead so you can get an objective view of the challenges and opportunities:
  - Key training sessions that might benefit from strategic nutrition support before, during and after
  - Busy periods when you will be running between commitments and have little time to obtain, prepare or even eat foods
  - Less hectic times when you can prepare for the busier times ahead.
- Rather than relying on the notional 'three square meals', consider how you can spread your food intake over a series of six meals and snacks suited to your timetable and training load. The possible advantages are:
  - Achieving nutrition support for key training sessions to ensure adequate fuelling, better performance and speedy recovery.
  - Achieving more even blood glucose levels rather than big peaks and troughs over the day. This may help to avoid 'flat spots' or afternoon fatigue.
  - Stimulating your metabolic rate. Each time you eat a meal there is a small rise in your metabolic rate. More meals means better stimulation.
- Avoiding the need to 'stuff' yourself to achieve a high kilojoule intake. It is more comfortable to follow a 'grazing' pattern: eat a little now and come back for more later.

- Avoiding 'hunger spots' when you are on a reduced-energy diet.
- Time your last meal before training (or competition) so that you can exercise comfortably yet achieve the right preparation for key workouts. It may be important to consume carbohydrate and protein in the period before the workout. This may mean stopping an hour before for a light snack or a liquid meal (low-fat milk smoothie or Sustagen Sport/Powerbar Proteinplus) and up to two to three hours before for larger or heavier meals.
- Promote recovery after key sessions (training or competition) by eating a carbohydrate and protein mix as soon as possible. Your next meal might be waiting for you as soon as you finish the workout. If not, start recovery processes by choosing a suitable drink or snack within 15–30 minutes of exercise, and continue to implement your nutritional plan at the next meal. Don't neglect your need to replace fluid or electrolytes, either. (Read Chapter 5 for more details on strategies to promote recovery).
- Achieve your hydration targets by maximising the retention of the fluids you drink. Drink with meals so that your fluid intake coincides with your intake of salt. It can also be useful to sip fluids over a recovery period rather than chug a large volume in one go.
- Having access to food and drinks when you need them will be an important factor in achieving your nutrition goals. If you live your life on the run, you will need to plan ahead. Having a portable food supply with you will help you to eat on the go. Think of some suitable snacks to store at work, in your locker, in your sports bag or in your car.

FIGURE 2.2
How to mix and match plant foods to complement proteins

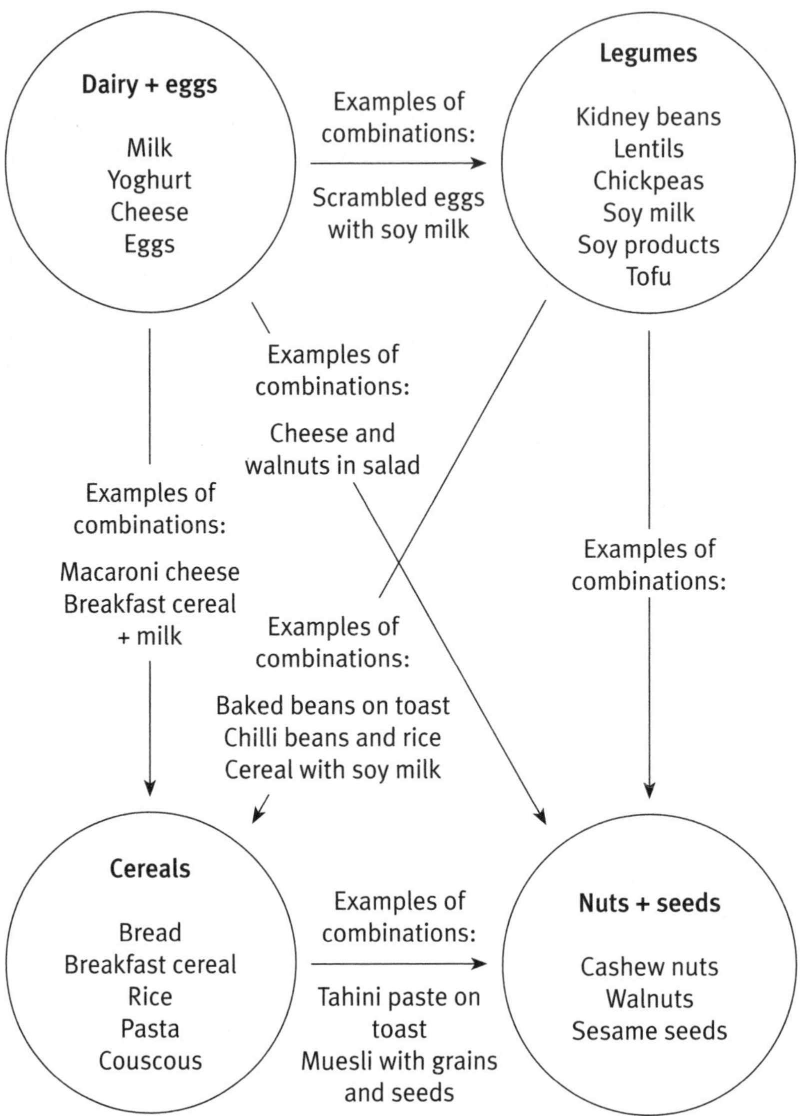

FIGURE 2.3

How to use weight checks before and after a workout to tell you about your sweat losses

Weigh in before training, after going to the toilet (kg)
Weigh in wearing minimal clothing—your underwear only, if possible
Weigh in after the session, in the same clothes and after towel-drying your hair and gear (kg)
If you have to wee during the session, weigh in before and after you go
Weigh your drink bottle before and after your workout to find out how much fluid you consumed. Or just estimate the amount of fluid consumed and convert ml of fluid into grams

Calculations (with example)
Your fluid intake (ml) = drink bottle before – drink bottle after (g)
e.g. 700 g – 400 g = 300 g or 300 ml

Your urine losses (ml) = your weight before – your weight after a toilet stop (kg) × 1000
e.g. 60.25 – 60.00 = 0.25 kg = 250 ml

Your fluid deficit (dehydration) (ml) = your weight before workout – your weight after workout (kg) × 1000
e.g. 60.50 – 59.00 = 1 kg = 1500 ml

Your fluid deficit (% body weight) = 100 × C in kg/body weight (g)
e.g. (100 × 1.5)/(60.50) = 2.5%

Total sweat losses over the session = Fluid deficit (g) + fluid intake (g)—urine losses (g)
e.g. 1500 + 300 – 250 = 1650 ml

Sweat rate over the session = sweat losses converted to ml per hour after training
e.g. Training lasted for 90 min
sweat rate = 1650/90 × 60 = 1100 ml or 1.1 L/hour

3
Achieving an ideal physique

Imagine designing opening ceremony uniforms for a whole Olympic team! They would need to be pretty versatile to suit all the different sizes and shapes that athletes come in. High jumpers: tall and lean with long legs; weight lifters: muscle-bound arms and short, muscle-bound legs for a low centre of gravity; gymnasts: small, light and lean; swimmers: wide shoulders. A designer could make these assumptions because physical characteristics such as height, weight, limb lengths and the amount and distribution of muscle mass or body fat help the performance of various types of exercise. So athletes, particularly at the highest level of competition, will tend towards the physique that favours the demands of their sport.

An athlete's physique reflects both the basic structure he or she inherited from Mum and Dad and the remoulding achieved by training and diet. Hopefully, you chose your parents well and selected the sport to which you are best suited! There's not much you can do about your height, and you will have inherited a potential for your muscularity and fatness. Nevertheless, at some point in your sporting career, you are likely to want to fine-tune your weight, body-fat levels or muscle mass.

3.1 What is a desirable body-fat level?

We require a certain minimum level of body fat to remain healthy. For men this is approximately 3–5 per cent of body weight, and for women about 10–15 per cent. Of course, most people carry considerably more body fat than this minimum. In terms of sports performance, extra body fat can improve flotation, provide insulation against the cold, and protect body organs from damage during contact sports. However, these benefits must be balanced against the increased effort required to move additional body weight. Being heavier increases the energy cost of movement. In particular, extra body fat causes a decrease in the ratio of body weight that is active to body weight that isn't—often referred to as your power-to-weight ratio. (At this stage, we should note that when we jump on the scales, we actually measure our body *mass*. However, since most people refer to it as *weight*, we will use that term throughout this book.) Participants in some sports will not be disadvantaged by a higher level of body fat, particularly if the sport is based on skill rather than aerobic fitness. Think of golf or archery. By contrast, a low level of body fat is crucial for athletes such as triathletes and marathon runners, who expend energy in transporting their own weight over long distances. Having a high power-to-weight ratio also helps in sports where body weight is moved against gravity—such as cycling up hills or high jumping. Athletes in sports that have weight divisions will be better served if muscle is at a maximum and body fat is sacrificed to reach a weight limit.

In some sports, athletes are concerned about their appearance. Body-builders, gymnasts and figure-skaters pursue a 'trim, taut and terrific' look to impress the judges in their sports. In some sports, such a physique can be an ally of skill: a gymnast or diver, for example, needs to be small and light to complete elaborate moves in a tight space. In body-building, by contrast, being 'ripped' is more about aesthetics (the 'look') than about body function or performance. Many athletes also become worried about their appearance because of the type of competition clothing they are required to wear. How would you cope if your competition uniform was a Lycra bodysuit, a skin-tight swimming costume or even a bikini? It's not surprising that some athletes become concerned about how lumps or rolls of body fat will look in competition photos, as well as how they'll affect the outcome of the game or race.

So what is an ideal physique for each sport? Sometimes, coaches or athletes set rigid criteria based on the characteristics of other successful competitors. Although such information is useful, it doesn't take into account that the physical characteristics of athletes vary, even between individuals in the same sport. It also fails to acknowledge that some athletes need many years of training and maturation to achieve their ideal shape and body composition. Therefore, it is dangerous to establish compulsory body-fat and body-weight targets for each sport. Rather, individual athletes should be monitored over their career and over the different parts of a season or specialised training to see the range of characteristics that are associated with good outcomes. Within this range, each athlete can probably find his or her own ideal weight and body-fat levels, guided by the following questions:

- At what weight and body fat level do you seem to train best?
- At what weight and body fat level do you seem to achieve your best competition performances?
- Can you also maintain good health at these levels?
- Can you achieve and maintain this weight and body fat level without unreasonable effort and without compromising other nutritional goals?

Be aware that some athletes will perform at a top level or at their personal best at a weight or body-fat level that falls outside the typical ranges. But then some top athletes don't fit the expected moulds in lots of ways—world-record holder Paula Radcliffe towers above most elite marathon runners, and many basketball teams boast a very short guard who is essential to their playmaking. So it isn't necessary to become the physical clone of a successful competitor, or to achieve minimal body-fat levels *per se*. Of course, some racial groups or individuals are naturally light and have low levels of body fat without paying a substantial penalty. In addition, some athletes vary their body-fat levels over a season so that very low levels are achieved only for a specific and short time. But pursuing the leanness goal above all else can lead to many problems. Athletes who become too lean are susceptible to fatigue, an increased risk of infection and intolerance to cold. Other penalties arise from the methods used to achieve such a low body-fat level, such as drastic dieting or excessive training. Bottom line: be sensible with your body-fat goals.

3.2 What is a desirable muscle mass?

Weightlifters, sprinters, rowers and rugby players all need to develop muscle mass so they can generate explosive power. In other sports, muscle mass is required to achieve the right 'look'—body-building exemplifies this need. Of course, some athletes, like rugby forwards and gridiron football players, simply need to be big for momentum and protection, and have some leeway for carrying body fat. An increase in muscle size and strength occurs naturally during adolescence, particularly in males. However, in sports where size, strength and power are important, athletes want to achieve specific muscle hypertrophy (growth) through a program of progressive muscle overload or resistance training. As is the case for body-fat levels, many athletes and coaches have unrealistic expectations about how muscular an individual can get, and how quickly. Genetics can make it harder or easier for any athlete to respond to a muscle-gain program, and it takes years for most athletes to achieve their ideal muscle mass.

There are still many false beliefs about how to gain muscle. Some athletes still think they should gain as much weight as they can by any means, then work on 'turning body fat into muscle'. This isn't possible, since fat and muscle are separate types of tissue and can't be interchanged. However, in some sports, the athlete needs to gain bulk as well as strength, so a high-energy diet that adds significant amounts of body fat as well as muscle mass will not be problematic. On other occasions, athletes set out to gain a lot of muscle mass while becoming very lean. This is achievable, but usually the leanness and the muscle mass need to be attained one at a time. After all, gaining muscle mass is more effectively done in an environment of energy surplus, while loss of body fat requires an energy deficit. All in all, gaining and maintaining ideal muscle mass requires not only a special program but a way to measure results so that weight gain or loss can be separated into its components of fat and muscle.

3.3 Measuring body fat and muscle mass

There are a number of high-tech ways to estimate body composition. We used to consider underwater weighing to be the gold standard, although it is cumbersome to do and it is available only in certain laboratories. These aren't the technique's main disadvantages, however. Weight readings taken underwater divide the body into estimated body fat and estimated 'lean body mass' based on the different densities of these tissues. The problem is that the densities of the bone and muscle of athletes (part of the lean mass side of the equation) are not uniform or accurately known. This can cause major errors in the estimates. There are some newer techniques that are now considered far more—but still not entirely—accurate. One of the best known involves a special X-ray machine known as a DXA, which can partition the body into bone, muscle and fat. However, this method is also expensive and relatively inaccessible. Of course, even with the latest equipment and tightest techniques, no method is perfect. All results need to be interpreted with this in mind.

When it comes to real-life work with athletes, we need a method for monitoring body composition that is portable, inexpensive and readily accessible without sacrificing too much accuracy. Many sports scientists believe that these characteristics are met by what we call anthropometry, or the measurement of body dimensions. The most popular type of anthropometry is the skinfold test, in which callipers are used to measure the amount of fat under the skin at various body sites (usually between three and seven). The traditional method then used a prediction equation to convert the results into an estimate of percentage body fat. More recently, there has been a move to get rid of this conversion, since it adds error to the process. Instead, the protocol is simply to add up the individual skinfold measurements. Athletes are now used to hearing about their fat levels as a skinfold sum of 42 mm or 74.2 mm rather than 4 per cent or 10 per cent body fat. Anthropometry doesn't stop there, though. Other measurements that can easily be taken on athletes, such as body lengths, circumferences and girths at various sites, can add to the picture of physique. In fact, when all these numbers are put together, we can get good estimates of muscle mass (overall and for different sites) and skeletal mass as well as body fat. This is the way many expert groups, such as the Australian Institute of Sport, monitor athletes' growth and development and their changes in physique in response to training and diet.

For this to be a useful practice for athletes, a number of boxes must be ticked:

- The sports scientist must be trained to undertake the measurements according to a standardised protocol. In fact, a body called the International Society for the Advancement of Kinanthropometry (ISAK) has established such protocols for measuring skinfolds, girths, circumferences and body lengths, and offers accreditation courses for professionals.

- Physique characteristics need to be measured over a range of body sites. The ISAK protocol recognises eight sites for the measurement of body fat (see Figure 3.1). However, the Australian protocol for monitoring the skinfold fat of athletes is usually based on seven sites (the iliac crest site is omitted). See Figure 3.1

FIGURE 3.1

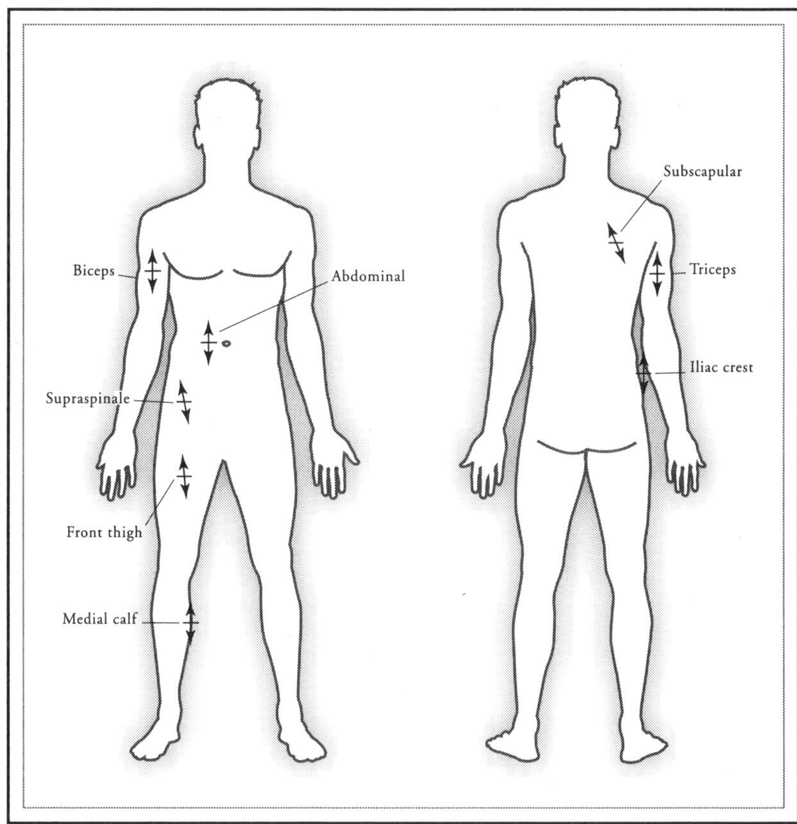

ISAK sites for measurement of skinfold fat

- Skinfold measurements should be taken using a good set of callipers (for example, John Bull or Harpenden calipers). The standard technique is to take readings on the right-hand side of the body; after each site has been measured once, the whole sequence should be repeated. Where the two readings differ by more than 0.5 mm, a third measurement should be taken.
- Sports scientists should know their own margin of measurement error. No one is 100 per cent precise. Part of ISAK training is to identify the size of your typical error so any measurements made on an athlete can be put into perspective. For example, if you measure an athlete's sum of skinfolds as 52.1 mm on one occasion and 49.8 mm on another, you need to know whether this is a real change or whether it could be ascribed simply to the way you take the measurement.
- If an athlete has skinfold measurements repeated over a period of time to monitor changes, it is preferable that the same sports scientist take the readings on each occasion.

As techniques such as this become widespread, we can build up profiles of the typical physique characteristics of athletes in various sports. Consider this useful information. However, the most useful information is the file of results that can be built up on the same athlete over time using careful and standardised techniques. This can help you to identify the answers to the questions asked about ideal body composition above.

3.4 Losing body fat

So your Lycra is bulging, or perhaps you have come back from injury to find that your skinfold sum has jumped by 20 mm. Maybe you need to lose 3 kg to row in the lightweight crew. At some point in their life or their sporting career, most people try to lose weight.

The bottom line for achieving loss of body fat is to eat fewer kilojoules than your body expends, creating an energy deficit (negative energy balance). This might sound simple, but in practice, most people's weight-loss attempts end in failure. Instead of taking a simple and consistent approach and focusing on long-term outcomes, some athletes seek a magical program that will require no effort and produce results within days. Some turn to grapefruit diets, herbal powders or 'fat-burning' supplements. Others take drastic measures, such as severe food restriction, dehydration techniques, diuretics and laxatives. Since these methods fail to achieve an energy deficit or consider the long term, they also fail to produce the desired fat loss. Some of them can actually depress the body's metabolic rate, lowering its energy needs and making it even more difficult to create an energy deficit. In the worst-case scenario, this may directly harm your exercise performance or your health.

While some people make a lifetime career of being on (and off) diets, there is only one successful way to approach weight loss—and that's once and for all! The first steps are to forget the magic and miracles and be prepared to invest a little effort and, above all, sufficient time. You can make the scales show a loss of a kilo in an hour (by sweating without replacing fluid) or a day (by not eating and letting your gut empty its usual contents). But—and we recognise that this is an oversimplification—to 'burn' off 1 kg of body fat, you must create a net energy loss of almost 30 MJ (~7000 kcal). Since most people can only afford to cut down by 2–4 MJ per day (500–1000 Calories), you will need a week or two to accumulate the energy deficit that creates the loss of 1 kg of body fat. On the bright side, once you have truly oxidised this body fat, it is gone—unless you revert to your old food habits and put yourself into an energy-gain situation.

What is the formula for a successful fat-loss plan? Checklist 3.1 summarises the key features that you should incorporate, with realistic goals and adequate time at the top of the list. It is best not to juggle a weight-loss program with a competition schedule. Rather, you should tackle your weight goals early in the training cycle or even in the off-season. Even then, you need to protect your intake of important nutrients so you don't sacrifice your health and exercise goals.

You may be able to work out a suitable fat-loss program for yourself or find the elements in a good sports nutrition book. On the other hand, a sports dietitian is an expert who can tailor a specific eating plan for you and help to monitor the results. There are different ways you can arrive at this plan together. One approach is to start from scratch and construct an eating program that contains all the right energy and nutrient levels at the right time of each day. Another is to take your existing diet and identify some changes in the quantity and type of foods and drink that will result in a useful energy deficit (see Checklist 3.2.) There are some advantages to an eating program that is simply an improvement on your old, familiar ways. Most people fail when they 'follow a diet' from a book or magazine—even when the nutritional ideas are sensible—because one-size-fits-all diets are usually too strict to suit their own special requirements and lifestyle for the long term.

Another angle again is to concentrate on the psychology of eating and the behavioural changes that will allow the athlete to eat well. After all, many of us know what we should be eating but for various reasons don't follow through (see, again, Checklist 3.2). In many situations, a combination of tactics will be needed to achieve a winning program. You will find a number of examples in the second part of this book. Don't underestimate the value of the ongoing input of a sports dietitian. You may need moral support for the long haul as well as a chance to fine-tune the plan according to the feedback from performance indicators and body-composition changes.

3.5 Restrained eating

Chapter 2 explained the laws of thermodynamics regarding energy balance. Simply speaking:

- Energy intake = energy expenditure = no change in body energy stores (body fat/body weight stays the same)
- Energy intake > energy expenditure = gain of body energy stores (gain of fat + muscle)
- Energy intake < energy expenditure = loss of body energy stores (loss of fat + muscle)

For years, however, athletes and scientists have been puzzled by an apparent exception to these laws. Exhibit A: Dietary surveys of serious female athletes—from swimmers, runners and basketball players to gymnasts and ballet dancers—often report energy intakes that are unexpectedly low. We're talking about group averages of less than 8.4 MJ/day (2000 kcal), with individual athletes reporting energy intakes below 5 MJ/day (1200 kcal). How can athletes sustain their exercise needs on the intakes expected of sedentary people? Exhibit B: The waiting rooms of sports nutrition practices are full of female athletes who claim that in spite of one to two hours of intense training each day, they simply can't lose weight. Others claim that they need to keep kilojoule intakes very low just to prevent a gain in body fat. Clearly, it's frustrating to do the same training as the guys in the next lane, and then watch them eat anything they want without a care in the world while you have to count every morsel. Of course, this problem doesn't exclusively plague female athletes: some males also seem to draw the short 'energy requirement' straw, and athletes may simply reflect the complaints of a large percentage of the female population. 'Restrained eater' is one of the terms used to describe people who have to watch everything they eat, rigidly keeping energy intake to a minimum.

So does this energy discrepancy really exist? Can a female runner cover 100 km a week in training and remain at a stable weight on less than 7.5 MJ (1800 kcal) a day? A number of recent studies have tried to examine the energy-balance characteristics of various female athletes by separately assessing energy intake and energy expenditure over a period of a week or so. For example, scientists at Indiana University monitored a group of elite female distance runners, measuring energy intake (estimated from seven-day food records) vs. energy expenditure recorded over the same period using the doubly labelled water technique. The results showed that average daily energy intake (8.5 MJ/day) accounted for only 70 per cent of average daily energy expenditure (12.5 MJ/day). Yet the athletes did not lose body weight or change body composition during that time. Other careful studies of energy balance in female athletes, using different techniques to measure energy expenditure, have reported similar findings. In some cases, the energy-balance oddity was particularly striking in athletes who had interrupted menstrual cycles compared to those with regular periods.

Chapter 2 briefly summarised some of the methods available to measure or estimate energy requirements and commented on the limitations of these techniques. Our present techniques for monitoring energy intake could be generously described as low tech, since they typically involve a paper and pencil! Traditionally, scientists have studied the energy intakes of athletes by making them keep detailed records of everything they eat and drink for periods of four days to a week. This is tedious for both the scientists and their victims. What's more, there are numerous inaccuracies, both in arriving at the kilojoule values of foods and fluids, and in making sure that what is described during the study period truly reflects the real-life situation. It is a well-known problem that most people 'under-record' their habitual food and drink intake when they are keeping a dietary diary. Consciously or unconsciously, they either forget to write down every morsel they consume or downsize their description of food portions. In other situations, they consciously or unconsciously eat less or make different food choices while they are being observed so that they consume less than their true energy intakes during the recording period. In such situations, you would expect them to lose weight, but sometimes the weight change isn't monitored adequately.

So there are two possible explanations for the energy discrepancy reported in studies and in the real-life complaints of athletes:

- First, the measures or calculations of energy expenditure are wrong, erring on the high side. Various components of total energy expenditure may be lower than expected, whether for basal metabolism or for exercise and other daily activities. In any case, the athlete is 'metabolically efficient' or adapted to the exercise program in some way that reduces total energy needs.
- Alternatively, the figures for energy intake are underestimates. If an athlete is not losing weight/body fat, he must be consuming as much energy as he needs. Therefore, he must be underreporting the food and fluid consumed—either by not writing everything down or by underestimating the size of the portions consumed. Sometimes the apparent discrepancy occurs because the athlete restricts his eating for a large part of the week, then has a brief but damaging splurge that more than compensates for the restriction.

Each of these explanations occurs in real life, and they often coexist in the same athlete. Both situations are problematic, but for different reasons.

Athletes who underreport and underestimate their true energy intake are in denial about their ability to meet their nutrition goals. Attempts to improve diet, whether for weight or fat loss or to optimise nutrition for training, will be hit and miss unless they are aware of their true eating habits. Creeping portion sizes, chaotic meal patterns, eating on the run, hidden energy in drinks, snacking that is unaccounted for . . . These are just some of the factors that interfere with the accurate monitoring of eating and drinking. The athlete may not be aware that a bigger drink or sports bar—25 per cent more at no extra cost!—has more kilojoules too, and it's easy to forget the little 'tastes' and 'nibbles' that come your way in the course of a day—especially when a series of these are substituted for a square meal or a single plate of food. Athletes who falsely consider themselves to be restrained eaters must face the facts before they can move to a better level of nutrition.

'Part-time restrained eaters' are those who follow a cycle of very restrictive eating followed by the inevitable binge. This is also easy to fall into unawares. After all, dieters tend to focus on the good days rather than the 'blips'. Many fail to realise that the energy surplus during even a brief binge on energy-dense fatty and sugary foods and alcohol may be equal to or greater than the deficit achieved during the restriction phase. In addition, the binge foods and drinks are of low nutritional quality. So while the binge may compensate for the energy deprivation, it may not pay back the nutrient needs that were forgone during the low-energy intake phase. This situation requires unravelling so that energy, fuel and nutrient intakes are modelled on the week's training requirements rather than a roller-coaster of alternating discipline and abandon.

The most problematic group are the true restrained eaters—athletes who limit the quantity, range and enjoyment of their food intake. Some of these athletes may have achieved unnaturally low body-fat levels as a result of their efforts, or be moving in that direction. However, others may still be carrying more body fat than desirable and may actually be in energy balance—that is, not losing weight. What both groups share is a low energy intake. One problem arising from this is a significant increase in the risk of nutrient inadequacies and failure to meet nutrition goals. This is because when the total energy budget falls below 5–6 MJ per day (1200–1500 kcal), it becomes difficult to fit in enough food to supply all needs for protein, calcium, iron and other vitamins and minerals. This is exacerbated if the athlete combines low energy with poor dietary variety.

In addition, we are now becoming aware of a phenomenon called 'low energy availability', thanks to Professor Anne Loucks, an American sports scientist who has dedicated her career to trying to understand this problem. She coined the term 'energy availability' to denote the energy that your body can tap into after your training/competition program has been taken into account—in other words, the energy left after you subtract the energy cost of daily exercise from your total kilojoule intake. This is the budget that your body draws on to look after itself, and Professor Louck's work has shown that if it's too low, your hormone health, your immune system, even your ability to burn energy will all be impaired.

We agree that there are athletes who really do have unusually low energy requirements. Some studies have shown that they have reduced BMRs, perhaps a higher efficiency (burning fewer kilojoules) in their training, and a smaller amount of incidental activity in a day. Studies in females have shown that just a couple of days' drastic cut in energy availability—either from exercising more on the same energy intake or cutting down kilojoules without exercise—causes changes in metabolic and other important hormones that might in turn explain or cause energy conservation or a disruption to reproductive function. We can't join all the dots yet to show a direct and single link. Indeed, faced with low energy availability, some individuals seem more predisposed to these hormonal and energy disruptions than others. Nevertheless, it seems clear that the low-energy path is a risky one.

Some consequences of inadequate energy availability may be reversible. And at least in the old days, we used to consider some of the issues to be small and inconsequential. For example, a disruption to menstrual periods in a hard-training female athlete used to be considered typical, but hardly problematic if you were a young person who wasn't planning on becoming pregnant in the near future. We now know, however, that other disruptions may be occurring that are silent, serious and irreversible. Bones may become fragile as a direct outcome of low energy availability, as well as an indirect result of disrupted levels of reproductive hormones such as oestrogen. Athletes who don't face chronic illnesses or injuries that interfere with their ability to train and compete may count themselves lucky. However, there may not be much to cheer about later, if their low-energy habits accelerate or exaggerate problems of ageing such as osteoporosis or frailty due to low muscle mass. It makes sense to make adequate energy a priority.

Professor Loucks has defined low energy availability descriptively, as the condition in which energy intake is inadequate for basic body maintenance. But her studies have also been able to define it numerically, in terms of the number of kilojoules that are consumed relative to lean body mass. At least, this number has been determined in women. There is probably a male equivalent, but it is less well defined at present. Calculating it can be a little tricky, but as a rule of thumb, low energy availability occurs when you cut back your energy availability by more than a third. The good news is that this does give you a bit of 'play' to create an energy deficit to promote fat loss. The bad news is that if you go too hard at this, you'll likely pay a price. The chapter on distance running provides a case history to further illustrate the concepts of energy balance and energy availability, the differences between them, and what these might mean to athletes in various sports.

3.6 Making weight

Weight-matched sports include boxing, wrestling, judo, weight- and power-lifting, horse-racing and lightweight rowing. There are two traditions in these sports that show an unfortunate side of athletic nutritional practices. The first is the desire to compete in a lower weight division than your normal training weight—theoretically gaining an advantage over a lighter, weaker opponent. The second tradition is to shed the excess weight fast—often 3–6 kg in as many days. This is when drastic techniques come into play, such as dehydrating in saunas or plastic suits, fasting, or using diuretics and laxatives. These methods may produce a loss of body weight, but the real loss is not of fat but of water, muscle and glycogen stores. Depending on the sport, there may be hours or a day of recovery between the weigh-in and competition. Also depending on the sport and the techniques used, weight-making can be associated with loss of performance and various health issues. The situations of most concern are:

- When the athlete has to lose a large percentage of his body mass—more than 2–3 per cent (i.e. more than 2 kg for a 70-kg athlete)
- When the athlete makes weight on top of a long period of heavy training and energy restriction, resulting in loss of fat and muscle
- When weight making is repeated frequently—for example, by jockeys who ride at meetings once or twice a week, and have to

weigh in for each race in the day's program, or wrestlers who take part in weekly competition series
- When the sport involves prolonged high-intensity exercise in the heat (e.g. a lightweight rower competing in mid-summer)
- When the athlete is young and growing—because making a weight target becomes more difficult as 'normal' body weight increases, and because restrictive dieting practices interfere with growth and development

The timing of the weigh-in is a double-edged sword. On one hand, when the weigh-in is only an hour before the start of the event, there is little time for recovery and the athlete will go into the event dehydrated and fuel depleted. However, a longer time for recovery may tempt some athletes to increase the amount of weight they are willing to try to 'lose'. In the case of horse racing, jockeys weigh in after the race, so there is no time for recovery.

A simplistic view of the ideal approach to weight making is that athletes would:

- Compete in a weight division that allows them to train at a healthy weight and with healthy eating patterns
- Be able to achieve their competition weight by simply fine-tuning their training weight—in other words, be within 2–3 per cent of their target weight
- Compete in their event with optimal nutritional preparation

How this occurs in a range of sports will be discussed in more detail in the second half of this book.

3.7 Bulking up

Many athletes dream of becoming bigger, stronger, or more buff: in other words, they dream of muscle. Often they try to buy these dreams with pills, potions, powders and three helpings at each meal. For all the magic and misconceptions, there are only a few real requirements for muscle gain. In probable order of importance, they are:

- Genetic potential—picking the right parents with the right body type

- Weight training—giving muscles the right stimulation
- Good timing with energy and protein intake—getting the best out of each training session
- A high energy intake—more of everything, including, but not exclusively, protein

In attacking this list, it is important to start with realistic goals based on the first two points. You may also need to seek expert advice—a strength coach to set a program of progressive muscle overload, and a sports dietitian to support this with a well-timed high-energy diet. Despite the great interest in this area, precious little is known about exactly what energy intake should be set for maximum muscle gain, or how much of this should be set aside for protein, carbohydrate and other nutrients. But the general approach should be to increase total energy intake and to distribute it before, during and after training sessions so there is plenty of fuel to support good training and plenty of building blocks for muscle. These issues are covered in more detail in Chapter 4 (Competition nutrition; use the same strategies for your training sessions) and Chapter 5 (Promoting recovery).

How hard you push these strategies may depend on how much you need to increase size and bulk, versus strength. Some athletes may need to boost their energy intake aggressively to cover the costs of training as well as those of laying down new muscle and body fat. Others' needs may be better served by a more strategic approach. Periodic measurement of body-fat levels and muscle circumferences will reassure you that any gains in body weight are from muscle, not fat. The next section provides advice on 'action-packed' eating.

3.8 The high-energy diet

Whether you are trying to gain muscle mass or simply maintain a strenuous training load, you may need to consume a lot of energy each day. To outsiders this may sound like paradise—and for some it can be enjoyable. But for other athletes it can range from a chore to a near impossibility. Hurdles to chewing through all the necessary kilojoules include:

- Lack of time, including time to buy and prepare food. Subtract your training time, your work, sleep and all the other

commitments in your day, and this probably leaves you with three hours to pack in 25 MJ (6000 Cals)
- The bulk of the food. A high-carbohydrate, high-fibre diet means lots to chew and digest
- Lack of access to food (or suitable food) at possible eating times
- The need to limit food intake before training to avoid discomfort during exercise
- Fatigue and loss of appetite after training

Athletes tackling a high-energy diet need to be organised to ensure that suitable meals and snacks are available and appropriately scheduled throughout the day. Poor planning will throw a big spanner in the works. If you are having trouble, a sports dietitian can help you to look over your daily schedule. Keep a record like that suggested in the fat-loss section. This will help you look for opportunities to increase your energy intake (see Checklist 3.4 for ideas).

CHECKLIST 3.1
Features of a weight/fat loss plan that's likely to work

Theme	Ideal features
Goals	• Realistic weight and skinfold targets, including short-term targets and a long-term aim
Time frame	• A realistic rate of loss: ~0.5–1.0 kg per week, or about 5–10 mm from your total skinfold measurement each fortnight • Realisation that this may not happen in a consistent and consecutive way, but can still be used to set your overall timeline
Energy intake	• A drop in habitual energy intake compared with your energy requirements that's sufficient to achieve the desired rate of fat loss

Theme	Ideal features
	• Adequate energy so that 'energy availability' stays above the threshold considered too low • Energy spread over the day to avoid 'low energy spots' and hunger
Carbohydrate intake	• Reduction in carbs as part of energy cuts, but enough muscle fuel to train effectively. Carbohydrate intake should fluctuate up and down over the week according to daily fuel needs • Allowance for some training sessions to be done without specific fuel support—for example, light sessions and recovery sessions may be done first thing in the morning before eating, or without the need for a sports drink • Protection of fuel supplies for key training sessions of the week—particularly high-intensity sessions. This might mean planning to eat carbohydrate before, during and/or after the session
Protein, vitamins and minerals	• Adequate but not excessive protein intake to allow needs to be met • Worthwhile intake of protein timed for recovery needs • Special attention to nutrient-rich food choices so that maximum nutrition is achieved for minimal kilojoules • Use of a low-dose broad-range multivitamin–mineral supplement if dietary intakes are restricted for prolonged periods
Flexibility and longevity	• Ability to suit your lifestyle and make use of foods that are readily available • Ability to be followed long-term

Theme	Ideal features
Social eating and food enjoyment	• Room for some treats and favourite foods—perhaps in smaller amounts, or for special occasions • Opportunities for eating out, or enjoying food in the company of others • Satisfaction and 'fullness' after eating meals—no need to experience uncomfortable levels of hunger or deprivation

CHECKLIST 3.2

Reducing energy intake for weight/fat loss without sacrificing sports nutrition goals

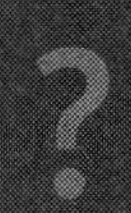

Show caution with portions

- Have a plan of meals and snacks, tailored to meet your energy needs over the day. Don't be distracted by what everyone else is eating.
- Know appropriate portion sizes for various food types in your plan and how to exchange one food for another. Be able to recognise your desired portion size in any situation—relate it to common items such as your palm size, a tennis ball, a pack of cards, your mobile phone or a match box.
- In a self-serve situation, fill one plate. Don't go back for seconds.
- Don't restrict yourself too much or allow yourself to get too hungry—plan meals and snacks to keep the edge off hunger and prevent binges.
- Avoid buying jumbo sizes of foods, which encourage overeating. It isn't a bargain if you eat it all at once!
- Be strategic with recovery nutrition. Rearrange meal schedules so that existing food intake is well timed to promote efficient

recovery after workouts. If a post-exercise snack is needed, choose nutritious foods and reorganise menus to take this into account.

- Enjoy your special or favourite foods, but in smaller quantities. For example, share a dessert in a restaurant, or have a chocolate frog rather than a family block.

Reduce excessive intake of energy-dense foods

- Target sources of fat, alcohol and sugar in your diet. These are generally energy dense but nutrient poor (see Chapter 1 for Checklists 1.3, 1.4 and 1.7).

Maximise the nutrient density of meals and snacks

- The other hints in this checklist will help you make sure you get maximal nutrients from each mouthful (see Checklist 1.2 for ideas on making the most of the fruits and vegetables you eat).
- Consider a low-dose broad-range multivitamin/mineral supplement when reducing your energy intake for prolonged periods.

Increase the satiety factor ('fillingness') of meals and snacks

- Use vegetables to increase the volume (and reduce the energy content per mouthful) of meals and snacks:
  - Add thick salad fillings to sandwiches
  - Increase the ratio of vegetables in recipes (e.g. in stir-fries, pasta sauces, pizza toppings)
  - Eat salad or add vegetables to the plate before serving meat and carbohydrate choices
- Choose fibre-rich versions of foods—wholegrain breads and cereals, whole fruits, and raw vegetables.
- Chew rather than drink your kilojoules. If you must drink juice, allow one glass daily and dilute with water. Consider milk as part of your allowance of 3–4 servings of dairy foods each day.

- Slow down the rate of eating by choosing foods that are:
  - Spicy hot (hard to overdo!)
  - Served piping hot (e.g. sip a skinny hot chocolate rather than chugging a glass of milk)
  - Served frozen (e.g. freeze a carton of yoghurt or fruit portions for a longer-lasting snack)
- Drink low-energy drinks with meals and snacks to increase the volume consumed on each occasion (water, tea or coffee, low-joule mineral waters and soft drink).
- Combine protein and carbohydrate at meals or snacks to enhance total satiety value (e.g. a skinny hot chocolate and a slice of toast rather than four slices of toast).
- Choose low glycemic index carbohydrate-rich foods (e.g. oat-based porridge or Bircher muesli instead of flaked-corn cereals; multi-grain breads rather than white bread).

Observe your eating behaviour

Keep a food record from time to time to consolidate your new eating habits and to identify when and why you eat without being hungry or really needing the food. Stop poor food behaviour by tackling the problem at its source:

- Eating when depressed or upset—deal with the problem that is making you depressed or upset. Have a list of ways to pamper yourself that don't involve food
- Eating when bored—find a non-food activity, as above
- Eating because the food is around—either remove yourself or remove the food. Don't rely on will-power!
- Eating while you are doing other things (e.g. watching TV, driving a car). Save your food and make eating a separate, focused activity
- Stop undereating or skipping meals. Restrictive eating usually ends in a binge, so don't start the cycle

CHECKLIST 3.3
Avoiding the pitfalls of restrained eating

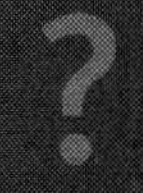

- Consult a sports dietitian to learn how to assess your situation and resolve eating problems.
- Establish whether you really are a low energy consumer by keeping a truthful food diary for a week. This will allow you to see:
    - If you are really nibbling or consuming more than you realised (and if those kilojoules can be better used to increase your intake of nutritious foods)
    - If you are eating more fatty foods and high-fat or sugary splurges than you realised (if so, find more appropriate amounts and choices of food)
    - If you lose weight while you are recording. Most people will consciously or unconsciously cut back when they are accounting for their food intake. This will not only tell you that your energy requirements are greater than you thought but you may lose some unwanted body fat as well!
- Look at ways of increasing your energy requirements, either by increasing the amount or intensity of exercise or by increasing/ preserving your metabolic rate:
    - If your program consists of skill- or strength training only, it may be possible to add some aerobic activities to increase the total energy cost of your training. Talk to your coach about this.
    - Spread your energy intake over the day. Do not skip meals, especially breakfast, if you want to keep your metabolic rate stoked.
    - Experiment with a small increase in energy intake, using carbohydrate-rich foods to provide an extra 800–2000 kJ a day (200–500 Cals) to fuel your training. You may be surprised—not only will you not gain weight, but the extra fuel will put more spring in your step and more quality in your training, and help you perform better in all aspects of your life. What's more,

a kick-start to training and metabolism can often result in a loss of body fat.

- Even when you are on a fat-loss program, beware of cutting your daily intake so much that you end up with low energy availability. This may cause insidious disruptions to health and bodily functioning. Although its figures are guesstimates, Table 3.1 is a guide to the threshold of low energy availability.
- Work hard to choose nutrient-dense foods so you get the most nutritional value from the fewest kilojoules:
    - You will probably need to take a multivitamin/mineral supplement. A sports dietitian can advise you on the best type and dosage.

CHECKLIST 3.4
Achieving a high energy intake

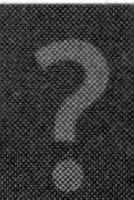

- Above all, be organised. You will need to apply the same dedication to your eating program that you apply to your training. A haphazard approach—eating what is available, when it is convenient—is no way to get the quality or quantity of food you need.
- Increase the frequency rather than the size of meals. A 'grazing' pattern of six to eight meals and snacks enables you to eat more, with less gastric discomfort, than the conventional pattern of three large meals.
- Plan to have food on hand for every eating opportunity. Identify a range of portable snacks that can travel with you on your busy day. It's also valuable to keep an emergency food supply in your car, sports bag or locker.
- Increase the energy content of foods by adding layers and toppings. For example, add jams and syrups to toast and pancakes, yoghurt and fruit to a bowl of cereal, and make two- or three-layer fillings in sandwiches.

- Avoid eating too much fibre, and make use of some 'white' cereal foods with less bulk (e.g. white bread, white rice). You may find it impossible to chew your way through a diet based on wholegrain and high-fibre foods.
- Support training sessions by eating before, during and after them. This may help you to train more effectively as well as boosting your kilojoule tally. Many sports foods and drinks provide a compact energy source as well as addressing the nutritional needs of training and recovery.
- Avoid 'wasting space' with low-energy fluids. Choose sports drinks at workouts rather than water, and drink juice or milk with meals and snacks.
- Make action-packed smoothies and shakes with skim milk, fruit and ice cubes. Low-fat ice-cream and non-fat yoghurt are optional extras for a creamy drink. Liquid meal supplements such as PowerBar Proteinplus or Sustagen Sport are also available.

TABLE 3.1
Examples of calculations of approximate threshold for low energy availability

Body weight	% body fat	Lean body mass (body wt kg—body fat kg)	MJ/day* The energy cost of training must be added to this figure	Cals/day* The energy cost of training must be added to this figure
50 kg	5	48 kg	6.0	1425
50 kg	10	45 kg	5.7	1350
50 kg	15	43 kg	5.4	1275
50 kg	25	38 kg	4.7	1125
55 kg	5	52 kg	6.6	1570
55 kg	10	50 kg	6.2	1485

Body weight	% body fat	Lean body mass (body wt kg—body fat kg)	MJ/day* The energy cost of training must be added to this figure	Cals/day* The energy cost of training must be added to this figure
55 kg	15	47 kg	5.9	1400
55 kg	25	41 kg	5.2	1240
60 kg	5	57 kg	7.2	1710
60 kg	10	54 kg	6.8	1620
60 kg	15	51 kg	6.4	1530
60 kg	25	45 kg	5.7	1350
65 kg	5	62 kg	7.8	1855
65 kg	10	59 kg	7.4	1755
65 kg	15	55 kg	7.0	1660
65 kg	25	49 kg	6.1	1465
70 kg	5	67 kg	8.4	1995
70 kg	10	63 kg	7.9	1890
70 kg	15	59 kg	7.5	1785
70 kg	25	53 kg	6.6	1575
75 kg	5	71 kg	9.0	2140
75 kg	10	68 kg	8.5	2025
75 kg	15	64 kg	8.0	1915
75 kg	25	56 kg	7.1	1690
80 kg	5	76 kg	9.6	2280
80 kg	10	72 kg	9.1	2160
80 kg	15	68 kg	8.6	2040
80 kg	25	60 kg	7.6	1800

Body weight	% body fat	Lean body mass (body wt kg—body fat kg)	MJ/day* The energy cost of training must be added to this figure	Cals/day* The energy cost of training must be added to this figure
85 kg	5	81 kg	10.2	2425
85 kg	10	76 kg	9.6	2295
85 kg	15	72 kg	9.1	2170
85 kg	25	64 kg	8.0	1915

*Notes:

1. These calculations are based on the theory that low energy availability occurs when daily energy intake drops below 125 kJ/kg (30 Cal/kg) of lean body mass + energy cost of training.
2. It is not necessary to know your exact percentage of body fat to get an idea of this threshold. Use this table and guesstimate where you fit between very lean (5 per cent body fat for men; 10 per cent body fat for women), and 'normal body fat' (15 per cent body fat for men and 25 per cent for women) for a sedentary person. The range of numbers given should allow you to find roughly which energy figures apply to you.

4
Competition nutrition

Competition is your time to 'seize the day' and push yourself beyond your best. Your training and taper should have prepared you well, but there's one final step: recognising the physiological issues that might slow you down and plotting nutritional strategies to keep them at bay. Each sport presents athletes with 'walls' to hit. Your strategies will help you avoid these through sound preparation before the big day as well as special practices during the competition. Of course, while this chapter is focused on the event itself, many of these strategies can be used in training—and may improve its outcomes.

4.1 An overview of fatigue factors

Most people use the word 'fatigue' to describe a feeling of tiredness. In sports science, fatigue has a more specialised meaning, describing an athlete's inability to sustain speed, strength, power, skills, even concentration and decision-making. Depending on the sport in question, all these aspects of performance might slump at once. The results can be dramatic—sights like a marathon runner staggering on the track or a tennis player collapsing with cramp tend to stick in our memories. Mostly, however, fatigue is subtle, and the reduction in your exercise output may not be noticeable to you as it is occurring. Fatigue is an inevitable part of sport or exercise, and dealing with it is partly a matter of pacing yourself appropriately for the event. What you want to do, however, is stay ahead of your competitors, the world record, or your PB. Ensuring optimal performance means reducing or delaying the onset of fatigue as much as possible.

Many physiological factors can cause fatigue during exercise. Our focus in this chapter is on the factors that are nutrition-related and changeable. Some of these revolve around fuel sources, while others relate to homeostasis, or the balance of our body's internal environment. Whether it's a case of hydration, body temperature, acidity, or sodium levels, our body has a narrow range (known as homeostasis) in which it functions efficiently. While we have inbuilt mechanisms to keep these levels within the safe range, exercise challenges these mechanisms and pushes us past our physiological limits.

We can identify the fatigue factors in a sport or event by considering demands it places on the body. The duration and intensity of the exercise dictate the type and amount of fuel that is needed, which needs to be balanced against our ability to supply that fuel. High temperatures can increase the rate of fluid loss or the accumulation of body heat, and even change the rate at which carbohydrate fuel is burned. They also exacerbate the perception of fatigue caused by all factors. Finally, our preparation—how well we are able to fuel and hydrate before an event or during events—must be considered. Sometimes it's a fact of competition life that the event timetable leaves insufficient time between events for a full nutritional recovery. But sometimes poor recovery is our own doing—for example, if we dehydrate and restrict food intake in the lead-up to an event to meet a weigh-in target.

As well as identifying the likely fatigue factors in principle (which we'll do below), it is important to include past experience in your assessment. You may be able to recall times when you have had symptoms such as headaches, heavy legs, light-headedness, confusion, or stomach problems. These symptoms may give clues to what is preventing your body from performing at its best.

In simplistic terms, in explosive efforts such as jumps and lifts, most of the fuel is supplied not by burning fat or carbohydrate fuel but anaerobically (without oxygen), via high-energy phosphate compounds within the muscle cell. Adenosine triphosphate (ATP) and creatine phosphate can power only several seconds of work, but they are quickly regenerated between efforts. Repeated short bursts tax the regeneration of creatine phosphate, though creatine supplementation can counter this. As the exercise effort is sustained, or repeated, metabolism continues anaerobically, but with muscle glycogen now providing the main fuel source. If you've started the event with extremely low glycogen levels you will by now be running out of fuel—and feeling the consequences. But more likely, it will be the build-up of acidity (the hydrogen ions accompanying the production of lactate) and other by-products of this fuel use that cause the burning sensation and fatigue. Aside from ensuring that you have adequate glycogen stores, you can limit these effects by finding ways to increase muscle and blood buffering of the hydrogen ions.

As the exercise goes on for longer—and necessarily at a lower intensity—aerobic metabolism becomes more important. For this, your muscles burn a fuel mixture of fat (relatively unlimited supply in the body) and carbohydrate (limited supply), with the proportions depending on factors like:

- the intensity of exercise (the carbohydrate contribution is greater at a higher workload)
- the duration of exercise (carbohydrate contribution typically declines over the duration of the event)
- your pre-event diet (consuming carbohydrate in the hours before exercise increases the carbohydrate contribution to fuel)
- your level of training (training allows you to exercise at the same absolute workload with a higher fat : lower carbohydrate mix)

Team sports usually involve a mixture of (anaerobic) high-intensity bursts, interspersed with (aerobic) recovery periods. Meanwhile, athletes in steady-state events, such as running or cycling, gravitate to a predominantly aerobic workload just below the threshold at which blood lactate starts accumulating. Of course, steady-state is a relative term, since even the longest races will involve periods of higher-intensity work as athletes stage breakaways, surge up hills or sprint to the finish. The bottom line in these sports is that 'race pace' can be sustained only as long as carbohydrate fuel stores last—which is typically about 60–90 minutes for continuous exercise at maximal aerobic effort.

Fatigue can be manifested in two ways, known colloquially as 'hitting the wall' or 'bonking'. The 'wall' refers to a feeling of heaviness or deadness in the exercising muscle that makes the athlete slow down or even stop. The likely cause is the exhaustion of muscle glycogen, which forces the muscle to turn to fat and blood glucose for energy. 'Bonking' is caused primarily by the lowering of blood glucose levels, and occurs when the muscles siphon glucose out of the blood more quickly than it can be replaced by the liver (or by eating/drinking carbohydrate during the event). This often happens in conjunction with muscle glycogen depletion, but in some sensitive individuals it may occur as an independent event. 'Bonking' produces a central nervous system fatigue—dizziness, mental confusion, and an overwhelming tiredness and desire to sleep. The smart athlete will try to avoid both of these consequences of carbohydrate depletion.

Dehydration occurs in sport in several ways. Some athletes may start an event with a fluid deficit—from deliberate dehydration to make a weight category or from failure to rehydrate in hot weather or after previous exercise. A deficit can also arise during exercise as athletes fail to replace the fluid lost in sweat when their bodies try to cool themselves. Just like a car, you produce heat as a by-product of work, and this must be dissipated to keep your body at its preferred temperature. The harder you work and the heavier you are, the more sweat will be produced to cool you down. Athletes who have heavy sweat loss, low fluid intake or both are at risk of incurring a fluid mismatch that will affect their performance and perhaps health. A body-fluid deficit has creeping physiological effects—increasing body temperature, increasing heart rate, and increasing the perceived effort involved in exercise. The environmental conditions contribute to the cause and effect of dehydration. If it's hot, sweat losses increase and the physiological effects of a fluid deficit are pronounced. If it's humid, the production of sweat achieves little relief, since it can't evaporate easily to produce the cooling effect. Therefore, body temperature increases at a faster rate. The symptoms of mild to moderate dehydration include headaches and confusion, dry mouth and cessation of sweating, even though it's hot.

There is still a lot of discussion about the true effect of dehydration on exercise performance. The following summarises current thinking:

- In laboratory studies, the effect of dehydration on prolonged exercise is related to the size of the fluid deficit. As the deficit increases, so do the effects on physiology and performance.
- These effects are more pronounced when exercise is done in hot conditions.

- Dehydration also affects mental functioning—decision-making, concentration and skill. It may thus be more detrimental to an athlete in an unpredictable, skill-based activity like a team game than to a runner who just needs to keep putting one foot in front of another!
- The effects of dehydration build continuously, so the point at which it becomes a disadvantage is determined by our ability to detect a difference. In lab-based studies, we can detect an impairment of endurance and the performance of prolonged aerobic or intermittent exercise with a fluid deficit of as little as 2 per cent of body weight. This equates to 1 L of fluid for a 50-kg athlete and 1.5 L for a 75-kg athlete. In real-life sport, the differences between winning and losing can be far smaller than our ability to detect differences in performance in the lab. So it is possible that on-field performance impairments result from smaller levels of dehydration, or have greater effects on competition outcomes, than is seen in our current studies.
- On the other hand, laboratory studies cannot mimic some of the things in real-life sport that might reduce the effects of dehydration on performance—ranging from the motivation of competition to the effect of wind and air flow out in the open. So we may be overestimating the effects of dehydration based on the results of our laboratory studies. Clearly, more studies of dehydration and performance need to be done in the field!
- The effects of dehydration on strength and power are unclear.
- Fluid loss of more than 3–4 per cent of body weight greatly increases the risk of gastrointestinal discomfort and upsets. This appears to be linked to a reduced rate of gastric emptying.

Changes in body temperature outside the range of homeostasis are dangerous to the body. A high core temperature deserves some discussion in this section of nutrition fatigue factors, both for what it isn't and what it is. Heat illness during exercise—generally described as heat exhaustion in its milder forms and heatstroke when it reaches emergency proportions—is sometimes confused with dehydration. Essentially, however, your body temperature rises as you accumulate heat from the environment and from exercise. Preventing heat illness is primarily about choosing a safe exercise environment (considering whether the heat, humidity and your clothing will make your body store too much heat), and an appropriate pace (considering how much of your own heat output you'll be able to dissipate). On a very hot day, athletes who are competing at a very high intensity may overheat well before they become seriously dehydrated. In cool conditions, athletes who have deliberately dehydrated to make weight can suffer effects of dehydration without an excessive rise in body temperature. However, heat illness and dehydration are linked, since in hot weather, athletes who are dehydrated will increase their body temperature more than if they were well hydrated. Some new studies that show that drinking cold or icy fluids might assist other techniques to cool overheating athletes, such as ice vests and cold baths or showers. Future work may see us recommending that hot athletes use their drinks to manage body temperature as well as nutrition and hydration. Whether cold beverages just make athletes feel better in the heat or actually drag down core temperature, and to what extent these outcomes might enhance performance, is not yet known.

Gastrointestinal disturbances are another fatigue factor which is interrelated with fuel and hydration—or the lack of them. Tummy upsets can arise because of poor food and drink choices before or during an event. They can directly impede performance—the athlete may have to slow down or stop owing to pain or the need to vomit or make a pit stop. However, they contribute to even more problems if the athlete is then unable to hydrate and refuel during the rest of the event—not to mention the extra loss of fluid and electrolytes through diarrhoea and vomiting.

The final fatigue factor to consider is low blood sodium (hyponatraemia). Although large salt losses from sweating might contribute to this, the biggest cause of hyponatraemia is overhydration. In fact, the condition is also called water intoxication. This can occur when people drink too much before and during the event. The early symptoms of this potentially fatal problem include headaches, confusion and a feeling of doom. If hyponatraemia is allowed to become severe, it can lead to collapse, coma and sometimes death. Because mild hyponatraemia tends to look like other sorts of fatigue, and because hyponatraemia and dehydration call for very different treatments, it also helps to have some other signs to tell the two conditions apart. A report that the athlete has been drinking large volumes of fluid, or an observation of weight gain over the exercise session or above normal training weight, is a good clue.

Now that we have an idea of the types of fatigue factors that we can expect during competition, we can examine some ways to minimise or delay them. These involve action to take before, during and after the event. Once you have read the rest of this chapter, and Chapter 5 (Promoting recovery), use Checklist 4.1 to make sure you have taken on all the information you need for your specific competition.

4.2 General preparation for competition

The days leading up to your competition are generally sufficient for setting and achieving your fuel and fluid targets for the event itself. How hard you need to prepare depends on the challenges of your sport, the importance of the event and the frequency of competition. A long, intense event like a marathon or Ironman triathlon will probably throw up more potential sources of fatigue, and if this is your biggest competition for the year you will want to leave nothing to chance. On the other hand, if you are involved in a team sport and play in a couple of leagues, you may have a game scheduled once or twice a week, so less preparation can go into each game.

In getting your fuel stores stocked up for competition, you can rest a little easier knowing that your training has given you an edge in this department. Aerobic endurance training teaches your muscles to store more glycogen and use it more sparingly during aerobic exercise by increasing the contribution of fat to the fuel mixture. With your everyday (increased) muscle glycogen stores intact at the start of an event, you will have enough fuel on board to see you through all but the longest competitions.

To reach this everyday potential for muscle glycogen storage, you require:

- 24–36 hours of rest or tapered exercise
- A carbohydrate intake reaching 7–10 g per kilogram of body weight

For many athletes, this might be as simple as scheduling a day of rest or light training before the event while continuing to follow high-carbohydrate eating patterns. However, not all athletes eat sufficient carbohydrate in their usual diets to maximise glycogen storage, particularly females who count kilojoules to control body fat levels. These athletes may need encouragement to loosen their dietary reins and make refuelling their top dietary goal on the day before competition. Similarly, some athletes may need to reorganise their training programs to allow lighter training sessions or rest on the day before their event, or to shift sessions that cause muscle damage into an earlier part of the week. Checklist 4.2 summarises ways to fuel up adequately for your event.

4.3 Carbohydrate loading for endurance events

Carbohydrate loading is one of the most talked about yet misunderstood topics in sports nutrition. For a start, all athletes, from darts players to ultramarathon runners, think they need to do it. Second, many athletes use carbo-loading as a euphemism for gluttony—never mind the quality of the food, it's quantity that counts. And finally, the technique has been refined since its introduction in the 1960s, but many athletes have yet to catch up with the news.

To remove the mysticism from what is a potentially valuable practice, you should first decide whether your sport requires you to have super-loaded muscle glycogen stores. If you are going to drive around the block, you don't need an extra petrol tank in your car—it would just mean extra weight to carry. If you are driving in an endurance rally, on the other hand, you'll have an opportunity to use the additional fuel. Typically, endurance sports that involve over 90 minutes of continuous high-intensity exercise, using the same muscle groups, will challenge the capacity of the athlete's normal fuel stores. Think about this definition carefully. Although your triathlon may take over two hours, it involves three separate sports and therefore different muscle groups. And while a game of basketball may also take 90 minutes to complete, the duration of any one player's activity may be considerably shorter. You may need to think back to past events—did your pace or performance drop off late in the competition, accompanied by symptoms of muscle-glycogen fatigue? If so, it may be helpful to face the starting gun with super-loaded glycogen stores. You won't run faster or work harder in the beginning, but you will be able to exercise at your optimum pace for longer. In the long run, you will finish faster because you have avoided the 'wall' that would otherwise make you slow down substantially before the finish line.

Once you have decided that you compete in an endurance sport and that carbohydrate loading could be useful, the next step is to forget everything you have read or heard about it—particularly about depletion phases and low-carbohydrate diets. In its place try the following modified—and simplified—technique. The original carbohydrate-loading program familiar to most athletes was developed by Scandinavian researchers, using healthy but essentially non-elite subjects. They found that a program that first stripped glycogen from the muscles for three days (hard training plus low-carbohydrate diet) then followed up with glycogen storing for three days (reduced training plus high-carbohydrate eating) achieved a doubling of glycogen stores over usual values.

We now know that well-trained endurance athletes are 'lean, mean glycogen-storing machines'. Every day in training they use up large amounts of glycogen, and every day their muscles rebuild the stores. In fact, this is a continuous mini-cycle of depleting and loading. With these storage techniques already well rehearsed, there is no need for a severe depletion phase to prime the muscles for extra glycogen loading. All well-trained athletes have to do to load up their muscle glycogen stores is to give their muscles the luxury of more time and a tapering-off of training while they meet the fuel targets for maximum glycogen storage. Again, a daily intake of carbohydrate in the range of 7–10 g per kg is a general guide. Which side of the range you target might depend on your total energy budget, how big you are and how much time you have to load up. Smaller athletes on a tight fuelling-up schedule might aim for the high end, while large athletes with plenty of time might start at the low end.

We stuck to a three-day storage phase for carbohydrate loading for years—until Australian sports scientists found that as little as 36–48 hours of rest and high-carbohydrate eating might be enough to max out glycogen stores—at least in well-trained athletes. This would allow a midfielder in Australian Rules football to practise a weekly loading strategy over the 48-hour period between the last key training session and the game. On the other hand, a marathon runner who is peaking for one or two events a year might be able to devote three full days to taper and carbohydrate-focused eating in preparation for running 42 km at best race pace. As well as meeting carbohydrate targets over the final days, many carbo-loading athletes like to switch to low-fibre foods over the last 24 hours before their event. Many like the feeling of going into the race with a light feeling and empty gut. This may reduce the risk of gut upsets or the need to get the morning pit stop out of the way before the event starts.

The bottom line is that it is no longer considered necessary (or useful) to undertake a severe depletion phase before carbo-loading begins. In fact, it can be a disadvantage, because trying to train hard on a low-carbohydrate diet is unpleasant. It may also risk a carry-over of fatigue and injury into the competition. While the principles of carbohydrate loading are now much simpler, the practice is still beyond many athletes. This is because carbo-loading used to enjoy a reputation of being all about junk food. We have been to pasta parties and carbo-loading banquets organised for athletes before a marathon or Ironman race where the menu has included greasy cheesy lasagnes, meat lover's pizzas, doughnuts, cream pies and other fatty fare. Make sure that your carbohydrate loading plans actually achieve your fuel targets by following Checklist 4.2 and the sample carbohydrate loading plan in Table 4.1.

4.4 The pre-event meal

The pre-event meal is another nutritional practice that has become shrouded in superstition and ceremony. Its value to performance can vary from positive (in the case of an athlete who is still carbohydrate-depleted from a previous event) to merely confidence-boosting (for the athlete who is already well fuelled and hydrated) to disastrous (for an athlete who chooses the wrong foods and has a gastric upset during the event). And even when the physiological effects of a pre-event meal are minor, the psychological ones can be great. During the last hours before an important competition, athletes need to feel focused and prepared, and most athletes and teams have a special eating ritual to suit their situation and needs.

The main goals of meals eaten in the 1–4 hours before an event are:

- to finish topping up glycogen stores in muscles and the liver. Liver fuel stores are important to consider if you are competing in morning events, since they may be low after an overnight fast
- to top up fluid levels, especially if dehydration is likely to be a problem during the event
- to leave your gastrointestinal system feeling comfortable during the event—not so empty that you feel hungry, but not overfilled or prone to upsets
- to leave you feeling confident and ready to perform at your best!

There are many different ways to achieve these goals, and planning will need to cover several practical issues. The first is to choose a meal that complements the athlete's overall preparation for the event—or more specifically, recovery from the last training or competition session. The importance of the pre-event meal in topping up fuel and fluid levels depends on the timing of the last major workout, the degree of depletion caused by this session, and the amount of carbohydrate and fluid consumed since. For example, an athlete who has been preparing exclusively for an event may have tapered down her training and eaten carefully in the day or days leading up to it. In this case, the role of the pre-event meal is simply fine tuning, since the main work has already been accomplished. On the other hand, if the athlete is competing in a tournament, or playing back-to-back games on a tour, the pre-event meal will be a crucial part of the cycle of recovery and preparation between tightly scheduled events. Similarly, an athlete who trains hard right up to the event, or restricts food and fluid intake to make weight, will need to rely on the pre-event meal to restore fluid and fuel to optimal levels.

The second consideration for the pre-event meal is the time of day when the event is scheduled. Athletes who compete early in the morning will have to weigh their need for sleep against the need for adequate time to digest pre-event meals and snacks. While muscle glycogen levels can be prepared in the days leading up to the event, liver stores are less stable and need to be restocked overnight. A moderate-sized carbohydrate meal on the morning of the event will be enough for this. However, if the event starts too early to allow 3–4 hours for a meal to digest, you may opt for a smaller carbohydrate meal 1–2 hours before the event. To compensate for this, you should pay more attention to carbohydrate intake during the event, thus supporting the liver's ability to maintain your blood glucose levels (see Chapter 4.7).

The final consideration is the risk of gastrointestinal discomfort or upset during the event. Factors such as the timing, the amount and the content of pre-event meals (e.g. too much fibre or fat intake) can increase the risk of upsets during exercise. Certain types of athletes are predisposed to such problems, and events involving running or bouncy movements are also more likely to be associated with gut trouble. Careful attention to pre-event meals will be important for athletes at risk.

With such a mixed bag of goals and practical considerations, timetables and individual likes and dislikes, it is no wonder that the pre-event meal takes so many forms. Some athletes prefer to keep to a meal plan that mimics their everyday eating patterns, while others prefer to have a special plan to make competition day feel important. When the event is away from home, the biggest challenge may be to find foods that feel familiar and comforting. The psychological and even superstitious overtones of pre-event rituals must also be considered. We often see athletes eating pre-event meals that fall well outside our guidelines in this book. Fortunately, in many cases the pre-event meal is just a matter of fine tuning, so departing from the rules won't make a significant difference. If the athlete has invested emotionally or psychologically in a pre-event ritual and the event does not make special fuel demands, it is often best to leave the issue alone. However, for high-fuel situations, carbohydrate-rich menus are still the name of the game. Suitable meal and snack suggestions are found in Checklist 4.3 and Table 4.2.

4.5 Low-GI carbohydrates and sugar—pre-event friends and enemies?

Despite the benefits, eating carbohydrate before a workout or event can have its drawbacks. Eating carbs causes a metabolic chain reaction that increases the rate of carbohydrate fuel use during subsequent exercise. These effects last even when a carbohydrate-rich meal is consumed four hours before a workout, but most of the focus has been on eating sugary foods in the hour before an event. In one study, when athletes consumed glucose an hour before prolonged cycling they fatigued *sooner* than when they cycled without eating. Possible explanations include a dip in blood-sugar levels after the start of exercise, or a faster depletion of muscle glycogen stores. These findings made some athletes wary of pre-exercise carbohydrate eating. You can still find sports nutrition books and articles that warn athletes not to eat sugary foods in a so-called 'danger period' before exercise.

On balance, however, the majority of studies show that fuelling before prolonged exercise improves endurance and performance. Although carbohydrate eating increases carbohydrate burning and may cause blood glucose levels to drop a little after the start of exercise, in most cases this is a temporary blip that corrects itself with no apparent harm. After all, the regulation and metabolism of blood glucose are vastly different during exercise than at rest. The key is to ensure that you end up with a net fuel gain. If you consume only a little carbohydrate and the price you pay for this is to make your muscles use carbohydrate faster, you may end up with an overall loss on the fuel-performance balance sheet. However, by putting a worthwhile amount of extra fuel into your muscles you will more than compensate for the richer fuel mix. The cut-off level for pre-event carb intake seems to be about 1 g per kilogram—50 g for a 50 kg athlete.

Nevertheless, a small group of athletes appear to have an exaggerated and negative response to carbohydrates eaten in the hour before exercise. These athletes show the classic symptoms of hypoglycaemia—shakiness and fatigue—after starting their exercise bout. Why they react like this is unclear. Risk factors identified in one study included consuming only small amounts of carbohydrate (<50 g), having increased sensitivity to insulin, and a mild to moderate workload in the exercise period. However, other studies have cast doubt on these conclusions, and even on the idea that a drop in athletes' blood glucose leads to symptoms of hypoglycaemia or a reduction in exercise performance. Some things in sport remain a mystery. Nevertheless, athletes who have clear-cut reactions when they consume carbohydrate before exercise could try to manipulate the timing or choice of carbohydrate in their pre-event meal (see Checklist 4.3). Consuming carbohydrate during exercise is important for all athletes in fuel-demanding sports, but will be critical for athletes who are sensitive to carbohydrates eaten before exercise.

It's been suggested that making up pre-event meals from low-Glycemic Index carbohydrate sources is a good idea for all athletes, not just those who suffer from blood-glucose fluctuations. The idea is that the low-GI carbs produce a smaller metabolic 'jolt', and thus reduce the degree to which the fuel mix increases in carbohydrates and decreases in fats. A couple of studies have shown that a pre-exercise meal of low-GI foods improves the capacity for prolonged cycling more than does a high-GI meal, or exercise without any carbohydrate intake. This was said to be because low-GI foods sustain the available carbohydrate supply during exercise. Several sports foods on the market claim to be performance-enhancing because of these results. However, the majority of studies haven't shown much difference in outcomes when low-GI and high-GI pre-exercise meals are compared head to head. Importantly, though, most of these studies miss a crucial piece of the sports-nutrition picture because they set the athlete the task of completing an endurance exercise bout without any fuel intake during the session. This is not the recommended practice for good performance, and it isn't the way things are done in real-life sport: scientists and athletes agree that an efficient way to stay fuelled during prolonged exercise is to consume carbohydrate throughout. According to one study that did include 'in-flight refuelling', carbohydrate is consumed during endurance exercise, it doesn't matter what type of carbohydrate is consumed in the pre-event meal.

All athletes must judge the benefits and the practical issues associated with pre-exercise meals and snacks in their own individual sporting situation. In cases where athletes are unable to consume carbohydrate during a prolonged event or workout, they may find it useful to choose a pre-event menu based on low-GI carbohydrates to promote more sustained fuel release throughout exercise. However, there is no evidence of universal benefits from such menu choices, particularly where athletes are able to refuel during the session or where favoured and familiar food choices happen to have a high GI. In the overall scheme, pre-event eating needs to balance a number of factors, including the athlete's food likes, the choices available, and gastrointestinal comfort.

4.6 Fluid intake during events

Some degree of fluid imbalance is inevitable in many sports because of the mismatch between the athlete's sweat losses and the capacity to replace fluids during the event. During events lasting longer than 30 minutes, it is worth checking the need and opportunity to drink to offset sweat losses. A range of factors influence fluid intake during events, but across a range of sports and exercise activities, high-level athletes typically drink at a rate that replaces only 30 per cent to 70 per cent of their losses. The following factors influence fluid intake during exercise:

- Individual variability—we can be genetically predisposed to being a 'good' drinker or a 'reluctant' drinker
- Being aware of sweat losses and the benefits of good hydration
- Having fluids available (aid stations, trainers or handlers with bottles, bidons carried on a bike)
- Having an opportunity to drink (aid stations, breaks between halves or quarters, time on the interchange bench)
- Palatability of drinks (sweet flavour, cool temperature, salt content)
- External cues or encouragement to drink
- Gastrointestinal comfort
- Fear of the need for a pit-stop
- Weight-control issues (fear of the kilojoule content of sports drinks, belief that change in body mass after exercise reflects weight loss).

These factors need to be built into any fluid plan.

At this point we should carefully note that fluid intake during exercise needs to be appropriate to the individual and the event—so, to get it right, some athletes will need to drink more and others might need to drink less than their current practice. We have already suggested that athletes try to keep the real fluid deficit over an event to less than 2 per cent of body weight, especially in hot conditions. Dehydration will continue to be the main issue faced in high-level sport. Nevertheless, some high-level athletes will probably manage to overhydrate during their event. Too much fluid can cause gut problems, unnecessary time spent at aid stations or for pit stops and, in some cases, an unnecessary weight gain. For example, if you are a high-jumper, it doesn't make sense to sit around the arena guzzling drinks between rounds, leaving you with an extra kilogram to haul over the bar on your final jump. Meanwhile, some recreational exercisers will overhydrate into the danger zone. The bottom line is that a fluid plan needs to be based on your real needs, not well-meaning advice to drink as much as possible at every chance. The overview in Figure 4.1 shows how fluid needs vary between athletes and situations.

In general, it is not always possible or even desirable to replace all of the fluid deficit caused by exercise. Once sweat rates exceed 800 to 1000 ml/hr it becomes difficult to drink enough to keep pace. In some events, such rates commonly exceed 2 L an hour. However, many athletes with high sweating rates (see Figure 4.1) can improve their fluid intake practices and reduce the fluid deficit that accumulates during exercise. Athletes who face the starting line already dehydrated should also consider themselves in need of a plan for more aggressive hydration during the event. Checklist 4.4 provides some advice on strategies to achieve this. Athletes who have smaller rates of fluid loss during exercise, and those who have hydrated or even overhydrated before the event, need to be treated separately. These athletes can or should be more circumspect about drinking during an event.

Hydration guidelines for athletes have evolved over the past 30 years. The most recent guidelines, including the 2007 position stand of the American College of Sports Medicine (*www.acsm.org*) recognise that needs to hydrate and refuel during exercise can be integrated successfully. In general, water is regarded as a suitable beverage for exercise lasting less than 60 minutes, although a sweet-tasting drink may encourage an athlete to drink more. Of course, this last needs to be weighed against the need to consume kilojoules (people who are trying to lose weight probably won't want any extra) and the fact that commercial drinks cost more than tap water. For events of an hour or more, the athlete should consider the potential benefits of adding a fuel source to the mix (see Chapter 4.7). Sports drinks are designed to replace fuel (4–8 per cent carbohydrate = 4–8 g per 100 ml) and salt (10–35 mmol/L) simultaneously.

Early fluid-intake guidelines focused on distance running and provided prescriptive advice about drinking practices in terms of recommended volumes to be consumed at aid stations or time points. We recognise that people like the security of definite recommendations—for example, 'drink 250 ml every 15 minutes' or drink '250 ml at every aid station'. However, such 'one size fit all' guidelines can't apply sensibly to all sports and athletes. Drinking a litre an hour, as suggested above, might sound reasonable and achievable. In fact, it may well be appropriate for a serious recreational triathlete who weighs 80 kg and is losing 2 L of sweat an hour in the heat of the Hawaii Ironman cycling stage. However, Haile Gebrselassie's attempts to break the world marathon record in cool conditions will not allow him to slow down enough to swallow such a volume—let alone tolerate it in his gut. At the opposite extreme, a slight female cyclist in a mass-participation bike event in cool weather may be drinking a litre of fluid an hour to balance actual losses of 250 ml. Over 5–6 hours, this could lead to a dangerous level of water intoxication. Therefore, despite the pressures to come up with a single answer, we suggest that each athlete take responsibility for developing an individualised fluid plan. Checklist 4.4 provides some help.

4.7 Refuelling during the event

Carbohydrate that is consumed during prolonged exercise has the potential to provide an additional source of fuel for the brain and muscles. Studies of running and cycling have found that fuel intake during exercise can improve endurance (how long you can go before you tire) and performance (allow you to finish the race faster). Other studies show improved skills and movement patterns in the second half of team and racquet games. Not all sports have been covered in these studies, and not all studies show clear advantages following carbohydrate intake. This says as much about the difficulty of doing sports-science research as it does about the strength of the evidence.

Information about the benefits of consuming carbohydrate during prolonged exercise is not new. At the Boston Marathon in the 1920s it was reported that runners performed better when they ate candy during the race. Tour de France cyclists certainly consumed some form of carbohydrate en route during the early years of this race, well before sports scientists demonstrated that it was a good thing to do. Today's guidelines for athletes offer some finely tuned advice regarding the type, amount and timing of carbohydrate refuelling during events (see Checklist 4.4), based on the following observations:

- During exercise lasting more than 60–90 minutes, carbohydrate can serve as a source of fuel to the muscle, a contribution that peaks after about 60 minutes.
- Performance benefits are seen when athletes consume around 30–60 g of carbohydrate an hour during these prolonged events; they will need to experiment with the amount that suits the fuel demands of their event.
- Amounts as much as 90–100 g of carbohydrate an hour may be beneficial in extended endurance events such as stage-race cycling (5–6 hours) or Ironman triathlon (8–15 hours). Where glycogen depletion in muscle is likely to impair performance, carbohydrate from fluids (i.e. sports drinks) and foods is a valuable source of fuel.
- Although the fuel contribution doesn't really 'kick in' until about an hour into the race, greater benefits are seen when fuelling starts early.
- The source of carbohydrate should be palatable, practical to consume and easy to digest. A range of carbohydrate drinks and foods of moderate and high GI appear suitable, and new studies show the benefits of mixing a couple of carbohydrate types together. Since different types of carbohydrates move from the small intestine into the body using different transporters, a mixture of carbohydrates leads to greater overall absorption and fuel availability to the muscle.
- There is puzzling evidence that carbohydrate intake also benefits performance in high-intensity events lasting about 1 hour. The puzzle arises because muscle carbohydrate stores aren't depleted in these events and because not enough time has passed for the muscle to be burning large amounts of carbohydrate from the refuelling course. We now think that performance benefits come from the brain rather than the muscle. Your brain feels better when it receives carbohydrate, allowing you to exercise at higher intensity.
- New research has shown that the carbohydrate doesn't even have to reach the brain to make it feel better. Swilling a sports drink around your mouth before spitting it out also leads to better performance where extra muscle fuel isn't an issue.

> Sports scientists think that receptors in the mouth and throat alert the brain to the incoming carbohydrate. Even if the fuel doesn't arrive, the brain behaves as if it did. We need more research to confirm and explain these findings because we can put them into effective practice. (Sports drink mouthwashes for those on weight-loss diets, perhaps?)

Whatever your competition plan, it should be practised and fine-tuned in training—particularly under conditions that mimic those of the Big Day. Often, practical issues will force you to adopt a plan that falls below (or even outside) the optimal guidelines. Do the best that you can—and follow what works for you. Many athletes perform well on practices that look less than ideal on paper!

CHECKLIST 4.1
Are you eating to compete at your best?

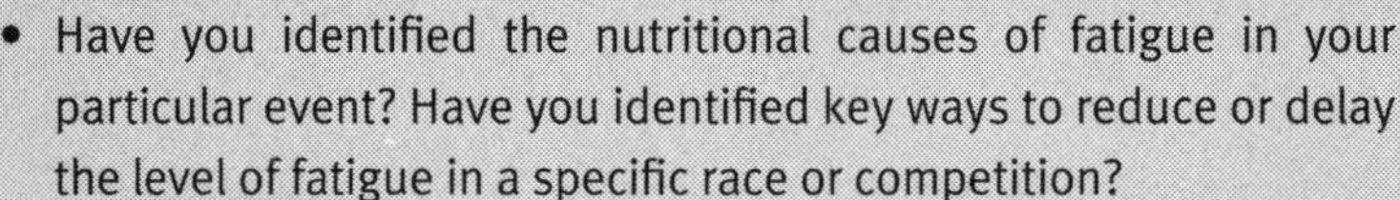

- Have you identified the nutritional causes of fatigue in your particular event? Have you identified key ways to reduce or delay the level of fatigue in a specific race or competition?
- Do you arrange your pre-event training taper and eating patterns to ensure that carbohydrate fuel stores (glycogen) are high enough in both your muscles and liver to meet the demands of your particular sport?
- In 'endurance' events, involving more than ~90 min of continuous or intermittent exercise, do you 'load' your muscle glycogen stores with a special program of eating and tapered training for 24–48 hours before the event?
- Do you top up carbohydrate stores with a pre-event meal or snack during the 1–4 hr before competition, especially in events where carbohydrate fuel is important?
- Do you keep hydration at an acceptable level during the event by drinking appropriate volumes of fluids before, during, and after the event? Do you have a flexible and well-practised fluid plan

that takes account of your likely needs and the opportunities to drink during your event?

- During events lasting 1 hour or longer, do you consume carbohydrate drinks or foods to supply an additional source of fuel to your brain and muscles?
- Have you found a plan for eating and drinking before and during the event so you won't risk gastrointestinal discomfort or upsets?
- Have you practised this plan during training sessions or smaller events to fine tune the details?
- In weight-class sports, can you achieve your competition weigh-in with minimal harm to health or performance?
- Do you follow nutritional practices that will promote recovery after the event, particularly during multi-day competitions such as tournaments and stage races?
- During a prolonged competition program, can you follow an eating plan that looks after your longer-term energy and nutritional needs?
- Do you make well-considered decisions about the use of supplements and specialised sports foods that have been shown to enhance performance or meet the physiological demands of your event?

CHECKLIST 4.2
Fuelling up for sports competition

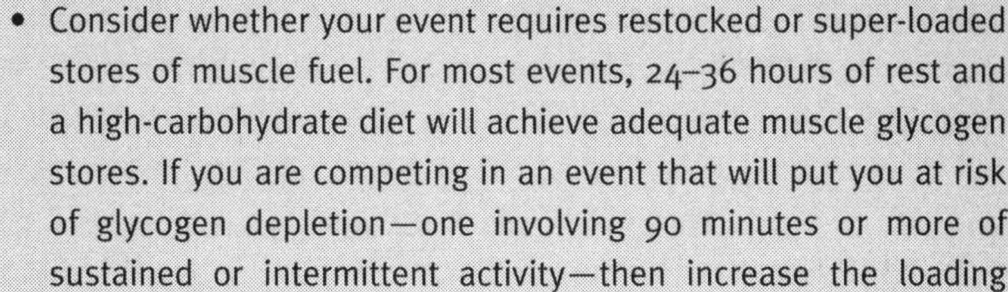

- Consider whether your event requires restocked or super-loaded stores of muscle fuel. For most events, 24–36 hours of rest and a high-carbohydrate diet will achieve adequate muscle glycogen stores. If you are competing in an event that will put you at risk of glycogen depletion—one involving 90 minutes or more of sustained or intermittent activity—then increase the loading period and loading targets. The theoretical activity requirements of the event may provide a clue to the need for aggressive fuelling up. On the other hand, your past experience of 'hitting the wall' during competition is a good indicator that carbohydrate loading could be useful.

- Consider whether you have given yourself enough time and opportunity to fuel up. If you are competing frequently—once or twice a week, for example—this may not always be possible. Try to achieve better preparation for your most important events.
- Schedule training so sessions that could potentially damage muscle fibres (for example, those involving hard running, body contact or eccentric weight work) are early in the week, allowing more time for recovery.
- For maximal refuelling in any time period, use a ready reckoner (Table 2.8) to make sure your daily diet achieves a carbohydrate target within the range of 7–10 g per kg of body weight. For example, a 50-kg athlete should aim to eat 350–500 g of carbohydrate over the day preceding competition, while an 80-kg athlete might aim for 600–800 g.
- If you need to follow energy restrictions for weight control, recognise that this will limit your capacity to eat carbohydrate and store glycogen. You may need to cycle your nutrition goals—changing them between periods when weight control is the priority and those when you should be more liberal with energy and carbohydrate intake.
- If you are carbohydrate loading for a specific important event, relax your total nutritional goals a little and place carbohydrate intake at the top of the list. For example, reduce the amount of protein in your meals to make more room for large serves of carbohydrate foods. In addition, sugar and sugary foods, including sports drinks and gels, provide a compact carbohydrate source despite their relatively low levels of micronutrients. Table 4.1 sets out a typical carbohydrate-loading menu.
- Don't get tricked into fuelling up with chocolate, rich desserts, fatty

pasta dishes and take-aways. Although these are favourites with many carbo-loading athletes, they are a rich source of fat rather than carbohydrate. You may not actually meet your carbohydrate targets.

- Over the final 24 hours before your event, consider switching to a low-residue diet to reduce your stomach and intestinal contents. Eat low-fibre foods and make extra use of compact sugary ones. You may even like to use liquid meal supplements or other formula foods to supply some or all of your carbohydrate needs over the last 12–24 hours. These are very low in residue and will leave you with an empty gut to race 'light'.
- Note that the amount of carbohydrate recommended and the dietary strategies suggested above are specific to carbohydrate loading and should not be applied to everyday eating.
- Finish off with a well chosen pre-event meal (see Checklist 4.3).

CHECKLIST 4.3
The pre-event meal

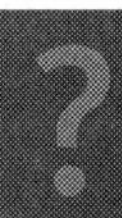

- Work backwards from your event to set up a series of meals or snacks over the day. The final meal should be eaten 4 hr before the event in the case of a larger meal, or 1–2 hr in the case of a snack.
- Consider carbohydrate-rich, low-fat foods to ensure easy digestion, but also for a final top-up of fuel supplies for demanding events. Typically, a carbohydrate target within the ballpark of 1–4 g per kg body weight will do the job (e.g. 50–200 g for a 50-kg athlete, 80–320 g for an 80-kg athlete). Many people find their normal breakfast choices are a great pre-event meal even when it is not breakfast time. Other suggestions are found in Table 4.2 (Pre-event meal ideas).

- Experiment with the type, timing and amount of food that works best for you. Practise in training or some minor competitions so you have everything right for the big day. Learn which foods, if any, cause you discomfort or upsets and avoid them. High-fat foods are often a problem, but you might also find that you need to reduce your normal fibre intake before an event.
- Take special care to consume carbohydrate before morning events, especially if you are competing in an endurance sport. If the liver's glycogen stores are low from an overnight fast, you may be less able to maintain blood glucose levels, especially late in the event. Experiment with a small snack or carbohydrate drink if time is short. In addition, compensate for low liver glycogen stores by consuming carbohydrate during the event (see Chapter 4.7).
- If you are one of the small group of athletes who experience fatigue during exercise after consuming carbohydrates, try some of the following techniques:
    - Experiment to find the critical period during which carbohydrate intake should be avoided.
    - Make sure your pre-event snack or meal provides more than 1 g/kg carbohydrate to compensate for your increased use of carbohydrate during the event.
    - Include some high-intensity bursts in your warm-up. This kick-starts your liver to release glucose into the bloodstream.
    - Try low-GI carbohydrate-rich choices in the pre-event meal (see Table 4.2).
    - Importantly, consume carbohydrate during the workout or event.
- If you are unable to consume carbohydrate in adequate quantities during the event, consider a pre-event meal based on low-GI carbohydrate-rich foods (see Table 4.2). Although most people won't specifically benefit from eating low-GI foods before an event, individual athletes may find some value in this.
- If you have a busy competition schedule (e.g. competing daily in a tournament or cycle tour), plan ahead to ensure that you restore

food and fluid levels between events. What you consume before, during and after an event are all equally important. Even if you are becoming tired, don't neglect any of these eating opportunities.

- If you suffer from competition nerves or need to eat quite close to your event, consider a liquid meal supplement or a fruit smoothie. These are high in carbohydrate and low in fat and bulk, and many athletes can drink them in comfort even up to an hour before an event.
- Drink adequate amounts before the event. If it's a hot day, or your sport provides little opportunity to drink during the competition, make sure you are well hydrated at the start of the event.

CHECKLIST 4.4
Fluid and fuel strategies during competition

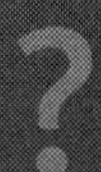

- Consider the need and opportunity to hydrate in events lasting more than 30 min, and add refuelling to the game plan for events of more than 60 min of continuous exercise. Not all events or situations will need or allow a plan, but it's worth considering the cost-benefit ratio for these events.
- Develop your own fluid plan based on previous competition experience and training observations. It should keep pace with most of your sweat loss (see Figure 2.3) but be flexible enough to adapt to the conditions and happenings of the day. Listen to your thirst, but also work with a plan that considers fuel needs and practical opportunities to consume foods and drinks during the event. They may not always match up.
- Neither overhydrate during the event nor allow yourself to fall into fluid deficit that reduces your performance. As a general rule, aim to keep total fluid losses to less than 2 per cent of your body weight, especially in hot weather. Know when to be stricter or more liberal with this goal.

- Identify the opportunities to consume fluids and foods, and their availability during your event. Build this knowledge into your race/match plan. Depending what your sport is, you may make use of aid stations, carry supplies yourself, or have trainers/handlers carry them. You may have scheduled breaks or you may need to eat or drink on the run. You may have a choice about what you consume or you may need to go with what is provided.
- Practise your plan in training sessions so it will all feel comfortable on the day. It may not at first. Practice will help you learn to tolerate foods and fluids and fine-tune your plan. Knowing how your body responds will be an advantage on race day.
- Note that water is a great choice in events shorter than 60 min. Balance the energy vs. money cost of other fluids such as sports drinks, cordial and defizzed soft drinks. Of course, there may be advantages in drinking what you enjoy, even if there isn't a real exercise benefit.
- Where possible, make sure that drinks are kept to a refreshing temperature (usually cool) and that any flavours are ones you like.
- For events lasting 60 minutes or more, build in a refuelling plan that matches the fuel demands of the sport. An intake of ~30–60 g of carbohydrate per hour is a good starting point. The low end of this range may be suitable for shorter events, where your brain will be the main beneficiary. The high end (or even higher) might be needed to meet muscle fuel needs and energy considerations in gruelling events like cycle tours, marathons and triathlons.
- Choose your carbohydrate sources from a range of easily digested foods and drinks (see Table 4.3). Prefer what you find affordable, palatable and well tolerated. Common or everyday foods often do the job well.
- Remember that ready-made products can make refuelling easier. Sports drinks replace fuel, fluid and salt in one go, and you may be able to adjust the concentration as your priorities change. Other sports foods such as gels and bars may also suit the practical

demands of your sport. Many new brands contain high levels of electrolytes for longer sports and salty sweaters, or a mix of carbohydrates to improve total absorption. Generally, these advances are supported by scientific research findings, but their convenience needs to be balanced against their cost.

- For longer events, expect flavour fatigue to set in after many hours of the same thing, and have a range of types or tastes (savoury and sweet) on offer.
- Consider some salt replacement in long events (especially if you are a salty sweater). This may help with thirst and appetite—salt makes drinks more palatable, and a salty or savoury snack may offer a complete flavour change.
- Make use of solid foods in longer events where you're likely to get hungry. Remember that these are also a more compact way to carry fuel on your bike or in your pocket.
- Plan to spread your fuel and fluid intake according to real nutritional needs over the event. It makes sense to start feeding early and try to prevent severe fuel depletion or dehydration rather than waiting till it causes fatigue. Note that your nutrition needs and priorities may change over the event or be different from what you anticipated. You may be able to change concentrations of drinks or add new supplies to manipulate nutrient levels either according to a prearranged plan or in response to the unfolding demands of the competition. It's good to have a Plan A and a Plan B. Of course, in some events you may have to compromise your ideal plan by fitting in with organised feeding opportunities and supplies.
- Try out different drink containers, sachets, bags and other devices that will allow you to carry and consume your race nutrition supplies with ease. Necessity will often be the mother of invention.

TABLE 4.1
A carbohydrate-loading menu

Day	65 kg male runner (~650 g/day carbohydrate)	50 kg female runner (~500 g/day carbohydrate)
Day 1 The menu focuses on the carbohydrate-rich foods; other foods can be added to balance the menu. An exercise taper should accompany this menu to optimise muscle glycogen storage. It is possible that carbohydrate loading can be achieved by 2 days of such a diet.	**Breakfast:** ¾ cup oats + cup milk with honey 2 slices toast with jam 250 ml sweetened juice **Snack:** Scone with jam **Lunch:** 1 large bread roll with fillings 200 g carton flavoured yogurt + banana 600 ml sports drink **Snack:** 2 crumpets + honey **Dinner:** 1 cup cooked pasta + ½ cup sauce 1 cup jelly 600 ml lemonade **Snack:** Cup low-fat milk with 2 tsp Milo Throughout the day—100 g confectionery	**Breakfast:** ¾ cup oats + cup milk with honey Slice toast with jam 250 ml sweetened juice **Snack:** Scone with jam **Lunch:** 1 large bread roll with fillings 200 g carton flavoured yogurt 600 ml sports drink **Snack:** 1 crumpet + honey **Dinner:** 1 cup cooked pasta + ½ cup sauce 1 cup jelly 250 ml lemonade **Snack:** Cup low-fat milk with 2 tsp Milo Throughout the day—100 g confectionery
Day 2	**Breakfast:** 3 pancakes with syrup Cup low-fat milk with 2 tsp Milo **Snack:** muesli bar 250 ml fruit juice **Lunch:** 1 large bread roll with fillings 200 g carton flavoured yogurt + banana 600 ml sports drink **Snack:** 2 crumpets + honey	**Breakfast:** 2 pancakes with syrup Cup low-fat milk with 2 tsp Milo **Snack:** muesli bar 250 ml fruit juice **Lunch:** 1 large bread roll with fillings 200 g carton flavoured yogurt 600 ml sports drink **Snack:** 1 crumpet + honey

Day	65 kg male runner (~650 g/day carbohydrate)	50 kg female runner (~500 g/day carbohydrate)
	Dinner: 3 cups noodle stir-fry 1 cup jelly 600 ml lemonade **Snack:** 1 cup liquid meal supplement Throughout the day—100 g confectionery	**Dinner:** 2 cups noodle stir-fry 1 cup jelly 250 ml lemonade **Snack:** 1 cup liquid meal supplement Throughout the day—100 g confectionery
Day 3 Many athletes like to increase the focus on low-fibre and low-residue eating on day before race, allowing them to reach the start line feeling 'light' rather than with gastrointestinal fullness. If a further focus on a low residue diet is needed, the athlete could exchange more of the food on this plan for liquid meal supplements and confectionery	**Breakfast:** 2 cups low-fibre breakfast cereal + ¾ cup milk 2 slices toast with jam 250 ml sweetened juice **Snack:** fruit bun +600 ml sports drink **Lunch:** 1 large bread roll with fillings 200 g carton flavoured yogurt 600ml sports drink **Dinner:** 1½ cups cooked rice + ½ cup sauce 1 cup jelly 600 ml lemonade **Snack:** 250 ml liquid meal supplement Throughout the day—100 g confectionery	**Breakfast:** 1½ cups low-fibre breakfast cereal + ¾ cup milk Slice toast with jam 250 ml sweetened juice **Snack:** fruit bun **Lunch:** 1 large bread roll with fillings 200 g carton flavoured yogurt 600 ml sports drink **Dinner:** 1 cup cooked rice + ½ cup sauce 1 cup jelly 250ml lemonade **Snack:** 250 ml liquid meal supplement Throughout the day—100 g confectionery

This menu provides carbohydrate intakes of ~10 g/kg per day for a 65-kg male and 50-kg female athlete before the event on Day 4. Athletes of differing sizes should scale this intake up or down according to their body mass.

TABLE 4.2
Pre-event meal ideas

General ideas

- Breakfast cereal* + low fat milk + fresh/canned fruit
- Muffins* or crumpets* + jam/honey
- Pancakes + syrup
- Toast* + baked beans* or canned spaghetti
- Baked potatoes with low-fat filling
- Creamed rice
- Rice based dish (e.g. risotto) from low-fat recipe
- Pasta* with tomato-based or other low-fat sauces
- Rolls* or sandwiches* with banana filling or lean salad filling
- Fruit salad plus low-fat yoghurt
- Liquid meal supplements
- Homemade fruit smoothie (milk, fruit, yoghurt, etc.)

Examples of low-GI carbohydrate-rich choices

- Sultana Bran with milk
- Porridge or Bircher muesli
- Low-fat fruit yoghurt
- Liquid meal supplements and flavoured milk drinks
- Multi-grain bread + baked beans
- Pasta meal

* Note: you may need to avoid high-fibre types if you are at risk of gut discomfort or problems during events.

TABLE 4.3
Common food and fluid choices used to refuel during sport

Choice	Amount required to provide 50 g carbohydrate
Gatorade (6% carbohydrate)	800 ml
Powerade (8% carbohydrate)	600 ml
Sports gel (40 g sachet)	2 sachets
Sports bar (60 g bar)	1.25 bars
Cereal bars or muesli bars	2 bars
Bananas	2 medium

Choice	Amount required to provide 50 g carbohydrate
Other fruit (e.g oranges)	3 medium pieces
Jelly beans or jelly lollies	60 g
Chocolate bar	80 g
Dried fruit	80 g
Cola drinks (11% carbohydrate)	450 ml
Bread/sandwiches	Medium roll or 2 thick slices of bread with honey/jam
Fruit bread or cake	100 g

FIGURE 4.1
How meeting fluid needs should be approached in endurance events

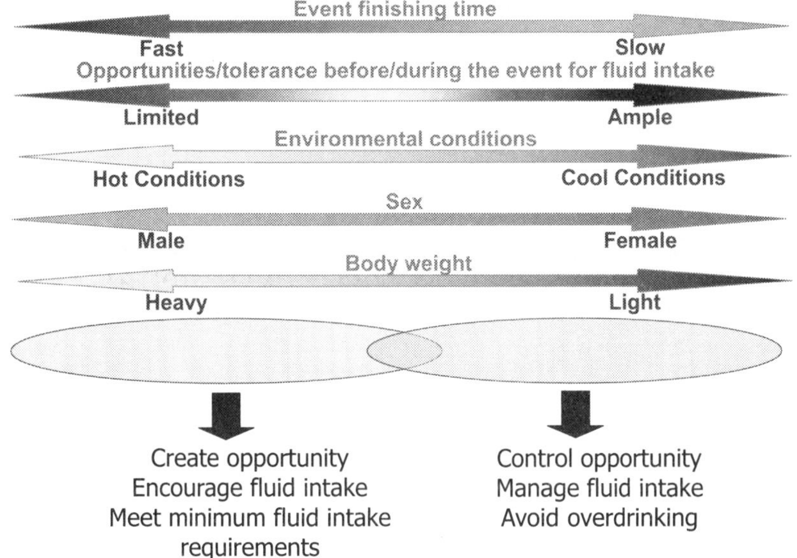

5
Promoting recovery

Being an athlete in the new millennium means pushing yourself hard and long—striving to go beyond your best, using training, science, will power, skill, everything you've got, and holding it all together until the finish. And then doing it all over again.

In many sports, you need to compete more than once to take home the gold medal, with anywhere from 30 minutes to 24 hours between events. For example, you may be racing in an athletics meet where you have to run in heats, semi-finals and even the final in the one day. In a basketball or tennis tournament you may be scheduled for one or two games each day. A cycle tour may involve one or two stages a day for a week or more. Such competition schedules make it difficult to recover fully between events. Training can be even more challenging, particularly, when two or even three hard sessions are planned each day. In all cases, your ability to recover from one session and present yourself at your best for the next will affect not just your training but your competition results. Your adaptation to training occurs during this recovery period—and it's that adaptation that you want to take to the next starting line or siren.

Over the past decade, recovery has become an integral part of training and competition. Athletes attend special recovery sessions and count the hours in their training programs. Sporting clubs and institutes have built dedicated recovery centres, invested in recovery equipment and employed recovery experts. All this tell us that recovery is not passive, and it's not something that happens by good luck or in its own good time. There are a variety of ways to speed recovery processes and ensure that athletes adapt to training or return to competition at their very best. These include massage, stretching, immersion in cold or hot-and-cold water, relaxation techniques and sleep. Nutritional aspects of recovery include:

- replacing the fluid and electrolytes lost in sweat
- replenishing muscle glycogen stores
- repairing any damage caused by the exercise and building new muscle as a response to the stimulus of exercise
- ensuring your immune system is working well.

An athlete's peak training diet will actively address recovery issues. There are three important components to optimal nutrition during the recovery phase. First, you need to establish what your main nutritional goal is post-exercise. Do you want to refuel, replace lost fluids or repair muscle damage? Next, you need to provide your body with building blocks to achieve your nutritional goals—carbohydrate, protein, water, vitamins and minerals. Finally, you need to time this nutritional support well—maximising recovery by supplying these nutrients when the body is most able to take advantage of them.

5.1 Rehydration

Even if you have consumed fluid exactly to plan before and during an exercise session—whether competition or training—you are still likely to finish the session with some degree of dehydration. This is particularly true for prolonged and intense sessions in a hot environment, where sweat losses exceed your fluid intake. However, dehydration may also be expected in short events during which you've had little or no opportunity to drink. Ideally, you should aim to fully restore such fluid losses by your next workout or event. This is difficult in situations where your fluid deficit is more than 2 per cent of body weight and the interval between sessions is less than 6 to 8 hours. In normal circumstances, thirst prompts us to drink enough to maintain fluid balance from day to day. However, in acutely stressful situations such as hard exercise or competition, or a sudden change in temperature and altitude, thirst may not prod us into drinking enough. In fact, after a dehydrating episode there can be a lag of 4 to 24 hr before body fluid levels are restored. The success of rehydration after exercise (or after dehydrating to make weight), depends not just on how much we drink but on how much water is retained and redistributed throughout our body compartments.

Since you can't count on your body to identify and repair an acute episode of dehydration on its own, it's useful to have an objective way of assessing and a definite plan of attack. Figure 2.3 provided a protocol for assessing your sweat losses during an exercise session and the resulting fluid deficit, but it assumed that you were in fluid balance at the start of the session. Generally, we equate 1 kg of weight loss with 1 L of fluid deficit. This won't be true if you were dehydrated or overhydrated before the workout. If you fluid loaded, assume that you stored an extra 500–1000 ml depending on your size. If you carbo-loaded before the event, subtract 1–1.5 kg from your pre-event weight to account for the extra glycogen and the water that is stored along with it, leaving you with your true fluid losses. If in doubt, go by your usual training weight. If your fluid deficit is 1 L or less, you may get away with drinking as you're inclined to for the day. However, if your fluid deficit is 2 per cent or more of your body weight, and you have less than a day, the best way to ensure that fluid balance is restored is to have a plan that covers what types of fluid you consume, how much and when.

Amount of fluid

Simply drinking a volume of fluid equal to the fluid deficit at the end of an exercise session won't fully restore fluid balance. After all, you keep on sweating and producing urine during the recovery phase. Depending on factors such as the type and timing of what you consume, you may be good at retaining this fluid or you may waste a lot in unnecessary wee stops. Typically, you need to drink a volume equal to 125–150 per cent of the post-exercise fluid deficit to compensate for these ongoing losses and ensure that fluid balance is restored over the first 4 to 6 hr of recovery. So already you can set yourself a general target for fluid consumption in this recovery period.

Type of fluid

On the face of it, any drink should help to restore fluid levels. In practice, some fluids are better at doing this than others—and in some situations, speed is the name of the game. Your net fluid gain is effectively the difference between the amount of fluid you consume and the volume of urine you produce afterwards. So when you want to rehydrate, you need to balance the incentive to drink a fluid against your body's ability to retain it.

What prompts us to drink is a topic on which drink manufacturers have, unsurprisingly, done considerable research. But it's also been pursued by scientists representing sport and the military, who want to know what athletes or soldiers feel like drinking in the heat of the contest or battle and afterwards. This type of research is done by unobtrusively observing what happens when subjects are given free access to different drinks. It's produced some interesting results. First, some people are simply better drinkers than others. Second, the palatability of a drink makes a difference to how much people drink, even when they know they are dehydrated. Typically, people like sweet drinks—with some cultural differences as to favourite flavours, and often a change in flavour preferences during exercise, or when people are dehydrated. Most people also like drinks to be cool (5–15°C) rather than icy cold or warm, especially when large volumes need to be consumed speedily. Adding some salt to a drink increases the volume consumed because salty drinks don't turn off the thirst drive as quickly. However, a common observation from voluntary-drinking studies is that even the best drink does not entice dehydrated athletes to drink a volume equal to their fluid deficit. Typically, athletes start off well, but reduce their rate of drinking over the next hours—even when drinks are freely available and a fluid deficit still exists. This speaks to the value of having a plan.

To study how well a drink is retained in the body, scientists first dehydrate their subjects then make them consume a given volume of various fluids and check how much urine is produced over the next hours. Such studies have shown that the best way to improve fluid retention is to consume sodium (salt) at the same time as the drink. After all, sweat losses involve the loss of electrolytes as well as fluid. Our bodies are designed to regulate the concentration (osmolarity) of blood as well as its volume. Replacing only fluid will lower the concentration even before volume is restored—and urine will be produced to protect against this. Adding salt to a rehydration fluid helps to restore osmolarity and volume in tandem, resulting in lower urine production and higher fluid retention from the same amount of drink. Figure 5.1 shows the effectiveness of different fluids at restoring fluid balance in a study in which athletes were dehydrated by 2 per cent body weight, then required to drink fluids containing different amounts of salt in volumes equal to 150 per cent of their post-exercise fluid deficit.

There are several details illustrated in this figure that are worthy of comment. First, as the amount of salt in the fluid increases, the output of urine decreases. A small amount of salt (25 mmol/L—equal to the concentration in the typical sports drink) is better than a negligible amount (in water). The best choice is a solution with >25 mmol/L, but once the sodium concentration hits ~50 mmol/L the benefits taper off. Not surprisingly, this is the concentration of salt in the oral hydration solutions used to treat dehydration following diarrhoea. Second, unless salt is replaced, people are unable to fully rehydrate. The subjects in this study drank volumes equivalent to 150 per cent of their fluid losses, but still ended up with a fluid deficit in cases where their drink had low or negligible salt content. Third, the experience of subjects in these low/no salt cases was probably confusing and disruptive to recovery. After all, they would have been producing large volumes of urine, and it would have been easy to take this as a sign that they were well hydrated. In addition, if (in 'real' life) their exercise bout (or recovery phase) had occurred at night, they would have had broken sleep owing to the frequent trips to the toilet. So, there are clear benefits to the strategic replacement of both salt and fluid. Adding salt to rehydration drinks is only one way to achieve this. Drinking fluids while eating salt-containing foods or salt added to meals is also effective.

Drinks can contain fluid-retention factors, but also urine-stimulating compounds. It is common to hear that caffeine 'dehydrates' you by increasing urine losses. We're often told by well-meaning folk to avoid caffeine-containing beverages such as tea, coffee, and cola or energy drinks during and after exercise or during air travel because of their (alleged) dehydrating effect. In fact, a review of a large number of studies in everyday situations concluded that low to moderate amounts of caffeine have a *minimal* effect on urine production and hydration status in regular caffeine consumers. Most importantly, caffeine-containing drinks don't dehydrate people *per se*, because they actually *add* fluid to the body. Although one study found that cola drinks weren't quite as effective as sports drinks at rehydrating people after exercise, the differences were small and probably not of practical significance. In addition, this study didn't consider that a tiny increase in fluid losses from caffeine-containing fluids may be more than offset by the increased voluntary intake of drinks that are well liked and part of social rituals. If you are asked to suddenly remove such beverages from your diet or post-exercise meals, you may not compensate by drinking an equal volume of other less familiar or well-liked fluids.

Alcohol has a more pronounced effect on urine production, especially when consumed at high doses. Funnily enough, it is one of the fluids that some athletes are quite prepared to consume in large volumes after exercise! One study (for which there was probably no shortage of volunteers) investigated the effect of rehydrating after exercise with various alcoholic drinks. It followed a similar protocol to the study we just mentioned. Figure 5.2 shows the results in terms of urine losses and total fluid balance after 6 hr of recovery. According to this study, a low-alcohol drink (1–2 per cent alcohol) may have minimal impact on urination and thus rehydration, but drinks with a higher alcohol content, such as regular beer, wine or spirits, will hinder rehydration. So a low-alcohol beer may have its place after sport—maybe as a shandy (adding lemonade for some carbohydrates) or with cheese and pretzels (for salt, carbohydrate and protein). Maybe the lawn bowls players have it right! However, spending too much time at the bar after exercise will interfere with rehydration and other recovery goals. Apart from any direct effects, excessive alcohol intake will distract the athlete from doing the right things and promote high-risk behaviours.

Timing of fluid intake

The final decision for the athlete is when to drink recovery fluids: all at once, or spread through the recovery period? A lot has to do with your schedule. How much time do you have until your next workout or race? What else do you have to fit into the recovery phase? Drinking large volumes early means that more fluid is restored in the first few hours. This could be useful if you don't have much time before the next session, although you will have to get the volume and timing right to avoid having fluid sloshing around in your gut when you line up again. If you have other commitments in the recovery period, you may want to get some of your rehydration out of the way early. In general, however, it's better to spread your fluid intake out over a longer period, because this minimises the urine lost—meaning greater fluid retention and more efficient rehydration.

5.2 Refuelling

As is the case for fluid balance, the length and intensity of your training session or competition event will determine how much glycogen was used and needs to be replaced before the next session. There are two main requirements for effective glycogen storage—carbohydrate intake and time. Roughly speaking, when conditions are favourable, muscle glycogen can be stored at a rate of about 5 per cent per hour. Thus it can take ~24 hours to fully replace muscles stores that have been depleted. This is one of the reasons why the training week should be broken into distinct periods. A good timetable will allow preparation before, and recovery after, key training sessions and competition. It will not matter that other lower-intensity sessions are undertaken without full refuelling—in fact, there may actually be some advantages to this (see Chapter 2.10). When you need to maximise glycogen storage, you should make sure you eat the amount and type of carbohydrate—and follow the timing—that promotes refuelling.

Amount and timing of carbohydrate

Table 2.4 in Chapter 2 provided a summary of the amount of dietary carbohydrate required to replenish muscle fuel stores, based on the fuel cost of daily training and competition. For times when full recovery is the challenge, we proposed a target amount of 7–12 g per kg body mass. This is actually quite a wide range—350–600 g of carbohydrate for a 50-kg athlete, or 560–960 g for an 80-kg athlete. Part of the reason for the flexibility in these targets is that, even for a given body weight, athletes have different-sized fuel tanks and different opportunities to fill them. You might need to consider how much of your body contributes muscle power for your sport—that is, how much of your body weight is active muscle in your event—and what constitutes the difference between depleted and fully fuelled. How many kilojoules you can devote to carbohydrate eating will also help determine where you fall in the range. In extreme cases, when athletes are exercising intensely for 6–8 hours or more each day (for example, the Tour de France), the high end of the range will be needed to cope with recovery and ongoing daily needs, as well as to meet huge daily energy (kilojoule) demands.

One of the important messages about glycogen storage is that it doesn't occur effectively until carbohydrate is consumed—the building blocks need to be available before the muscle can store them as fuel. This is the key reason why we might encourage athletes to consume a recovery meal immediately after their session is finished. Some studies have shown that there is a secondary benefit to an early timing of fuel intake. In the 1–2 hours after strenuous exercise, your body is primed for blood glucose to be delivered to the muscle, taken up, and stored. So when carbohydrate is consumed in this 'window of opportunity', it will promote a refuelling at the high end of the normal storage range. This is worth taking advantage of when recovery time is short and refuelling needs are high.

Rather than getting hung up on smallish variations in glycogen storage rates, however, it is easiest to observe the following rule of thumb: If you have less than ~8 hours for recovery and you need fuel for your next encounter, you should make every moment count by kick-starting your refuelling as soon as is practical after your first session. If you have a longer recovery period, or refuelling isn't a high priority, you can choose to hold off on eating/drinking carbohydrate sources until they are better appreciated. When or why might food be better appreciated later on? Sometimes you might finish a workout feeling so fatigued, lacking in appetite or upset in the gut that the very thought of forcing down food or concentrated fluids is too much to bear. In these situations it can make sense to wait. In other situations, the choices available straight after an event or workout may all be unappetising or of low nutrient density. If you have energy restrictions and plenty of time to refuel, it also makes sense to wait until you can consume foods that will better contribute to your overall nutritional goals and eating enjoyment.

How much is enough to kick-start the refuelling process? It appears that around 1 g of carbohydrate per kg body weight, or just over, is enough to have you refuelling at the maximal rate. If you want to continue at this rate, you'll need to consume the same amount hourly for 4 hours of recovery or until you are back into a normal meal pattern. What does this mean in practice? Some athletes may go straight to their next meal after finishing a workout or event, merely moving its usual time to better accommodate recovery. If fuel needs have been properly accounted for in the daily meal plan, this meal should provide enough building blocks for the early hours of refuelling until it's time for the next meal or snack. Alternatively, you may choose to start with a quick-recovery snack that ticks the box of providing ~ 1g/kg carbohydrate to buy some time before the next substantial carbohydrate-rich meal. Table 5.1 provides some ideas of suitable snacks or light meals.

What is the best pattern for the rest of the day—small meals or a couple of large meals? Most studies say that over a full day of recovery it doesn't appear to matter whether the muscle receives its carbohydrate supply in big meals or as a number of small snacks—at least from the glycogen synthesis point of view. As long as you can eat your way through your total carbohydrate needs each day and have considered the benefits of an early start, the timing details are up to you. For some people, a 'grazing' pattern is less filling and more fun. However, you may not have access to food or the opportunity to eat it at any time of day, in which case fewer, larger meals may be more suitable. If your recovery time is short and refuelling is very important—for example, in the 4 hours between tennis matches when you are playing singles and doubles in a tournament—there is some evidence—so far inconclusive—that small, frequent snacks might actually do the best job.

Types of carbohydrate foods

Not all carbohydrates have the same effect on glycogen storage. Fructose, a sugar found in many fruits, fruit juices and some sports drinks, is not very effective at restoring muscle glycogen stores. However, it does enhance glycogen storage in the liver, and is therefore a useful ingredient of recovery meals and snacks. Studies from the Australian Institute of Sport have shown that carbohydrate-rich foods with a low GI are less effective at recharging the muscles than those with a high GI (see Chapter 1.3 for a description and identification of low- and high-GI foods). For this reason, some nutrition experts have recommended that such foods should not dominate the meals and snacks eaten after exercise. However, we tend not to worry about specifically warning athletes away from low-GI foods. If you are eating a varied Western diet, you are likely to be leaning more towards high- and moderate-GI foods anyway. All in all, enjoying a variety of carbohydrate foods is probably the best way to ensure that both muscle and liver glycogen stores are looked after.

A special note about refuelling and muscle damage

Muscle damage, either through direct body contact and bruising or through eccentric loading (activities that make you sore a day later), causes a delay in the replenishment of muscle glycogen stores. In fact, some studies of runners who have completed a marathon show that their muscle fuel stores are still below par nearly a week later. Running involves eccentric muscle contractions, and a single hard or long running session may cause significant disruption of the muscle fibres, which physically interferes with their glycogen-storing capability. Furthermore, the white blood cells that rush to the area as part of the immune system's 'mopping-up' brigade use glucose, glycogen's precursor, as their own fuel. The principal detriment to muscle stores appears to occur 24–48 hours after the exercise session.

Some studies have shown that problems with glycogen storage following muscle damage can be at least partly overcome by increasing carbohydrate intake even further during the first 24-hour period after exercise, before the main effects come into play. Therefore, athletes who have completed a hard race, contact sports, or other events in which bruising or other muscle damage has occurred, should pay extra attention to their eating strategies during the first 24 hours of recovery and remember that additional high-carbohydrate eating may help to compensate for the storage delays.

5.3 Building new proteins

Athletes who undertake resistance training to build bigger and stronger muscles are understandably focused on synthesising protein during recovery from the workout. However, many other processes of recovery and adaptation between exercise sessions involve building protein. These proteins include new muscle cells and other protein components that were damaged during the exercise, as well as small blood vessels, hormones, enzymes and the signalling proteins that tell the cell how to respond to a stimulus. Whether you are a strength, endurance or 'stop and go' athlete, you will want your key training sessions and competitions to be followed by protein synthesis. The beauty of following a specific training program is that it tells your muscle cells what proteins to rebuild. That's why the muscle cells of body-builders know to build more of the muscle fibres that contract and produce power, and why the muscle cells of marathon runners know to build more of the proteins that transport fat and glucose or otherwise enable fat to be burned as an exercise fuel.

In Chapter 2 we explained that the latest thinking in sports nutrition is that total intake is not the most important protein issue for athletes. Rather, the clever athlete focuses on *timing* protein intake immediately after key training sessions. But be aware that you don't need a lot of protein (10–20 g) to provide all the building blocks for post-training protein synthesis. In fact, if you eat too much you will end up increasing the use of protein as a fuel. That's not smart use of a relatively expensive nutrient.

As pointed out in Chapter 2, we still have much to learn about protein and recovery, but the information we do have allows us to make the following recommendations:

- Strategic intake of a protein-rich food or snack after key training sessions or competitive events promotes recovery and adaptation. It is the most effective way for an athlete to address the increased protein requirements imposed by exercise.
- 10–20 g of a good-quality protein seems the ideal size of a protein recovery snack. There is a substantial increase in protein synthesis with a 10 g protein serve, but the response seems to level out at 20–25 g. In fact, more than 25 g of protein will lead to increased use of protein as a fuel source, which negates the

purpose of consuming protein. The protein ready reckoner in Table 2.9, and the recovery snack ideas in Table 5.1, show that it is relatively easy to incorporate 10–20 g into a recovery snack or meal. Case histories later in the book will give examples of ways to achieve this.

- We don't really know if there is an ideal protein type or what the best protein-rich food is. We do know that essential amino acids are important, so the best advice for now is to choose quality protein, either from an animal source like dairy, meat or eggs, or a combination of vegetable proteins (see Figure 2.2).
- There may be a small benefit from combining a carbohydrate source with your recovery protein snacks. This is a bit controversial, because not all studies show such benefits. However, even if it doesn't boost protein synthesis, some carbohydrate will enable you to refuel via the same snack (see Table 5.1).
- The ideal timing and pattern of a recovery snack is not known. However it makes sense to start protein intake within the hour after a key workout or event. If you have large energy needs, you may want to add a recovery snack before and after a weights workout.

5.4 Staying healthy and other recovery outcomes

Staying healthy and injury free is a key goal in sport. If you want to perform at your best, you need consistent training—not patchy periods between colds or stress fractures. And you can't afford to come down with a virus on the eve of competition. One of the down sides of training hard to promote maximal adaptation is that it puts your immune system and bones under stress. Recovery eating should therefore give your body the nutrients it needs to stay whole and healthy. This is a less well-developed area of recovery nutrition, so we can't offer absolute rules. However, we can give some general guidelines:

- Your immune system functions best when carbohydrate is available. Generally, strenuous exercise suppresses immune function and gives viruses a 'window of opportunity' after a workout, when you are most vulnerable to attack. Making sure you're well fuelled before, during and after a session helps to reduce this immune-suppressing effect.

- If you don't have adequate fuel, your immune system and bone health will suffer (see Chapter 3). Try to avoid energy restriction during periods of key training or competition, whether from weight loss diets or simple lack of planning. The greater your needs are, the more important it is to follow a plan rather than trusting it to luck.
- Choose nutrient-rich foods in your general diet so you have a wide range of nutrients as well as fuel and protein.
- New research is looking into the effects of probiotics/prebiotics, vitamin D and other nutrients on the immune and bone health of athletes in heavy training. Stay tuned.

5.5 Putting it all together—practical considerations

We have seen that the prompt intake of nutrients after hard exercise can help you recover more efficiently. The period immediately after such a session is crucial. This might sound great in theory, but in real life this is usually just the time when you have the least desire or opportunity to consume foods or fluid.

There are many factors that mitigate against good recovery nutrition:

- There may be no food or fluid available at the track, pool, field or velodrome, or perhaps the catering facilities serve only high-fat foods rather than nutritious high-carbohydrate choices.
- You may have other commitments and distractions—e.g. your stretching and warm-down program, meetings with coaches or officials, collecting or cleaning your equipment, press conferences, driving to your next appointment. These may make it difficult to find or eat a recovery snack.
- You may have no appetite. Many athletes feel nauseated or disinterested in food after a hard exercise session. Or you may be too tired to chew anything, let alone go home and prepare a meal. After a game or match you may be in celebration mode and figure you can party tonight, then pick it up again at the beginning of the week.

This is where good planning and organisation come into play. The first thing to consider here is what you need to recover and how important it is to be proactive with consuming fluid, carbohydrate, protein and other nutrients. As in many areas of sports nutrition, one size doesn't fit all. Each session or event will impose different priorities and different requirements for recovery. The questions you need to ask yourself in drawing up recovery strategies include:

- What do you need to recover? Are you dehydrated? Fuel depleted? Do you need to repair damaged tissue? Grow new muscle? Is your immune system under threat?
- How much time do you have before your next session?
- Can you speed up or enhance the recovery process? Will that be of benefit?
- What is your kilojoule budget? How can you manage recovery needs within that budget?
- Can you just concentrate on a few nutrients—such as carbohydrate and water, or do you need a bigger-picture approach to your total nutritional goals?

The answers to these questions will help you to focus on the sessions that need special recovery tactics. Checklists 5.1–5.4 provide some strategies for these key sessions.

The second part of your planning is to consider the practical challenges of getting food and drinks at the right time. You will need to think ahead to spot the obstacles and ways to overcome them. Bringing your own food and drink to a training session or event may help, especially if there's no catering at the venue, and there are likely to be big demands on your time and attention. Many carbohydrate-rich snacks and drinks are portable and non-perishable—check the list in Table 5.1. At worst, some choices need minimal preparation time and a little thought to storage—an Esky can be a great investment if there are no fridges or lockers around. With a few minutes to grab your drink bottle, your package or your bowl, you may be able to attend to your next commitment while munching on your recovery supplies.

For those who finish the session feeling hot, tired and a bit queasy, a drink may be more suitable than solid food. A cool carbohydrate drink, such as a sports drink, fruit juice, soft drink or cordial, will appeal to even the tiredest athlete. For additional nutrients, try a fruit smoothie or a commercial liquid meal supplement. Some of these can be bought in ready-to-go cans or Tetra Paks. On the next rung are high-fluid foods that don't take much chewing: yoghurt, Frûche and fruit pieces can be appetising when you're hot and sweaty, while hot soup or hot chocolate (with extra skim-milk powder or powdered liquid meal supplement) can be a boon when you come in wet and freezing. In general, bite-size pieces or finger foods are most practical. When you're too tired to chew, sandwich quarters or a kebab with fruit chunks look far more manageable than a triple-decker super roll or a huge plate of pasta.

When you've finished a hard match or event, it's understandable that you would want to celebrate or commiserate by taking some time out from your training diet. This may not create any problems if this is the end of the season or a one-off competition. However, if you're playing in a weekly competition or a tournament, you need to live to fight another day. And the next hours will be crucial to your recovery process, especially if you are severely dehydrated, fatigued or injured. Put first things first and get recovery happening. Refuel and rehydrate aggressively—a well-organised team will have suitable post-event recovery snacks and drinks waiting in the change rooms or club house. This makes it easy to get the right things happening quickly and without fuss. Perhaps, once you have the recovery processes under way, there will be time to have some fun. But do take care with alcohol intake—excessive drinking is not a good recovery plan (see Chapter 1.6).

Finally, when you get home after training or competition you may be looking to boost your fuel intake again. When it's late and you're tired, or a lot of time has passed since your session finished, you need to be organised enough to prepare a quick meal. Breakfast-type meals are quick and easy. Sandwiches and toasted sandwiches/jaffles are also speedy—provided you have some tasty and nutritious fillings available. It's usually the evening meal that takes time to prepare if you're in charge of your own cooking. However there are many quick recipe ideas and convenience ingredients that can see a meal on the table in 20–40 minutes. Many organised athletes cook ahead so that on busy nights after late training or competition they need only reheat. Of course, you can always have a snack as soon as you walk in the door, to keep you going until the meal is cooked. It doesn't have to blow your kilojoule budget, if that's a concern. You can always start with your dessert first—have some yoghurt and fruit immediately, then eat your main course when it's ready.

Getting recovery right in the competition setting is probably the toughest challenge, since there seems to be more at stake, and the practical difficulties of getting foods and fluids at the right time can be exacerbated by red tape. There is probably no single perfect system, but there are two abiding rules:

1. Experiment until you find the system that works for you and your sport. Practise in training to be sure.
2. Be prepared to organise your own supplies to make it happen on the day. Don't leave anything to chance or to the event organisers. Be in control.

CHECKLIST 5.1
Integrated recovery from key training sessions or competition: endurance and 'stop and go' sports

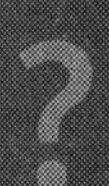

- If a session has emptied your glycogen tank and you have less than 8 hours until the next workout or event, maximise effective recovery time by consuming a high-carbohydrate meal or snack within 30 minutes of completing the session. Effective refuelling begins only after a substantial amount of carbohydrate has been consumed.
- Kick-start refuelling by consuming foods or drinks providing 1 g of carbohydrate per kg body weight straight after exercise. Repeat this every hour until regular meal patterns are resumed (see Table 5.1 for ideas).
- Count these recovery snacks and meals towards your total daily carbohydrate targets. Make sure that these targets are individualised (Chapter 2.2).
- Add protein to recovery snacks and meals to enhance the synthesis of new proteins for repair of damage and for adaptations to the workout:
  - 10 g of high-quality protein will have a worthwhile effect on protein synthesis

  - 20 g of high-quality protein will probably achieve the maximal stimulus to protein synthesis
  - We do not yet know if there is an optimal type of protein food. However, animal protein sources (dairy, meat, poultry, eggs, fish) and milk-based liquid meals and sports supplements are considered high-quality proteins and thus rich sources of essential amino acids.
- Remember that nutritious carbohydrate foods and drinks can also provide vitamins and minerals while also addressing refuelling/recovery goals. These nutrients contribute to overall dietary targets. Further research may show that consuming them early after exercise could speed other processes of repair and rebuilding, as well as strengthening the immune system.
- Consider compact forms of carbohydrate with a low fibre content when carbohydrate needs are high and you have a suppressed appetite or gastrointestinal problems. These include sugar-rich foods and sports bars.
- Choose carbohydrate-containing fluids (also low in fibre) if you are fatigued and dehydrated. These include sports drinks, soft drinks and juices, commercial liquid meal supplements, milk shakes and fruit smoothies.
- Organise small, frequent meals to achieve high carbohydrate intakes and meet protein goals without the discomfort of overeating. Frequent snacking (e.g. every 30–60 min) may enhance recovery during the first hours after exercise. However, in long-term recovery (24 hr), it doesn't appear to matter how food is spaced over the day, so organise eating patterns to suit your own preferences, timetable and appetite/comfort.
- Don't consume high-fat foods or excessive amounts of protein at the expense of carbohydrate when stomach comfort or total energy requirements limit your total food intake.
- Don't overdo low-GI carbohydrate foods such as lentils and legumes in recovery meals, since these may be less suitable for speedy glycogen storage.

- Don't drink excessive amounts of alcohol. Although it can directly impede refuelling and recovery, alcohol exerts its main effect on recovery through indirect means. If you are intoxicated, you are unlikely to follow sound nutritional practices and more likely to undertake high-risk behaviours.
- Restore fluid balance through a pre-planned fluid-intake program. When the post-exercise fluid deficit exceeds 2 per cent of body weight, follow special rehydration strategies (see Checklist 5.3).

CHECKLIST 5.2
Integrated recovery from key training sessions: resistance training

Post-exercise:

- Consume protein in the hour after resistance training to enhance the synthesis of new proteins to build muscle size and strength
  - 10 g of high-quality protein, providing ~3 g of essential amino acids, will have a worthwhile effect on protein synthesis
  - 20–25 g of high-quality protein (~6–8 g of essential amino acids) will probably achieve the maximal stimulus to protein synthesis
  - We do not yet know if there is an optimal type of protein food. However, animal sources (dairy, meat, poultry, eggs, fish) and milk-based liquid meals and sports supplements are considered high-quality proteins and thus rich sources of essential amino acids
  - Add carbohydrate to protein-based recovery snacks for refuelling and perhaps to enhance protein synthesis (see Table 5.1)
- When strength-training sessions are prolonged, or undertaken in conjunction with aerobic exercise, it makes sense to take steps to promote rapid recovery of depleted muscle glycogen stores. These issues are discussed in more detail in Checklist 5.1.

- Avoid excessive amounts of alcohol in the hours following a strength workout, since there is some evidence that alcohol impairs protein synthesis. Limiting alcohol intake benefits all aspects of post-exercise recovery.
- Remember that adequate energy intake is important for your muscle size and strength goals. In terms of daily protein requirements, the maximum intake likely to be needed is ~1.5–2.0 g per kg body weight. Intakes greater than this are not likely to confer any additional benefits for muscle gain.

CHECKLIST 5.3
Special recovery strategies for the dehydrated athlete

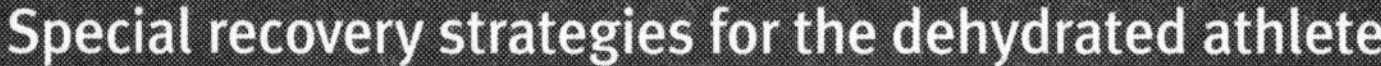

- Make rehydration a priority during recovery. Dehydration may impair your performance in subsequent exercise sessions. However, severe fluid deficits increase the risk of gut upsets and discomfort, potentially limiting your ability to eat and drink. When gut problems are present, consume water or diluted sports drinks before worrying about refuelling and protein recovery.
- Don't rely on thirst or a chance encounter with some fluids to treat significant dehydration. A 'hit and miss' approach may be acceptable when fluid deficits are 1 L or less, but when fluid losses are greater than that, you will do better with an organised rehydration schedule.
- Monitor weight changes during the workout to gauge the success of your drinking strategies and the residual fluid deficit that must still be replaced. A loss of 1 kg is equivalent to 1 L of fluid, but you will need to drink a volume equal to ~125–150 per cent of your post-exercise fluid deficit over the next 2–4 hours to fully restore fluid balance.
- Make sure drinks are available. This may be difficult when you're at a remote competition venue or travelling in a country where you need to drink bottled water.

- Encourage your intake with palatable choices
  - Most people prefer sweet-tasting drinks and will drink these in greater volumes than plain water
  - Keep drinks at a refreshing temperature to encourage you to drink more. Cool drinks (10–15°C) are preferred in most situations.
- Although it can be difficult to drink very cold (0–5°C) or icy fluids in large volumes, note that they may also help to reduce an elevated core temperature arising from a hot environment, high-intensity exercise or a combination of the two.
- Use carbohydrate-containing and nutrient-rich drinks to provide fuel and nutrients while you are rehydrating (see Checklists 5.1 and 5.2).
- Replace sodium (salt) to help you retain more of the fluids you ingest by minimising urination, especially if you are trying to cover a moderate-to-large fluid deficit (e.g. > 2 L). This will speed up the restoration of fluid balance and reduce the need to wake up from sleep and rest periods to wee. Options include:
  - Salty foods (bread and crackers, salty spreads, breakfast cereals) or salt added to post-exercise meals. Note that drinking with meals is a convenient way to combine fluid and salt, and should form the basis of a good hydration plan
  - High-sodium sports drinks (e.g. Gatorade Endurance, or commercial oral rehydration solutions (e.g. Gastrolyte) are a good choice as drinks consumed in the absence of food
- Choose a pattern of fluid intake (volume and frequency) that will balance gastrointestinal comfort and minimise urine loss. Spreading fluid intake over a period is probably more effective than chugging large volumes.
- Make decisions about caffeine-containing fluids based on sleep considerations rather than hydration issues. If you normally drink cola drinks, tea and coffee at a given time, allow them to contribute to your fluid plan—at least at meals when food is taking care of salt replacement.

- Wait until your fluid plan is nearly implemented before you consider alcohol, and if you do drink it, do so in moderation. Low-alcohol beers may be OK for fluid replacement, but anything above 2 per cent alcohol is not. Of course, this is just one of the many reasons to drink in moderation in your recovery phase (see Checklist 1.7).
- Be wary of using urine as a guide to the success of your rehydration. In the hours after drinking a large amount of fluid, you may produce lots of clear urine even when you are still dehydrated. Early-morning samples are usually the most reliable urine checks. Weight checks may provide back-up information about fluid balance in the morning and at other times.
- Where possible, avoid post-exercise activities that exacerbate sweat loss—for example, long exposure to hot spas, saunas or sun. Where ongoing fluid losses are unavoidable, make sure they are accounted for in your fluid plan. Always look at the big picture of recovery. Sometimes it's best to prioritise gut comfort and undisturbed sleep before trying to fully rehydrate. You can always finish that job in the morning.

CHECKLIST 5.4
Special recovery strategies for the athlete with a restricted energy budget

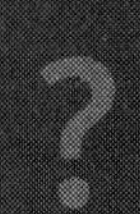

- Don't let recovery snacks contribute unnecessary additional energy to a restricted energy budget. When rapid recovery is desirable, change the timing of your session or meals so you can eat your normal meal as soon as possible after the workout. Where this is not practical, take a small snack from your usual meal plan to consume immediately after training or before resistance training (e.g. fruit or flavoured yoghurt usually eaten as a dessert), then have the rest of your meal at the usual time.
- Choose recovery foods with high nutritional value—you'll be taking in protein and micronutrients as well as fuel. Nutrient-rich

choices (e.g. fruit, flavoured milk drinks and dairy foods, sandwiches with meat and salad fillings) are more valuable for the Big Picture than lower nutrient choices (e.g. lollies, soft drink, bread with jam or honey).

- Choose recovery foods that promote satiety (a feeling of fullness) while reducing unnecessary energy intake (see Checklist 3.2):
    - Choose foods that add fibre, volume, low-GI ingredients and a little protein
    - Be consistent with low-fat eating strategies
    - Avoid energy-containing fluids other than those needed for sporting goals
- Recognise that a low energy budget may not be able to cover the guidelines for optimal intake of some macronutrients (e.g. carbohydrate for optimal daily glycogen synthesis).
    - Specialised dietary advice from a sports dietitian is valuable in ensuring that you have realistic goals and a meal plan to target them
    - Be prepared to cycle between nutritional goals—i.e. restrict energy during periods when you can afford to lose body fat, then liberalise energy and carbohydrate intake to promote better fuelling and recovery for key sessions or competition

TABLE 5.1
Ideas for recovery snacks and light meals

Carbohydrate-rich snacks (50 g carbohydrate serves) providing at least 10 g of protein

- 250–350 ml of liquid meal supplement (e.g. Powerbar Proteinplus drink or Sustagen Sport)
- 250–350 ml of milk shake or fruit smoothie
- 500 ml flavoured low-fat milk
- Some sports bars (check labels for protein and carbohydrate content)
- 60 g (1.5–2 cups) breakfast cereal with ½ cup milk
- 1 round of sandwiches including cheese/meat/chicken filling, and 1 large piece of fruit or 300 ml sports drink

- 1 cup of fruit salad with 200 g carton fruit-flavoured yoghurt or custard
- 200 g carton fruit-flavoured yoghurt or 300 ml flavoured milk and 30–35 g cereal bar
- 2 crumpets or English muffins with thick spread of peanut butter or 2 slices of cheese
- 200 (cup or small tin) of baked beans on 2 slices of toast
- 250 g (large) baked potato with cottage cheese or grated cheese filling
- 150 g thick-crust pizza with meat/chicken/seafood topping

FIGURE 5.1
Effect of salt (sodium) replacement on rehydration

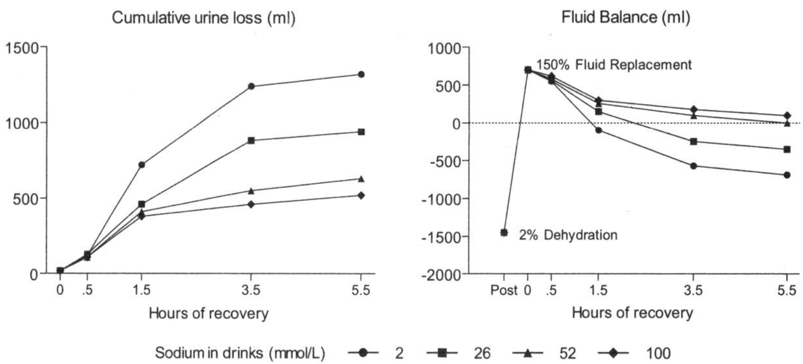

Subjects sweated 2 per cent of their body weight, then drank a volume of fluid replacing 150 per cent of this deficit in the first 30 mins of recovery after exercise. Over the next five hours, urine losses and total fluid balance were monitored. The fluid contained differing amounts of salt (sodium). Redrawn from Shirreffs *et al. Med Sci Sports Exerc* 1996; 28: 1260–1271.

FIGURE 5.2
Alcohol and rehydration

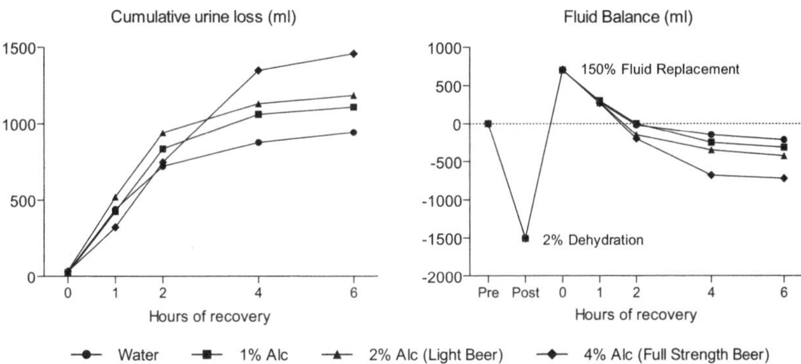

Drinking alcohol equivalent to a 'light' beer after dehydrating exercise did not affect urine losses or overall hydration in this study. However, regular-strength beer (and more concentrated alcoholic drinks) will increase urine losses and delay rehydration. In this study, despite drinking a volume larger than their sweat losses, subjects were still dehydrated when beer was the rehydration fluid. Redrawn from Shirreffs and Maughan, *J Appl Physiol* 1997 83: 1152–1158.

6
Pills and potions

Google 'sports supplements' and within a second you'll be presented with more than a million links dedicated to telling you about—and selling—special preparations targeted at athletes. The last decade has seen an exponential increase in the number of pills, potions and powders promising to make you bigger, stronger, leaner and faster. How can you refuse such tempting offers? Or, more compellingly, how can you afford to let your competitors get an advantage you don't have? Each year, people spend billions of dollars in the hope that the 'winning edge' can be found in a bottle or packet. We would love a dollar for each time we've been asked 'Do athletes need to take supplements?'

Our answer varies.

There are many reasons for this. One of the first things to ask is, What do we mean by supplements? Just vitamins, minerals, and the other products you'll find on the shelves of a health-food store? Or all the hardcore body-building products with names that sound like steroid drugs? What about all the special foods made for athletes, like sports drinks, gels, bars and protein drinks? Since these products vary widely in composition, price and level of scientific credibility, it makes sense that there can't be a single viewpoint about their value. The other question we need to ask is, Who is the athlete? Athletes come in many shapes and forms, and here different needs and goals. No product will have the same value to them all.

So our failure to give a black-and-white answer is not a reflection of our quality as sports dietitians. Rather, it reflects our recognition of the complexity of the situation and the need to find an individualised decision for each athlete. The aim of this chapter is to provide you with the tools to assess your own needs for supplements and sports foods. It will be a matter of weighing up the pros and cons in your specific situation (Figure 6.1). You should note that your judgement might change as products alter, more scientific research about supplements emerges, and your needs as an athlete change. The Australian Institute of Sport has spent a considerable amount of effort developing a flexible, individualised and evolving Sports Supplement Program. Because it makes some of this program's resources available to the public (*www.ausport.gov.au/ais/nutrition*), it makes sense to base your own approach around these tools.

FIGURE 6.1. The cost-benefit ratio for supplements

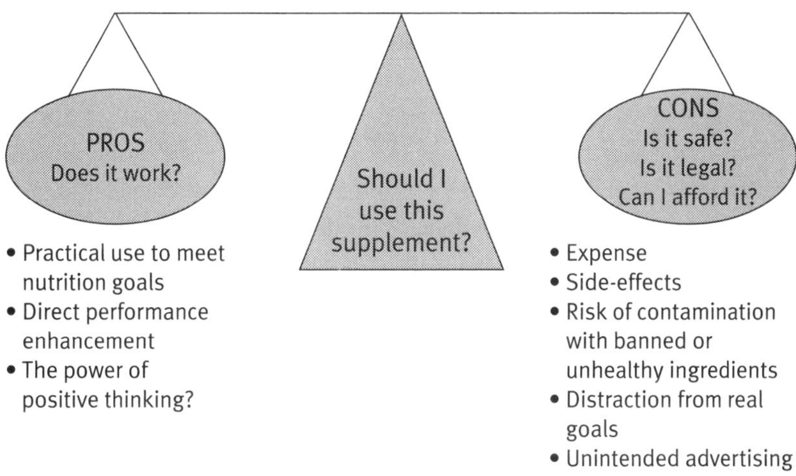

Before looking at the elements of a supplements balance sheet, we should share our definition of a supplement. We think this should take in all the pills, powders, potions and tailor-made foods for athletes, because they all exist in the sporting environment, seeking your attention and cash. Therefore, our definition of supplements includes products that are technically foods and others that are technically and legally 'therapeutic goods'. It includes products that can be bought in pharmacies and supermarkets, health-food shops, gyms and sporting retailers, from your aunt or next-door neighbour who has become an independent distributor for a multilevel marketing company, and from online stores. The modern athlete has access to all these sources, and thus to products from all over the world.

A common feature of all these products is that they lack the quality control that is expected of pharmaceutical agents like anti-inflammatory drugs or headache tablets. Although many supplements are packaged to resemble such products, the regulations that cover their manufacture are much less rigid and also less often enforced, particularly in certain countries overseas. And although companies are not supposed to market supplements using claims that are not supported by rigorous scientific studies, this is often ignored and also rarely enforced. One of the reasons for the lax policing of unsupported advertising claims is that a lot of them are made outside official, public channels, such as product labels and TV commercials. Instead, the claims are spread via word of mouth, the Internet, magazine articles and advertorials, and underground material circulated among sports participants.

6.1 The pros of supplements and sports foods

There are a number of sound reasons for athletes to consider adding supplements and sports foods to their nutrition plan. An important caveat on the following information is that it applies to specific situations in sport and specific products, rather than across the board.

Practical assistance to meet nutrition goals

In the last five chapters we have outlined the science of sports nutrition. As you've seen, many areas of our knowledge are well-defined and are supported by rigorous research. However, in many situations, the guidelines for sports nutrition recommend that an athlete consume energy and nutrients in amounts beyond most people's desire or gastrointestinal capacity, or at times when it can be difficult to find or consume everyday foods. Under such circumstances, a sports food that allows the athlete to consume a specific nutrient mix in a convenient form is a bonus. A sports food that is tailor made for a common challenge or common nutritional need in sport might have some of the following features:

- Comes in a portion size that provides enough of a key nutrient or nutrients to meet a certain sports nutrition goal, and makes it easy for the athlete to meet their needs for the key nutrient(s)

- Has a long shelf-life and minimal need for specialised storage facilities, so athletes can take it to as many destinations as their sport takes them
- Is packaged so that it can be accessed easily, especially during exercise or sporting activities. Some sports foods come in special bottles or packets that are easy to open or consume in mid-cycle or stride
- Is palatable and easy to swallow
- Is easy to 'stomach' during or after sport, when the athlete is at high risk of gastrointestinal upsets and discomfort. This will generally mean being low in fibre, fat and perhaps other components that can irritate the gut
- Can provide a nutrient that is at risk of neglect in the diets of many athletes, helping to prevent or treat a deficiency, at least until the diet can be adjusted.

Table 6.1 provides a summary of the sports foods and supplements that achieve these goals, and the situations in which they are commonly used. It should be noted that the nutritional effects of these products are often very well documented and make a detectable difference to performance. Therefore, there is a good level of scientific proof that the smart *use* of these products (rather than just the products themselves), can enhance the athlete's performance or help her to achieve her sporting goals. Of course, this assumes that the athlete is correctly educated about such smart use.

Direct enhancement of sports performance

The marketing hype that surrounds many ingredients in sports supplements sometimes obscures the fact that a few do enjoy sound scientific support for their claimed benefits. These ingredients are often called ergogenic, or work-enhancing, aids. (Actually, the unproven ones are also often called ergogenic aids, so take this label with a grain of salt.) The most credible ergogenic aids are identified below. Again, it is important to recognise that it is the correct use of the product in the appropriate scenario that achieves the outcome, rather than the product alone. In addition, it seems that there are 'responders' and 'non-responders' to these products' effects—in other words, they don't work for everyone. Sports scientists and sports dietitians need to work with athletes and coaches to find the individuals and situations in which ergogenic aids produce a true benefit.

We recognise that it is difficult to prove that a single ingredient or product enhances performance—or not. The case history in the body-building chapter illustrates this. It's for this reason that the AIS Sports Supplement Program doesn't actually say Product X does or doesn't 'work'. We think that for many substances there are probably shades of grey. Instead, the program establishes a probability that a supplement or supplement ingredient can benefit an athlete, and creates three categories according to the current strength of evidence. Note that we have a fourth category, since some supplements are banned according to anti-doping codes such as the restricted list of the World Anti-Doping Agency.

- Group A—there is good evidence that these products can be used to directly or indirectly achieve a performance benefit in specific scenarios
- Group B—there is current interest because of a good theory or some preliminary results that hint at a performance benefit, but it's really too soon to tell
- Group C—there's no proof, meaning it's less likely that these products provide a worthwhile benefit or that any benefits are too small to be really cost effective
- Group D—the product is either banned outright or is at high risk of being contaminated with banned substances

Various supplements can change category according to the current strength of support for their claims in the scientific literature. Table 6.2 provides a brief summary of some of the popular supplements and the scientific evidence behind their placement within the AIS classification system at the time of writing. You can check for updates at *www.ausport/gov.au/ais/nutrition*.

The placebo effect

When people receive special treatment, special supervision or special information, they usually respond by doing a better job with the tasks they are undertaking. Wikipedia defines a placebo as 'a substance or procedure a patient accepts as medicine or therapy, but which has no specific therapeutic activity. Any therapeutic effect is thought to be based on the power of *suggestion*.' Several clever studies have demonstrated that belief in the power of a dummy product can lead to a measurable improvement in exercise performance. For example, Dr Chris Beedie asked some cyclists to do a 10-km time trial in the lab on three occasions, each time giving them a different set of capsules. They were told that one treatment would be a placebo, one a moderate dose of caffeine, and the other a large caffeine dose—and that they would all receive these treatments in a different order. Once they had completed the three trials, the subjects were asked to say which treatment they thought they had received at each trial. Their performances were examined and compared to those in time trials done before the experiment began. This analysis found that the cyclists produced about 1 per cent less power in the 'placebo trial', but had a 1.3 per cent increase in power in the 'moderate caffeine trial' and a 3.1 per cent improvement in the 'high-caffeine trial'. They also described various symptoms associated with caffeine use. In fact, the whole study involved sham treatments—all the capsules contained a dummy powder. The results occurred because the cyclists had preconceived ideas about what caffeine did and their beliefs allowed them to 'produce the goods' with performance enhancement without consuming any caffeine at all! They even imagined themselves getting a better effect from caffeine when they thought the dose was larger. This really is the power of positive thinking.

Scientists believe that the placebo effect is real. In fact, when they do studies and experiments, they take care to remove its bias from their results by ensuring that subjects take a placebo as well as the treatment they are interested in. They assume that the subjects believe equally in each treatment, so any difference in outcomes is the true effect of the treatment.

Despite this recognition, scientists have really done very little to exploit the placebo effect fully. It probably doesn't work the same way for everybody—some people might be more or less 'suggestible' than others—and it may work for only a certain period or may change over time, Also, it's not yet known how to present a treatment to maximise the power of positive thinking about it. In fact, the placebo effect is often an afterthought—a blanket explanation for the great results an athlete ascribes to the latest cool supplement, diet or training idea, especially one that scientists don't really believe in. The placebo tends to be dismissed as somehow less 'valuable' than a physiological effect—a second-class-citizen of performance enhancement. But if an athlete truly does go faster, simply as a result of self-belief, perhaps this view needs rethinking.

The placebo effect needs to be factored into a cost-benefit analysis of any supplement. But because it is less well-known and harder to measure, it can be harder to assign a 'benefit' value to—and the cost of relying on a placebo if this has no effect can be significant. But it does make sense to learn more about the placebo effect, and to look for situations where it might enhance a physiological effect.

6.2 The cons of supplements and sports foods

There are several potential disadvantages to the use of any sports supplement, and these too need to be assessed objectively.

Cost

Some supplements come with a weekly price tag of $50–$60 (each!). We also know of some athletes who use several similarly pricey products: sometimes they spend more on supplements than on food. For example, according to legal documents presented in a court case, Australian 400-m runner Cathy Freeman spent nearly $3500 on vitamin and mineral supplements from health-food shops in the four months leading up to her gold-medal run at the 2000 Olympic Games. The issue of expense is compounded for coaches or dietitians looking after a whole team or program.

Cost obviously becomes even more of an issue when there is little scientific support for a product's claims. But it must be weighed soberly, even where benefits to performance can be shown. Supplements or sports foods generally provide their nutrients or food constituents at considerably higher cost than do everyday foods. This price might be justified because the supplement's maker is targeting a niche market, and has the added costs of special preparation and packaging or research and development. On the other hand, it might be inflated by the cost of advertising, or plain exploitation. There are various ways to keep a lid on the costs of your chosen supplements. Instead of automatically chomping on a sports food on every sports-related occasion, you can save such foods for important times or for situations where there's no good alternative. Lower-cost versions are often available—for example, the pharmacy-brand multi-vitamin rather than a similar formula that is 'taking America by storm', according to its distributor's marketing spiel; or a smoothie with added skim-milk powder rather than the protein powder marketed to body-builders.

Distraction

A more subtle issue with supplement use is that it can distract attention away from strategies that are really important in enhancing performance. We often see athletes who are side-tracked by the search for short-cuts from a bottle or packet. Success in sport is the product of superior genetics, long-term training, optimal nutrition, state-of-the-art equipment and a committed attitude. These things cannot be replaced by the use of supplements, but the enthusiastic claims of marketers often cast them into the shade. Even among supplements, there is often an inverse relationship between the hype associated with the product and the scientific support for its benefits. Yet all too often, athletes opt for the latest fad supplement over tried and true products that are backed up by years of scientific research.

We get particularly worried when the focus on short-cuts over sound practices involves younger athletes. Young athletes can look forward to substantial improvements in performance as they grow and mature and build experience in their sport. The impact of supplements is minor in comparison to this potential—although some children and adolescents will develop sufficiently in their sport to justify the careful use of sports foods to meet high-level nutritional needs. In fact, some expert groups like the American Academy of Pediatrics and the American College of Sports Medicine recommend that ergogenic supplements such as caffeine or creatine shouldn't be used by children and adolescents. Sometimes these warnings are based on the unknown health consequences of some supplements. Others feel that taking supplements speaks badly of the ethics of sport or the morals of a young athlete—or even that it might make the athlete more likely to take more 'serious' compounds, including prohibited drugs, down the track. We are not sure that there is any evidence to back these last claims, but we do agree that it's best for young athletes to develop the 'basics' before they look to more specialised sports nutrition strategies.

'Unintended advertising'

Did you ever consider that your words or behaviour might become an advertisement to other people? A lot of the 'proof' that keeps the supplement industry so profitable is the observations and recommendations of other athletes. Many athletes regard a high-profile performer's reported use or endorsement of a product as more convincing than a whole stack of scientific studies. What did you think when you read about Cathy Freeman's supplement purchases just now? Did you think, Wow, is that what it takes to win a gold medal? We would be surprised if you had no reaction at all. (To provide balance on this matter, Ian Thorpe, another gold-medal hero from the Sydney Olympics, went on record to say that he chose not to take supplements because he didn't want his performances to be attributed to factors other than his hard work.)

Of course, some supplements and sports foods do have value, and people should be free to endorse them, whether for a fee or not (though hopefully sticking to the facts). After all, the Australian Institute of Sport has some arrangements with sponsors to provide certain products to its athletes. But we and other people take seriously our influence on others right across the board. We often hear it said of some product that doesn't even have a good theoretical basis, let alone scientific support, that 'everyone' is using it so it must be good. We understand that athletes may feel afraid to miss out on something that their competitors might have. But if this is the only reason you take a product, you might consider whether by buying it you are adding to the problem rather than solving it. Popular support for a product should promote the need for research into its effects, not replace it.

Side-effects

We have already mentioned that people can react differently to a product—there are responders and non-responders to many strategies in sports nutrition, including supplements. Some non-responders even show side-effects—from discomfort to performance interruption and real ill-health. Because most supplements are considered by governments to be relatively safe, many countries do not require their known side-effects to be registered, as they do for drugs. So it's likely that the side-effects we hear about are only a sample of what really occurs. Nevertheless, public-health risks have been reported for the use of some supplements and herbal products. For example, nearly twenty years ago there was a scare that led to supplemental forms of tryptophan (an amino acid) being withdrawn from the market. More recently, makers of over-the-counter weight-loss supplements containing ephedrine (legal in the US but not Australia) have been in and out of American courts over their products' alleged involvement in the deaths of some athletes.

Side-effects can arise from toxicity; intolerance, allergies and other reactions to the supplement itself; and exposure to contaminants in it arising from poor manufacturing practices.

Inadvertent doping outcomes

High-level sports competition is usually governed by an anti-doping code that bans the use of substances or methods judged to be hazardous to health or against the spirit of sport. The 'prohibited' list of the World Anti-Doping Agency (WADA), for example, includes a number of products that can be found in supplements, though few of them are readily available in Australia. These banned substances include 'pro-hormones' (chemicals related to anabolic steroids that were recently permitted to be sold over the counter in the US and other countries) as well as stimulants such as ephedrine. Education programs from national anti-doping agencies such as the Australian Sport Anti-doping Agency (ASADA) warn athletes that supplements and sports foods can potentially contain banned substances, and urge them to read the labels of such products very carefully (*www.asada.org.au*). Clearly, you don't want to suffer the stigma and consequences of a positive drug test simply because you aren't paying attention to what you put in your mouth.

Unfortunately, we now know that careful label reading is not sufficient to avoid a doping 'positive' from supplement use. We started becoming aware of this around 2000, when a bewildering number of high-profile athletes started to return positive tests for nandrolone, though vehemently denying that they had used this banned steroid. Of course, denial is the usual route taken by drug cheats. However, some supplement studies undertaken by WADA- or International Olympic Committee-accredited laboratories provided an alarming explanation for these positive findings—that it is possible, and even likely, for supplements to contain banned substances that aren't declared on the label. The most highly publicised report, known in the trade as the 'Cologne study' because it was carried out by a laboratory in Cologne, Germany, covered an analysis of more than 600 supplements. These products were sourced from 215 suppliers across thirteen countries via retail outlets, the Internet, and telephone sales.

Although none of these supplements declared banned pro-hormones as ingredients, 94 products (15 per cent of those tested) were found to contain hormones or pro-hormones. A further 10 per cent of samples presented technical difficulties in analysis, which prevented the lab from being able to guarantee that they were hormone-free. Of the positive supplements, 68 per cent contained pro-hormones of testosterone, 7 per cent contained pro-hormones of nandrolone and 25 per cent contained compounds related to both. Forty-nine of the supplements contained only one steroid, but 45 contained more than one, and eight products had five or more. The steroid concentrations ranged from tiny to small, but it was noted that only a minute amount of nandrolone or related substances needs to be consumed to trigger a positive urine test.

Other findings of this study show how difficult it is to give iron-clad rules to athletes about how to avoid the types of supplements that are most likely to cause a positive doping test. Products could be purchased from one country and manufactured in another. Where products were made by companies that also made other products containing pro-hormones, just over 20 per cent contained undeclared pro-hormones (which could indicate cross-contamination occurring in the factory), but 10 per cent of products from companies that did not sell steroid-containing supplements were also positive (which could indicate that the ingredients used to make the products were contaminated). The brand names of the positive products were not provided in the study, but they included amino acid supplements, protein powders and products containing creatine, carnitine, ribose, guarana, zinc, pyruvate, hydroxyl-methyl butyrate (HMB), *Tribulus terrestris*, herbal extracts and vitamins/minerals.

Other studies have since found banned stimulants, banned designer steroids and other problem ingredients in supplements. In general, the amounts are small, but as we've seen, in the case of steroids even tiny amounts will trigger a positive test. The blame has generally been laid on accidental contamination or poor labelling in the course of slack manufacturing processes. However, there are some recent examples where supplements have been found to contain steroids in amounts larger than standard medical doses of such drugs. This would suggest they were a deliberate addition—perhaps to generate word-of-mouth reports of amazing results among its target audience. It must be remembered that most athletes in the world do not undergo drug testing—their participation in sport is recreational rather than elite, they train but don't compete, or their sport doesn't have an anti-doping code. Therefore, some athletes may not be concerned about the issue and some might even consider a little steroid or the like a bonus. Indeed, although many agencies in the world have declared their concern about inadvertently positive doping tests and what they say about manufacturing practices, the issue is not seen as a particularly pressing one for public health.

Of course, such contamination remains a big concern for serious athletes who do compete under anti-doping codes, since most such codes make athletes 'strictly liable', that is, ultimately responsible, if they are found to have consumed a banned substance, regardless of the circumstances or where the substance came from. There have been a number of cases where an athlete has received a full or substantial penalty despite evidence that the banned substance found in their urine came from a contaminated or poorly labelled supplement. Even where penalties have been reduced in such circumstances, the athlete is still left with the stigma of a positive doping record. This situation is discussed in more detail in the chapter on weight-lifting. Athletes should contact their national anti-doping agencies for information about the specific risks identified with supplement use and any initiatives being undertaken to reduce that risk.

6.3 The bottom line

Whether you're an athlete, a coach or a parent, no doubt you still want us to provide a simple and single answer to the question 'Do I need to take supplements and sports foods to perform at my best?' But our answer will continue to depend on the strict definition of each of the words in the question. Ultimately, the decision has to be made on an individual, personal basis, but we hope that this chapter has given you a fuller knowledge of the issues involved.

TABLE 6.1
Sports foods and supplements used to meet nutritional goals

Product	Description	Examples	Main sports-related uses	Chapter
Sports drink	• Powder or liquid providing 4–8% carbohydrate from a variety of sources (maltodextrins, sucrose, glucose, fructose) • Also contains electrolytes including potassium and sodium • Sodium content of most sports drinks is 10–25 mmol/L. • Some specialised sports drinks for endurance events have higher sodium content (30–35 mmol/L) • Range of flavours usually tested to be palatable during exercise	• Gatorade • Powerade • Gatorade Endurance	• Balanced hydration and refuelling during exercise • Post-exercise rehydration • Contribution to post-exercise refuelling	4 5 5

Product	Description	Examples	Main sports-related uses	Chapter
Sports gel	• Easily opened sachet providing a measured dose of concentrated carbohydrate syrup (25–35 g) with honey consistency • New brands moving to multiple carbohydrate sources for better intestinal uptake • Some brands have added electrolytes (similar amounts to sports drinks) • Some brands or flavours contain added caffeine (25–50 mg)	• Powergels • Gu • PB gels • Clif shot • Carboshotz	• Fuelling during exercise (note: if consumed with water, can be used to address fluid and electrolyte replacement needs) • Post-exercise refuelling • Supplement high-carbohydrate training diet or carbohydrate loading plan • Caffeine supplementation during exercise	4 5 4 6 Road cycling
Electrolyte supplements	• Powder sachets or tablets providing sodium, potassium and sometimes other electrolytes	• Gatorlytes • E-shots • Nuun electrolyte tablets	• Replacement of large sodium losses during ultra-endurance activities or by salty sweaters • Rapid and effective rehydration following moderate to large fluid and sodium losses through exercise	4 5

Product	Description	Examples	Main sports-related uses	Chapter
Electrolyte supplements contd			• Rapid and effective rehydration following dehydration undertaken for weight-making	3
Liquid meal supplement	• Powder (to mix with water or milk) or ready to drink liquid • Usually provides 50–70% of energy as carbohydrate or 30–50 g per single serve • Usually provides 20–40% of energy as protein or 15–25 g of protein per serve • Usually low-moderate in fat • Usually provide 25–50% of recommended dietary intakes of key vitamins and minerals in a single serve	• PowerBar Proteinplus • Sustagen sport • Gatorlode	• Compact nutrient-rich energy supplement in high-energy diet • Low-residue nutrition for weight-making diet • Low-bulk pre-event meal/ snack • Post-exercise recovery drink—refuelling and adaptation • Portable nutrition for travelling athlete	3 3 4 4 Tennis
Sports bar	• 50–60 g bar with easily chewed texture • Usually provides 35–45 g carbohydrate	• PowerBar Performance Bar	• Compact nutrient-rich energy supplement in high-energy diet	3

Product	Description	Examples	Main sports-related uses	Chapter
Sports bar contd	• Usually provides 5–15 g protein • Often provides 25% of recommended dietary intake of key vitamins and minerals in a single serve • Usually low in fat and fibre • Note that some sports bars are higher in protein and lower in carbohydrate and do achieve the sports-related uses as well		• Refuelling during exercise when solid form is needed • Low-residue nutrition for weight-making diet • Low-bulk pre-event snack • Post-exercise recovery—provides carbohydrate, some protein • Portable nutrition for the travelling athlete	4 3 4 5 Tennis
Vitamin /mineral supplement	• Capsule/ tablet • Provides 1–4 x Recommended Dietary Intake of vitamins and minerals	• Centrum • Pluravit • Cenovis or Blackmores Multivitamin/ mineral ranges	• Micronutrient support for low-energy or weight-loss diet • Micronutrient support for restricted-variety diets (e.g. vegetarian diet) • Micronutrient support for unreliable food supply (e.g. travelling athlete)	3 Tennis

Product	Description	Examples	Main sports-related uses	Chapter
Iron supplement	• Capsule/tablet providing ferrous sulphate/gluconate or fumarate, usually with ~100 mg per recommended therapeutic dose • Sometimes contains other nutrients such as folate or vitamin C	• Ferrogradumet • Fefol	• Supervised management of iron deficiency (including treatment and prevention)	2 Distance running
Calcium supplement	• Tablet providing calcium carbonate/phosphate/lactate with 300–600 mg as recommended therapeutic dose	• Caltrate	• Calcium supplementation in low-energy or low dairy food diet • Treatment/prevention of osteopaenia	2

Note that these products are all in Group A of the AIS Sports Supplement Program when used for these purposes (*www.ausport.gov.au/ais/nutrition*)

TABLE 6.2
Summary of some popular so-called ergogenic aids

Product	Description and protocol of use	Proposed benefits and summary of scientific proof	Concerns

Caffeine
 	
AIS Supplement Program Group = A
	• Caffeine is a plant-derived drug that is socially accepted and widely used
	• Major dietary sources, such as tea, coffee, chocolate, and cola drinks, typically provide 30–200 mg per serve
	• Some over-the-counter medications contain 100–200 mg per tablet (e.g. NoDoz) while energy drinks/shots with caffeine or guarana can contain 50–500 mg per serve.
	• Many sports foods now contain 25–50 mg caffeine per serve
	• In 2004, caffeine was removed from the WADA list of banned substances, allowing athletes to consume it, in their usual
		• Caffeine has numerous effects on different body tissues, making it hard to study—or at least to detect the reason for any observed effects.
		• The major effect of caffeine on sports performance, as in general life, is probably to change perceptions of effort or fatigue, thus maintaining a work rate or activity
		• Caffeine can be used as a training aid or to enhance competition performance
		• There is sound evidence that caffeine enhances the performance of
		  ○ Prolonged endurance or intermittent sports
		  ○ High intensity events lasting
			• The current caffeine intake practices of athletes are ad hoc and unsystematic. We see athletes using large or unmeasured doses of caffeine without appreciating new information about the emerging information about low-moderate caffeine doses
			• At higher levels of intake, caffeine can increase heart rate, impair fine motor control and technique, and cause over-arousal (interfering with sleep.
			• Interruption to sleep is a problem in sports in which the athlete needs to compete over several days
			• Although evidence of specific

Product	Description and protocol of use	Proposed benefits and summary of scientific proof	Concerns
Caffeine contd	diet or for specific performance enhancement, without fear of a positive drug test. Urine levels are still checked to monitor abuse. • Traditional protocols involve intake of ~5–6 mg/kg (e.g. 300–500 mg) 1 hr before exercise • New research shows that caffeine is beneficial when taken in a variety of protocols ○ Before and during exercise, including just before the onset of fatigue ○ 2–3 mg/kg seems the dose above which no greater benefits occur	1–20 mins • The effect of caffeine on strength, power and sprints is unclear • More sports specific research is needed to detect which events and individuals will benefit	problems are unclear, health authorities generally discourage long-term intake of large amounts of caffeine (>500 mg/day) • Some anti-doping codes (e.g. the National Collegiate Athletics Associations) ban the use of large amounts of caffeine, leading to urinary caffeine levels above a certain threshold • It is not appropriate for young athletes to use caffeine as an ergogenic aid
Bicarbonate	• High rates of anaerobic carbohydrate use during high-intensity exercise are associated with build-up of	• An increase in extra-cellular (blood) buffering capacity may aid an athlete's capacity to produce power during sports	• There have been reports of bloating and diarrhoea following bicarbonate loading • Special protocols are needed

AIS Supplement Program Group = A Bicarbonate contd	lactate and acidity (decrease in pH) • Increasing blood pH, by consuming a buffering agent, can mop up excess muscle acidity and prolong the time that high-intensity exercise can be sustained. This is known as extra-cellular buffering (buffering outside the cell) and requires the acid to move out of the cell into the bloodstream, where it is neutralised. • Bicarbonate and citrate are common buffering agents—available as household product (e.g. bicarb soda), pharmaceutical treatment for urinary tract infections (e.g. Ural) or special supplements (e.g. Sodibic) • Typical doses for acute loading are 0.3/kg bicarbonate and 0.3 to 0.5 g/kg citrate, taken 60–90 min before exercise.	or events limited by excessive build-up of hydrogen ions. ○ high-intensity events lasting 1–7 min ○ repeated high-intensity sprints (e.g. team and racket sports) ○ prolonged high-intensity events lasting 30–60 min • There is good scientific proof that bicarbonate loading can assist high-intensity events lasting 1–7 min • More sports specific research is needed to detect which events and individuals will benefit • Some research suggests benefits to prolonged or intermittent sports in which high lactate levels are generated, or to the training adaptations achieved by interval work in which high lactate levels are produced	for repeated use for multiple events (e.g. heats and finals) over single or several days • Bicarbonate tends to be a stronger buffer than citrate but may have a greater risk of side-effects

Product	Description and protocol of use	Proposed benefits and summary of scientific proof	Concerns
Bicarbonate contd	Should be consumed with 1 to 2 L of water to reduce risk of diarrhoea. • Longer ('chronic') bicarbonate loading (0.5 mg/kg spread out over the day for 3–5 days) may sustain the increase in blood pH, with benefits being maintained for at least 1 day following the last dose. This may ○ Replace multiple acute loading in athletes who compete in a series of events spread over a couple of days ○ Allow an athlete who suffers gut problems following large doses to spread the doses out and stop the day before their event		

Creatine AIS Supplement Program Group = A	• Naturally occurring compound found in the muscle; in the form of creatine phosphate it provides a rapid but short-lived source of fuel phosphate • Naturally occurring compound found in the muscle; in the form of creatine phosphate it provides a rapid but short-lived source of fuel • Daily turnover of ~2 g provided by dietary intake (meats) and synthesis in the body from amino acids. Muscle levels may be lower in vegetarians • Since 1990s we have been aware that increased dietary intake can raise muscle creatine stores by ~25% to reach ceiling level • Scientifically supported protocols for creatine use: 1. Rapid loading (5 days x 20 g per day spread into 4 x 5 g doses)	• Potential situations of benefit from creatine supplementation: ○ Single high-intensity sprint/bout dependent on creatine ○ Repeated sprints/bouts of high-intensity exercise, separated by short recovery intervals, limited by resynthesis of creatine phosphate stores between bouts. —Resistance training to increase lean body mass and strength. —Interval and sprint training —Training and competition in intermittent sports (e.g. team and racquet sports) • Creatine may enhance carbohydrate-loading for endurance exercise. • Well studied (>200 studies since 1992)	• Many creatine users are either unaware of correct doses or persist in using unnecessarily high doses. Higher doses of creatine do not further enhance creatine stores • Weight gain of 0.6–1 kg occurs with loading (water retention?). Weight gain may be counterproductive to sports where power-to-weight ratio is important or the athlete makes weight for a weight division • Long-term consequences of creatine use are unknown. —there are anecdotal reports of muscle cramps, strains, and tears, but studies haven't found an increased risk of these events —Creatine use in the suggested doses has not been seen to alter kidney function in otherwise healthy people.

Product	Description and protocol of use	Proposed benefits and summary of scientific proof	Concerns
Creatine contd	2. Slow loading (1 month x 3 g per day) 3. Maintenance after loading (3 g per day) 4. Depletion takes ~4 weeks after stopping supplements • Consuming creatine with carbohydrate (i.e. with a meal or snack) increases muscle uptake • Creatine monohydrate is the most common of creatine supplements. • Individual variability with response to creatine supplements—athletes with high starting creatine levels may not show a further increase	• Has therapeutic uses for some medical problems • Good support for benefits to repeated high-intensity sprints • Further sports specific studies needed to translate from the laboratory to the field • No benefits to endurance exercise have been found (in fact, decrease due to weight gain) but situations limited by glycogen haven't been studied	• There are many 'special' creatine supplements on the market claiming special uptake. This is not supported. • In fact, 'serum' (liquid) creatine products are unstable and may not contain any creatine
Colostrum	• Protein-rich substance secreted in breast milk in the first few days after a mother has given birth. Colostrum	• A small number of studies have found performance improvements with chronic supplementation. These	• There is no indication of the potential situations or athletic populations that might benefit from colostrum

AIS Supplement Program Group = B Colostrum contd	supplements are typically produced from bovine (cow) sources. • Rich in immunoglobulin and insulin-like growth factors (IGFs). The gut of a baby has 'leaky' junctions that allow it to absorb such proteins, thus developing its own independent immune system for survival after birth. The adult gut is not believed to absorb significant amounts of intact proteins • Colostrum supplementation is claimed to improve exercise performance and recovery • Typical colostrum supplementation involves 20–60 g of colostrum powder or liquid each day: the literature indicates that at least 4 weeks of supplementation may be required to induce a benefit	findings are interesting but have generally not been replicated in other studies of the same supplement • Equivocal effect on blood and salivary levels of immune system parameters • Pooling of data from several studies of 8-w colostrum supplementation has reported reduced incidence of upper respiratory tract infections. • Findings were not replicated in another study of 12 weeks' supplementation	supplementation. Therefore it is hard to target research or use • There is no clear mechanism by which colostrum supplementation benefits athletic performance • Colostrum supplements can be expensive. A 20–60 g/day protocol typically costs $20–60 per week. There is a need to investigate whether benefits can be achieved with smaller doses • Not all colostrum supplements are the same; even if some can be shown to provide benefits to athletic performance, this finding may not apply to all products

Product	Description and protocol of use	Proposed benefits and summary of scientific proof	Concerns
Colostrum contd	• Some recent studies show benefits from using low colostrum doses (10–20 g/day) in some athletes or situations		
B-alanine AIS Supplement Program Group = B	• Carnosine is a dipeptide (2 amino acids—β-alanine and histidine—joined). It is found in large amounts in the muscle, especially fast-twitch muscle, where the availability of β-alanine is believed to be the limiting factor in its production • Carnosine accounts for ~10% of the muscle's ability to buffer acidity produced by high intensity exercise • Recent studies have shown that daily supplementation with 65 mg/kg (4–6 g/d) β-alanine can increase muscle	• Increasing muscle carnosine levels may be an alternative strategy to bicarbonate/citrate loading to increase buffering capacity for high-intensity exercise. It may also be an additive strategy, since muscle carnosine is an intracellular (inside the cell) buffer, while bicarbonate/citrate raise extracellular (outside the cell) buffering • There is preliminary evidence that it might benefit athletes undertaking exercise that might be limited by the lowering of pH (build-up of acidity) in the	• Studies on β-alanine are too new to be certain about side-effects from taking β-alanine. • To date, the major side-effect that has been described is a prickling or 'pins and needles' sensation—occurring for ~60 mins about 15–20 mins following a dose. This is apparently related to the rate in the rise of plasma β-alanine concentrations and may be blunted by consuming a sustained release supplement or consuming it with carbohydrate foods • It is too soon to know if

B-alanine contd	carnosine content by ~60% after 4 weeks and ~80% after 10 weeks of supplementation by about 80% • We don't yet know how long to continue supplementation to maximise muscle carnosine concentrations, or how long muscle carnosine remains elevated if supplementation is stopped	muscle in association with high-intensity exercise • Competitive events lasting 1–7 minutes • Repeated bouts of high-intensity work (sprints, lifts) which cause an exercise-limiting increase in H+ ions over time • It has potential as an alternative or additive strategy to bicarbonate/citrate loading	athletes will benefit from β-alanine supplementation, which athletes or events should be targeted and how to periodise the use of β-alanine
Ribose AIS Supplement Program Group = B	• Pentose (5 carbon sugar) naturally found in the diet. It provides the backbone of DNA, RNA, and the fuel source ATP. The pathway that handles the production or scavenging of these important substances is limited and may be enhanced by increased availability of ribose • Some diseases in which the pathway is limited respond to ribose supplementation • Supplementation protocols	• Repeated sprints of high-intensity exercise reduce ATP pool in the muscle cell by ~20%, which may persist for several days. In such a situation, ribose supplementation may enhance synthesis and recycling of ATP and related chemicals and enhance training performance • Ribose supplementation studies have targeted athletes undertaking intermittent high-intensity exercise programs	• Oral intake of ribose is well tolerated, but there are insufficient studies conducted with large doses over long time-frames to allow full discussion of side-effects • Ribose supplements are expensive. At a recommended price of $70 for a 100 g supply, a daily dose of 10 to 20 g of ribose would cost $50 to $100 per week. It may take larger doses than this before benefits are seen

Product	Description and protocol of use	Proposed benefits and summary of scientific proof	Concerns
Ribose contd	in recent studies of athletes typically involve daily doses of 10 to 20 g of ribose	(weight training, interval training). • There is only one study that has reported a benefit from ribose supplementation in athletes (resistance training). All other fully published studies have failed to find any performance effects from ribose supplementation, or that ATP is limiting in such training protocols	
HMB AIS Supplement Program Group = B	• β-hydroxy β-methylbutyrate (HMB) is a breakdown product of the essential amino acid leucine, and is proposed to influence muscle protein metabolism and cell membrane integrity • Claimed to act as an anti-catabolic agent, minimising protein breakdown and the	• HMB supplementation is claimed to decrease protein breakdown associated with heavy training, thus enhancing development of muscle size and strength • A meta-analysis of several studies suggests a small benefit from HMB supplementation when combined with resistance	• Supplements aimed at enhancing the results of resistance training may be at greater risk of inadvertent contamination with prohormones

HMB contd	cellular damage that occurs with high-intensity exercise • Typical dose = 3 g/day in three divided doses of 1 g. Higher doses have been proven to be ineffective	training, but this has been criticised since all the studies come from the same researchers • HMB might be most valuable in the early phases of a new resistance training program when it is able to reduce the large catabolic response or damage produced by unaccustomed exercise. However, once adaptation to training occurs, reducing the residual catabolism and damage response, HMB supplementation no longer provides a detectable benefit. This theory explains why HMB tends to produce favourable results in novice resistance trainers rather than well-trained participants and why positive results are reported in shorter studies (i.e. 2–4 weeks) but not at the end of longer studies (i.e. 8 weeks).	

Product	Description and protocol of use	Proposed benefits and summary of scientific proof	Concerns
Glutamine AIS Supplement Program Group = B	• Glutamine is an amino acid that provides an important fuel source for immune cells. It plays a major role in protein metabolism; in some circumstances it provides an anti-protein breakdown effect • Studies in the early 1990s identified lowered blood glutamine levels as a marker of overtraining and fatigue in athletes, but a consensus has not yet been reached on how best to use this information. • Daily glutamine supplementation of 0.1 to 0.3 g/kg of body weight appears to be safe	• Glutamine supplementation is promoted as a nutritional supplement for athletes to maintain or boost immune function or to maintain muscle protein levels during periods of intensive training. It is claimed to prevent or lessen the severity of illness, particularly in susceptible athletes • To date there is no conclusive evidence demonstrating that glutamine supplementation lowers incidence of illness in healthy athletes who consume adequate levels of protein, or stops protein breakdown following resistance training	
Coenzyme Q10	• Coenzyme Q10, or ubiquinone, is a nonessential fat-soluble nutrient found predominantly in animal foods	• Coenzyme Q10 supplementation is claimed to enhance energy production and reduce the oxidative damage of exercise	• The issue of antioxidant supplementation is complex and as yet unsolved. Studies of vitamin C oxidation have also

AIS Supplement Program Group = C Coenzyme Q10 contd	• Is found in skeletal and heart muscle, where it is an anti-oxidant in the mitochondria and part of energy production • Some patients with diseases featuring low blood coenzyme Q10 concentrations improve their exercise capacity following supplementation • General marketing campaigns for coenzyme Q10 supplements promote increased vigour and youthfulness as a benefit of their use • Typical dosage for supple-mentation is ~100 mg/day	• One study has reported a benefit to exercise performance following Coenzyme Q10 supplementation. However, the majority of studies report no performance benefit • In fact, several studies have shown a consistent negative effect of CoQ10 supplementation on high-intensity training and performance outcomes in previously untrained people. Supplementation was associated with increased oxidative damage and reduced training adaptations	shown a negative effect on training outcomes • Supplementation with single antioxidants may unbalance delicate systems and turn the supplement into a pro-oxidant. In addition, the antioxidant may quench some of the oxidative changes that are positive (e.g. the signalling pathways that stimulate adaptation to training)
L-carnitine AIS Supplement Program Group = C	• Non-essential nutrient, found in dietary sources and manufactured in the liver and kidney from amino acid precursors (lysine and methionine) • Stored in large amounts in the heart and skeletal muscle • Is part of enzymes that	• It has been suggested that carnitine supplementation might enhance fat transport and oxidation—enhancing endurance performance and the loss of body fat • Carnitine is a popular ingredient in many fat-loss supplements	

Product	Description and protocol of use	Proposed benefits and summary of scientific proof	Concerns
L-carnitine contd	transport fatty acids into the mitochondria for oxidation • In some disease conditions in which muscle carnitine levels are reduced, patients have abnormalities of fat oxidation and poor exercise capacity	• Research does not support any benefits of carnitine supplementation on exercise performance • Loss of body fat following carnitine supplementation has not been studied in athletes, but studies in sedentary populations do now show any benefits • Part of the lack of effect can be explained by the failure of carnitine supplements to increase muscle carnitine levels. However, a recent study has shown that carnitine stores can be increased if high levels of blood carnitine are teamed with insulin stimulation (e.g. carbohydrate consumption). This needs further study	

Ginseng AIS Supplement Program Group = C	• There are several species of ginseng—American, Siberian, Korean, and Japanese. Although most of these ginsengs belong to the same Panax plant species, Russian or Siberian ginseng is extracted from a different plant (Eleutherococcus senticoccus) • Long history as a health supplement. Ginseng has been used widely in herbal medicines of Asian cultures to cure fatigue, relieve pain and headaches, and improve mental function and energy. • Has been described by Eastern European scientists as an adaptogen—a substance that is able to return physiology to normal after exposure to stresses • The chemical composition of commercial supplement products is highly variable	• Ginseng is claimed to reduce fatigue and improve aerobic conditioning, strength, mental alertness, and recovery • A few studies have reported enhanced exercise capacity with ginseng supplementation. However, the majority of studies have not found any benefits from ginseng use	• Some studies of commercial ginseng supplements have found very little active ingredient • Even if ginseng could be proved to enhance work capacity, athletes could not be sure of what they were receiving in a commercial supplement

Product	Description and protocol of use	Proposed benefits and summary of scientific proof	Concerns
Ginseng contd	because of differences in plant source, variation in active ingredients, and differences in preparation methods		
Oxyshots AIS Supplement Program Group = C	• Brand of oxygenated water—water containing dissolved oxygen • Proposed to provide 'massive amounts' of oxygen to body via the gut • Recommended dosage is 10–20 ml, 15–30 min pre-exercise	• Proposed to promote increased strength, endurance and aerobic power by supplying additional oxygen to body • No studies of Oxyshot supplement have been published, but studies of other oxygenated waters fail to find evidence of performance enhancement • Relies solely on testimonials from athletes	• Could be expensive if used for every training session—250 ml bottle costs $45–50
Glycerol	• A naturally occurring compound that forms part of the fat molecule • When consumed, it is rapidly	• Potential situations of benefit from glycerol hyper-hydration • An endurance athlete training or competing in hot humid	• Side effects in some individuals include headaches and gastrointestinal problems, particularly when glycerol is

AIS Supplement Program Group = D Note: at the time of writing this book, oral intake of glycerol was noted by WADA to be a plasma expander, and thus added to its list of prohibited substances. This situation is likely to be considered again—see *www.wada.org*	absorbed and distributed throughout the body's fluid compartments, until gradually excreted over the next 24–48 hr. While in the body, it acts like a sponge for additional fluid • A fluid loading protocol involves 1–1.5 g/kg glycerol consumed 2 hours pre-event with a fluid load of 25–35 ml/kg • This generally allows a hyper-hydration with ~600 ml of fluid more than a fluid load alone	conditions, where excessive fluid losses cannot be replaced sufficiently during the exercise and a limiting fluid deficit will otherwise occur. • Enhancement of rehydration after dehydration—such as weight making strategies • Studies are not universal in their findings, however, glycerol hyper-hydration has been shown to enhance performance in hot conditions when it makes a difference to the fluid deficit that otherwise accumulates.	consumed after a meal. • Experimentation is required to ensure that performance is not impaired by additional body mass attributable to water loading. • Use of glycerol as a hyperhydrating agent is considered to contravene the WADA anti-doping code

Product	Description and protocol of use	Proposed benefits and summary of scientific proof	Concerns
Tribulus terrestris AIS Supplement Program Group = D	• Derived from a weed (also known as puncture vine). Part of ancient Indian medicine • Claimed to increase testosterone concentrations by stimulating the production of another hormone (luteinising hormone) • Promoted as a herbal testosterone supplement	• Claimed to enhance testosterone levels—with alleged benefits being increased training vigour and increased response to resistance training • There is no evidence of increased testosterone concentrations nor enhanced training outcomes • Apparently, the doses taken 'on the street' by athletes are higher than the manufacturers' recommendations or doses that have been tested	• Although *Tribulus terrestris* is not banned, supplements purporting to increase testosterone concentrations should be considered high risk for containing undeclared prohormones and other banned steroid-like compounds. Several studies have identified *Tribulus* preparations as contaminated with these banned agents.

*For more information on these and other supplements see *www.ausport.gov.au/ais/nutrition*

Part II

SPORTS NUTRITION IN ACTION

Introduction

In this section we will turn theory into practice, looking inside a number of sports to see the nutritional challenges faced by athletes and identify the nutritional issues they face, depending on their sport, level and lifestyle.

These sports were chosen to represent a variety of different nutritional issues. If your sport has not been covered, you will probably find that you can identify with another sport or with the issues that arise in a combination of sports. Think about the features of your sport, both the characteristics of competition and the way that you train. The brief description at the beginning of each chapter may help you identify another sport (or group of sports) that makes similar demands to yours.

Of course, you may already have a list of nutritional issues that interest and concern you. Use the lists at the front of this book to look up a case history or a relevant checklist. For example, loss of body fat is a goal shared by athletes in many sports, and even if you are a lacrosse player you may be able to identify with the weight-loss efforts of Paula the netballer or Robbie the AFL player. Similarly, if you are interested in a nutritional assessment, you will find track athlete Michael's experiences of interest, and the hints for the travelling athlete in the tennis chapter will be valuable whatever your sport.

Finally, appreciate that each chapter covers typical issues and is by no means complete or exclusive. Your nutritional goals and interests may be a little different from those covered in the chapter on your sport. Hopefully, however, you will find something that addresses you personally and individually. Above all, enjoy this section for the chance to think about the practical and human aspects of nutrition for sport. It should help you to convert science into food choices and eating habits, and thus help you to take your sport as far as your ambitions reach.

Triathlon

Triathlon, described as the boom sport of the 1980s, had its Olympic debut at the 2000 Games in Sydney and delivered Australia a gold medal, won by Emma Snowsill, at the 2008 Beijing Olympics. In this multi-sport event, competitors complete a swim, cycle and run in immediate succession, with races broadly categorised as follows:

- Sprint distance: 500-m swim/20-km cycle/5-km run
- Olympic distance: 1.5-km swim/40-km cycle/10-km run
- Half Ironman ('Ironman 70.3'): 1.8-km swim/90-km cycle/21.1-km run
- Long course: 4-km swim/130-km cycle/30-km run
- Ultra distance/Ironman: 3.9-km swim/180-km cycle/42.2-km run.

In many triathlons, all competitors race alongside each other, with prizes for the top males and females, and the champions in each age group. There are not too many sports that allow everyday athletes to toe the starting line with their heroes!

Training

It is not surprising, with three sports to master, that triathlon training is time-consuming. Even recreational triathletes can spend more than ten hours a week in training. Typical weekly totals for a serious Olympic-distance triathlete are 10–15 km swimming, 200–300 km cycling and 40–60 km running; elite competitors do more. According to the website of the Ironman race series (*www.Ironmanlive.com*), the typical Ironman competitor undertakes seven months of preparation for a race, with a weekly commitment of 18–22 hours and a mean total of 11.3 km swimming, 373 km cycling and 77 km running.

The bulk of triathlon training is aerobic, with interval training included in some sessions. Many triathletes include transition training in their schedules, following up one sport immediately with another (usually a cycle followed by a run). Strength and conditioning sessions are often included during the off-season, when time and facilities permit.

The most important fuel for training is muscle glycogen, and intense daily training will challenge the recovery of stores in the various muscle groups involved in each sport discipline.

Competition

The official triathlon season in Australia extends from late spring to early autumn. Events are held on weekends (usually Sundays), typically early in the morning to avoid the heat. During winter, when open-water swims are impractical, triathletes may compete in run-ride-run races (duathlons). Sprint-distance and Olympic-distance events are non-drafting events for age-group athletes. This means they must avoid riding in the slipstream (draft) of another athlete during the cycle leg of the event. Elite competitors may race these distances in either a 'draft-legal' or non-drafting format. Long-course racing such as half-Ironman and Ironman events are raced as non-drafting events.

On the international circuit, age-group and elite triathletes can race all year round, with a schedule of Olympic-distance, half-Ironman, long-course and Ironman racing that culminates in world championship events. The International Triathlon Union (ITU) manages a schedule of international races (World Championship races) for elite competitors with a draft-legal race format. Half-Ironman (70.3 series) and Ironman (Ironman series) races are also held throughout the world, providing opportunities for elite and age-group athletes to race side by side. Ironman racing enjoys high participation rates worldwide and culminates at the Ironman World Championship in Hawaii.

Triathletes' competition schedules vary. Elite competitors specialise in a set distance (either short- or long-course racing), while it's common for age-group athletes to compete over all race distances. Some athletes compete most weekends during the competition season—up to twenty times a year—but select a handful of key races to focus on. Others choose to spread their races over the season. Juggling competition and training schedules can present a great challenge.

Triathlons are predominantly an aerobic event, but the physiological demands of each event require athletes to undertake sport-specific training. Short-course races may take as little as 45 minutes, and elite competitors complete Olympic distance events in approximately 1 hour 45 minutes. Ironman races take eight hours at best, considerably longer (up to 17 hours) for age-group competitors.

The intensity of exercise tends to remain constant for the longer non-drafting races, when athletes peg themselves against the clock. In draft-legal events however, the intensity varies considerably during the cycle leg as athletes repeatedly try to break away from the pack. A triathlon can be conducted at a higher intensity than a single sport of the same total duration, and competitors are less likely to be limited by the depletion of fuel stores, since the work is spread over a larger number of muscle groups. However, in longer triathlons the individual distances in each sport will challenge the fuel stores in the muscles involved, as well as the body's ability to maintain blood-glucose levels.

The duration of triathlons and the environment in which they take place also affect fluid loss and temperature regulation. While some triathlons can expose competitors to cold and possible hypothermia, in most cases dehydration and heat stress are greater risks. The Ironman championship in Hawaii each year challenges athletes not only with the long distances but with strong winds and ground temperatures of over 40°C.

Physical characteristics

The only spare tyres elite triathletes carry are under their bike seats in case of a puncture! Like distance running, triathlon performance is advantaged by a low level of body fat, so elite triathletes have skinfold thicknesses comparable to those of elite marathon runners. However, because swimming makes active use of upper-body muscles, the total muscle mass and body weight of a triathlete will be greater than that of the marathon runner, with most of the extra muscle around the chest, arms and shoulders. Interestingly, the race rules (drafting versus non-drafting) and distance of the event also influence the physiques of elite competitors. Elite Olympic-distance triathletes are typically lighter than their Ironman counterparts, since Ironman racing requires athletes to be strong and maintain form over a longer distance.

Common nutritional issues

Dietary extremism

Triathletes are renowned for their enthusiasm and self-discipline. They don't do things by half measures, and that includes diet. Many triathletes read widely about nutrition, and triathlon and multisport magazines are littered with articles on the subject, as well as advertisements for dietary supplements and nutritional ergogenic aids. Some triathletes become skilled trackers of 'bad foods', which they then single-mindedly eliminate from their diets. The result of this excessive strictness is a restricted dietary range, causing a number of problems and missed opportunities. The most important rule for a peak training diet is to include a variety of foods. Read Chapter 1.1 to see how this can be achieved while meeting all other nutritional goals for training.

Excessively low body-fat levels

Also on the 'you can have too much of a good thing' theme, a current fashion in triathlon is to strive for the lowest level of body fat possible. This sometimes happens as a consequence of nutritional extremism, but it's often pursued as a goal in itself. Triathletes should recognise first that optimum body-fat levels are individual, and that it is not necessarily an advantage to have the body-fat levels of Emma Snowsill or Chris McCormack—unless you are Emma Snowsill or Chris McCormack. Second, for all triathletes, the definition of optimum in regard to body-fat levels includes the issue of good health. If your body fat drops to a level that causes problems with cold intolerance, loss of immune function, and loss of strength/muscle mass, as well as menstrual disturbances and other penalties of restricted energy intake, then this level is not optimum for you—even if it does mean less 'dead weight' to carry over the course (see Chapter 3.1).

High energy requirements

The intense training program of a triathlete, especially a full-time or elite athlete, can require massive intakes of energy, which explains why most triathletes achieve low body-fat levels naturally. However, sometimes when a triathlete begins a training program, trains at altitude, or increases his training load, body weight can fall to an undesirable level. There are a number of reasons athletes don't automatically adjust their food intake to meet the increased requirements of training. A narrowly restrictive diet has been mentioned; other factors include being too tired after training to cook or even eat. An increased fibre intake associated with eating nutritious carbohydrate foods often means the athlete feels too full to overeat, especially when squeezing eating into gaps between work and training. (See Chapter 3.8 for smart ways to increase energy intake by eating 'compact' kilojoules and by increasing the number of meals rather than their size. See also the case history of Nick in the next chapter, 'Swimming').

Some male triathletes take a haphazard approach to eating because their intense exercise programs let them eat whatever they like and still maintain their physique. However, the timing of food before, during and after training sessions can influence training performance and recovery, and ultimately competition performance. Therefore, although athletes with high energy budgets can afford to include some less nutritious food choices, they should still make sure they maximise nutrients and match their meals and snacks to daily training sessions.

Loss of body fat

Sometimes, despite heavy training, a triathlete will need additional help to reduce body-fat levels. For some, this is a constant struggle. Females in particular seem to need to eat less kilojoules than their training loads would predict. If this applies to you, you may find it frustrating when fellow athletes eat twice as much as you, or enjoy the feeding frenzies otherwise known as carbo-loading banquets, without gaining a gram.

Chapter 3.3 will show you how to arrive at a weight-loss program and an energy intake level that are suitable for you.

Low iron levels

Triathletes, especially females, are at relatively high risk for iron deficiency. In its early stages, this may reduce the ability to recover between training sessions even before full-blown anaemia causes a definite reduction in exercise performance. As discussed in Chapter 2.5, hard-training triathletes may have a greater need for iron, perhaps because of iron losses from gut bleeding and red-blood-cell loss. However, the factor most likely to contribute to iron deficiency is the low level of readily absorbed iron in the typical triathlete's diet. Read Chapter 2.5 to make sure you aren't overlooking iron in your nutritional goals, and have your iron status checked periodically to pick up low levels early.

Amenorrhoea, low bone density, and stress fractures

An irregular menstrual cycle is a frequent result of the heavy training and often restrictive diet of the female triathlete. Insufficient energy (kilojoule) intake to cope with the added demands of daily training is the primary cause of such problems. Studies show that menstrual irregularity and its associated factors can in turn lead to low bone density and an increased risk of stress fractures. These problems, either singly or together, are complex in nature and treatment. See your sports doctor early in the picture—and for more information read Chapters 2.6 and 3.5, and the profile of Lola in the distance running chapter.

Daily recovery

With a twice-daily training program, it is not surprising that recovery is regarded as a magic word in triathlon circles. The faster the recovery, the sooner or harder the next session can be completed. Triathletes often walk precariously along the fine line between hard training and overtraining. During the competitive season, recovery is important for those who want to race each weekend or pick up their training straight after each event.

Your peak training diet should supply all the nutrients required for recovery between sessions, with emphasis on fluid strategies (Chapter 1.4) and carbohydrate intake (Chapters 1.3 and 2.2). Chapter 5 has special notes on rapid replacement of fluid and carbohydrate stores after prolonged exercise sessions.

In planning your training schedule, order your sessions to allow maximum recovery time for the specific muscle groups involved in each sport. Also note that hard running causes some muscle-fibre damage and will require more time to restock muscle glycogen stores, so give yourself adequate recovery time and extra carbohydrate after intense running sessions or races.

It's also important to maintain dietary balance when meeting the added demands for daily training. Foods and fluids consumed either in preparation for, immediately before, during or after training sessions should not be seen simply as fuel. As well as carbohydrate, they should contain adequate protein to facilitate muscular repair, and vitamins and minerals to support immune function and general well-being.

Dietary periodisation

A new idea in sports nutrition is to adjust your eating plan to the time of year. Just as athletes periodise their training into preparation and peak, so they sometimes alter their diet. This is covered in more detail in Chapter 2. A number of intriguing protocols have emerged. One involves a twist on pre-race carbohydrate loading known as 'fat adaptation and carbohydrate restoration', which aims to make the endurance athlete burn fat more effectively while keeping carbohydrate stores full. In theory, this might be useful for an Ironman triathlete whose event would be expected to deplete muscle glycogen levels. However, as explained in Chapter 2.10, scientists haven't been able to measure any performance gains from this protocol. One reason for its failure to live up to its potential is that the fat loading actually impairs the muscle's ability to burn carbohydrate as fuel. This would deprive the triathlete of a 'top gear'—and even when your race lasts 8 hours or more, it is still important to be able to power up a hill or sprint to the finish line. Therefore, we can't recommend this strategy for race preparation.

The other topical dietary periodisation protocol is called 'train low, compete high'. This refers to strategies to deliberately train with low glycogen levels to promote a greater training adaptation in the muscle, then switch to full fuel stores for the competition phase. Again, it sounds good on paper and has reinvigorated the interest in low-carbohydrate diets. However, current studies on this topic have manipulated glycogen levels by changing training patterns rather than by restricting carbohydrates. Instead of training for one session each day, subjects in 'train-low' studies do two training sessions on every second day and have a rest day in between. As pointed out in Chapter 2.10, it is important to stop athletes running too far ahead of the science or misunderstanding what is really involved. More studies are needed, but it is likely that the best training outcomes occur when triathletes train with a mix of sessions where they're fuelled up and sessions that deplete their fuel stores. This is the reality for most triathletes in hard training, whether through good management or accident. For the moment, the best approach to training periodisation is the trial and error involved in finding a protocol that suits you.

Preparation for an event

Race preparation depends on the length of the race, the training state of the athlete, and race aspirations. Pre-race strategies are covered in Chapter 4 and should involve preparation of adequate fuel and fluid stores. You may also try to manipulate an empty gut to start you racing 'light'.

For short events, a well-trained triathlete is able to store sufficient muscle glycogen with a 24–36 hour preparation of rest/tapered training and an increased carbohydrate diet. If it's your big race for the year, you might want a longer tapering period. Others who are training for longer events later in the season may not want to sacrifice even one day of exercise. Plan your preparation according to your short-term and long-term priorities.

Long-course and ultra-distance events challenge muscle glycogen stores and therefore deserve a modified carbohydrate-loading preparation. In this situation, the last 36–72 hours before a race should be devoted to packing glycogen stores, with a significant reduction in exercise and a higher-carbohydrate diet. Since most races start early in the morning, the typical pre-race meal is small and light and eaten on rising, about two to three hours before the event.

Food and fluid intake during the race

For sprint races and events up to the Olympic distance, fluid needs are of greatest importance to competitors, with sports drinks and water the most widely used fluids. Race organisers typically provide fluids at aid stations in the transition areas, and during the running leg. While those who are out for long hours in the heat of the day are reminded to stay hydrated, even top athletes should be warned about the dangers of failing to drink adequately while cycling or running. Chapter 4 explains that moderate fluid loss can reduce performance, and on hot days severe dehydration added to heat stress is a real threat to health.

Drinking pouches consisting of a pressurised sack with a plastic tube that runs along the bike frame and can be lifted to the triathlete's mouth (e.g. the Camelbak) can provide easy access to fluid for those who worry about wasting precious seconds by reaching down to the bidon cage. Of course, in elite competitions such as the Olympic Games, race rules may not allow the use of such devices.

More recent research has highlighted that some triathletes, particularly those competing in Ironman events can actually drink too much. Some who do so may go on to develop the life-threatening condition hyponatraemia (low blood sodium). Female athletes who compete at the back of the pack in cold conditions are at most risk of drinking more than they lose in sweat. It's important for triathletes to develop an individual fluid-intake plan for each race based on previous fluid-balance observations conducted in training sessions under similar environmental conditions (see Figure 2.3 and sections 4.6, 4.7 and Checklist 4.4 in Chapter 4).

As events become longer, the advantages of consuming carbohydrate during the race become more obvious. This practice will improve performance in long-course and ultradistance events by supplying additional fuel sources for trained muscles once glycogen stores have been exhausted. You might like to experiment with sports drinks in Olympic distance races also, particularly for races in which your 'fuelling up' may not have been optimal. In ultradistance races, there is usually a well-organised network of aid stations at which athletes are offered a range of carbohydrate-rich food and fluids, including sports drinks. See the account of the Ironman race below, and read Chapter 4.7 for guidelines to a well-organised feeding schedule. Most importantly, practise your intended strategies in training.

Ergogenic aids and dietary supplements

Triathlon magazines are littered with advertisements and advertorials promoting the benefits of consuming nutritional supplements and ergogenic aids to enhance performance, optimise recovery and maintain health. Read Chapter 6 to see which supplements can have an important and useful role in your training and competition and which ones are still awaiting scientific study. Make up your own mind once you have the facts to hand.

Profile: Natalie

A 226-kilometre picnic

Natalie stood on the pier at Kailua-Kona and thought of the race before her. This day had been the focus of her attention for the past twelve months. Natalie qualified for the Hawaii Ironman World Championship Triathlon early in the year, and she was determined to give her all to the gruelling event: a 3.8-km swim, 180-km cycle and 42.2-km run. On her first attempt at this challenge two years earlier, she had made a couple of rookie mistakes. This year that wouldn't happen again: she was making a run at the medals in her age group.

Her preparation had left nothing to chance. She trained diligently throughout a cold Canberra winter and practised her race nutrition plan to support her throughout long training sessions. In her previous attempt at Hawaii, her lack of attention to fluid and fuel intake during the race had let her down. This time around, Natalie had consulted an experienced sports dietitian to ensure she could meet her hourly fluid and fuel needs for the race.

On her last visit to the Big Island, Natalie had found that the supermarkets and health-food store at the top of town had the same kinds of foods as she ate in Australia. But her usual diet was hijacked at the 'all-you-can-eat' carbo-loading parties. She found herself 'pigging out' on foods she wasn't used to or which she'd barred from her diet. Her approach had been—it's Hawaii, it's a holiday! This time was different.

Conscious of the traps, she had come armed with a plan, yet she was also flexible with her approach and attitude.

During the race Natalie planned to use a combination of her favourite foods and drinks along with those provided by race organisers at the aid stations on the cycle and run courses. Her race instruction booklet outlined where these would be and what they would be offering:

- Bike leg: aid station every 7 miles (12 km)
- Run leg: aid station every mile (1.6 km)
- Additional stations at race start and transition areas

Menu:

- Gatorade Endurance Formula (sports drink)
- water
- defizzed cola drink
- ice and ice sponges
- bananas, oranges
- Fig Newtons (similar to fruit pillows)
- PowerBar Performance Bars
- PowerBar Gels.

Natalie had set up her bike to carry enough fluid and food, so she wouldn't need to collect a special-needs bag at the halfway mark on the bike course. Her nutrition priorities were to match her hourly sweat losses with a sufficient intake of fluid, and supply herself with a constant intake of carbohydrate.

She knew from past experience she would tolerate more carbohydrate on the bike, so her goal on the cycle leg was about 70–80 g of carbohydrate an hour. On the run, her tolerance for food or drink would be lower, so the goal was about 40–60 g of carbohydrate per hour.

Her race nutrition plan, devised in collaboration with her sports dietitian, was based around sports drinks, as these have the distinct advantage of simultaneously supplying fluid and carbohydrate. Theoretically, at least, the drinks should be rapidly digested and their elements quickly transported to her working muscles. Sports drinks would be complemented by gels and solid foods. She knew she would get hungry on the bike, since she was racing through the lunch period, so she planned to rely more heavily on solid foods throughout the cycle leg.

Natalie often felt uncomfortable if there was food in her stomach when she was running, so during the run she would focus more on carbohydrate fluids and gels. She realised this was her personal preference, since many of her training partners could eat a range of foods, from bananas to muesli bars, without difficulty during a run.

Natalie bought some Gatorade Endurance Formula and started using it in training. She planned to drink a consistent amount of sports drink each hour during the bike leg, manipulating her total fluid intake by varying the amount of water she drank. This way she was guaranteed a known amount of carbohydrate. She planned to consume a 750-ml bottle of sports drink every two hours. She calculated that this would supply ~25 grams of carbohydrate each hour, about a third of her hourly carbohydrate needs. Half a Vegemite sandwich (10 g), a Fig Newton (10 g) and a PowerBar Gel (27 g) each hour in addition to her hourly sports drink intake would provide the rest of the carbohydrate she needed to meet her target.

Of course, 375 ml of sports drink an hour would not cover her fluid needs entirely. In Hawaii's extreme heat, she anticipated that she might lose ~800 ml of sweat per hour. She planned to drink extra water each hour throughout the cycle leg to keep pace with her sweat losses.

One important thing she'd learned from other triathletes was to be flexible. What if she got to an aid station and missed the 'right' drink? What if she got hungry? What if she got sick of the taste of the Gatorade? Common sense told Natalie that her plan might need to be altered as she went. She might need to drink extra fluid at times; at other times, as her pace and the day's heat subsided, she might sweat less and need to drink less. If she got hungry, increasing her intake of solid food should allay the discomfort. A drink of Coke could give her a 'change of scenery' now and then. There had been plenty of time in her six months of training to think and experiment.

Natalie arrived in Kailua-Kona ten days before the race to acclimatise—to the weather, to the race atmosphere, and to the course itself. The last three days were spent carbo-loading, resting, and drinking adequate fluid. On race morning, she got up at 4.30 a.m., had a light breakfast, and found herself at the race start with 1700 other competitors just as excited and nervous as she was.

This time around, the race was all that she thought it would be.

It was tough, but they don't just give away the title of Ironman! After the swim, she stopped briefly in transition for a drink, then sped off on the bike. She had two bidon cages mounted on its frame, holding a bidon of Gatorade and another of water, which she replaced at aid stations along the way. She judged her intake to be about 600–900 ml per hour. Her intake of water steadily increased as the day heated up, but she drank three bottles of Gatorade over her six-hour ride, just as she had planned.

She found the Vegemite sandwiches a relief from the sweet-tasting fluids and gels. During the run, she alternated her drinks at each aid station—iced water, Gatorade and then Coke. She managed a PowerBar Gel each hour and found herself nibbling on a Fig Newton towards the end of the race as she started to feel hungry. When the finish line loomed ahead at last, her weary legs felt as if they were being forced to run a four-minute mile over the final flood-lit stretch. But she ended the race knowing she'd done well and with a big grin on her face. She didn't feel like drinking a Gatorade cocktail to celebrate, but Natalie would remember this race for the rest of her life—long after the marker-pen numbers stencilled onto her arms by sunburn had faded.

Profile: Adam

Yes, master!

Adam, an eighteen-year-old elite development triathlete, was keen to make his mark in his first ever Olympic-distance triathlon race (1.5-km swim, 40-km bike, 10-km run). The 16–19-year-old category of world championships follows a sprint distance format, but under-23 and open world championships involve the longer Olympic distance. The race was in Adam's home town, and it seemed a perfect time to test his mettle over the full distance against Australia's best senior-level athletes.

Adam was faced with several new challenges. Not only was this distance twice as long as he was used to, but the race timetable was different. Adam was used to the starter's gun sounding at 7–8 a.m., but the longer race started at 11.00 a.m. How good was this, he thought—a sleep in! Adam's coach felt that he was not approaching the step-up in race distance and intensity with the respect it deserved, so he suggested that Adam talk with a couple of the more experienced athletes in his training group to see what they did in their final preparation.

On a long training ride a couple of weeks before the race, Adam found himself sharing a wheel with Paul, the current Australian Olympic-distance champ and an Olympic Games veteran. Paul was well liked and was considered the ultimate professional. He had won triathlons all over the world and was very generous with his time towards the young guns in the squad.

Not wanting to sound like a novice, Adam said the coming race would be good because he could sleep in. He was done with early-morning race starts! Much to Adam's surprise, Paul said he was generally up at 6 a.m. on race morning to ensure he had time for a light 30-minute run before breakfast. He said he'd learnt early in his career that sleeping in meant he wouldn't have time for breakfast and a pre-race snack. 'Given that you're racing through lunch, you can't afford to start with your fuel tank half full,' Paul said.

Adam concluded that Paul must be one of those guys who can never relax.

As they were riding, Paul noticed that Adam had only one drink-bottle cage on his bike. He suggested that Adam carry both water and sports drink in the coming race: 'You will need two cages for that, so you should get down to the bike shop and have them attach a second cage.' As much as he valued Paul's advice, Adam had never used a sports drink in a sprint race, so couldn't really see the point of carrying the extra weight of a second drink bottle.

Late in the ride, Paul pulled out a carbohydrate gel from the back pocket of his jersey. Adam had never tried a gel before, as he didn't have a sponsor providing it for free. Paul mentioned that he always strapped a gel to his handlebar stem and typically used it midway through the bike course, particularly if it was a hilly one. He added that when he first started racing Olympic-distance events, he often took a spare gel to have during the run—just in case. 'When I first stepped up to racing Olympic-distance events, I found that having the gels on the bike and run gave me extra carbohydrate—and did I need it!' Now, of course, he was a ten-year veteran of such distance races. Adam appreciated the advice of a long-term champion. But he believed the upcoming race would signal a changing of the guard in the event and even felt a little guilty that he would have to be the one to show Paul's generation that they'd had their day.

On race day, Adam slept until around 8.45 a.m., which left him just fifteen minutes for breakfast. He had only a small bowl of cereal and a glass of juice, as he was a little nervous and didn't have much of an appetite. He left the hotel at 9.30 and noticed Paul having some raisin toast and juice at a café on his way to the starting area.

He had taken Paul's advice and bought some gels. They were expensive, though, so he had brought only two for the race. It seemed a waste of money to trial them first in training.

Adam got off to a flying start in the swim, and was cheered on by the local crowd. On the bike leg he found himself in a leading group of ten riders, including Paul. They took turns at the front of the group to ensure they got well ahead during this leg. Towards the end of the 40-km ride, Adam started feeling the effects of racing at such a speed and remembered he had a gel strapped to his handlebar stem. In one quick motion, he consumed the gel and reached for his lone drink bottle. It was empty. Surely, he thought, he hadn't drunk a full bottle already!

Paul noticed that Adam had run out of water and offered him a drink to wash down his gel. Adam began to wish he'd taken Paul's advice about carrying an extra water bottle. Despite the mishap, Adam managed to stay with the other leading riders as they entered the transition area for the run. Adam was first to leave after a lightning-fast transition. But after setting the early pace, he started to lose speed and rhythm.

Feeling that he was running out of gas, Adam now reached for his second gel. It wasn't in his pocket—he had left it in the transition, next to his running cap. There was nothing he could do but tough it out for the rest of the run. If only I'd paid more attention to Paul's advice, he thought. If only I'd given more attention to my race plan! The other leaders began to pass him. As his pace slowed further, more and more of the other athletes passed him too. In a thrilling sprint to the finish line, Paul edged out one of the other favourites. Adam struggled across the line in 27th place. As he thought over his hard-learned lesson, he began to appreciate how the Pauls of the world managed to win. No matter how good you were, he told himself ruefully, you still needed to respect the challenge of the race.

Swimming

Swimming is a popular sport in Australia. Most children attend learn-to-swim classes and our swimming champions are household names, having been responsible for more Australian Olympic medals than athletes in any other sport. Swimming is a highly technical sport, and serious swimmers usually begin a training program in their early teenage years. Indeed, it's an unusual feature of elite-level swimming that swimmers as young as 14 can achieve world-class performances in open races. Until recently, elite swimmers tended to retire in their early 20s. However, improved funding and rewards encourage many swimmers to extend their careers for another decade. The list of Olympic and world championship swimming medallists since 2000 includes Dara Torres, Alex Popov, Inge de Bruin and Jenny Thompson—all in their 30s and even 40s.

Competitive swimming opportunities range from school carnivals to masters races, and from mass-participation swims to the Olympics. In pool swimming, races are held in a number of strokes (freestyle, breaststroke, backstroke, butterfly and medley), over distances ranging from 50 m to 1500 m. Open-water swimming, in which a swimmer may complete an individual time-trial or group race in open water, has a smaller but growing following; 5-km, 10-km and 25-km races have been included in the world championships since 1991, and a 10-km swim was held at the Beijing Olympics in 2008. This chapter, however, is about pool swimming.

Training

By the time they are 12 or 13 years old, many top swimmers have already made a serious commitment to training. Typically, training sessions are held in the early morning (e.g. 5–7 a.m.) and late afternoon (e.g. 4–6 p.m.) to fit around school or work and allow maximum recovery time between the day's workouts. The number of a given swimmer's training sessions will vary depending on their age, the events for which they are preparing, and the stage of the season.

The training year is divided into phases, with weekly micro cycles within longer macro cycles. The emphasis shifts gradually from conditioning to race-intensity preparation, and there is a defined tapering-off period before competition. Most swimmers periodise their training so it peaks for one or two international meets a year (plus the qualification trials that most countries hold to select their national teams). However, it is becoming more common for swimmers to race regularly throughout the training season, at international World Cup and Grand Prix series as well as locally organised events. In such cases, specific peak training is not undertaken.

Typically, a swimmer does six to twelve pool sessions a week, with a workout consisting of an aerobic warm-up and swim-downs, drills to improve technique and practise race tactics (e.g. starts and turns), and interval sets with repeated bouts of swimming over varying intensities, duration, and recovery periods. The distance covered in each session ranges from 1000–2000—of quality work for a sprinter in a pre-race taper phase to 10 km for a distance swimmer in the base phase of training. Overall, an elite swimmer typically covers 30 to 70 km a week in the pool—although some coaches still build up to a 'hell week' where 100 km is the target!

'Dry-land' sessions are also built into the training program; these include stretching and flexibility work as well as resistance/weights training (typically two or three sessions a week). Some swimmers do other forms of cross-training such as running and cycling, particularly during the early conditioning phase of the season or as a means to lose or control weight/body fat levels. In total, the elite swimmer may spend 20 to 30 hr in training each week. Clearly, such training calls heavily on muscle glycogen stores, and swimmers who fail to replenish their stores on a daily basis may be unable to complete such high training volume or high-intensity sessions.

There has been much discussion between scientists and coaches about the need for such high volumes of training when the longest event on the race program is 1500 m. One argument used in favour is it helps swimmers develop an efficient technique or 'feel for the water'. However, other coaches have had success with lower training volumes, more race-pace or event-specific swimming, and a greater focus on resistance training. At the club or school level, of course, training commitments are considerably less, and swimmers may not train all year round.

Competition

Swimming races are undertaken in both long-course (50 m) pools and short-course (25 m) pools, but long-course swimming is better recognised and included on the Olympic program. Within swimming circles, races are typically divided into sprint (50–100 m), middle-distance (200–400 m), and distance events (800–1500 m), although these terms are used differently than in other sports. Times range from just over 20 seconds for the shortest sprint (50 m), to 7–8 min and 14–16 min for 800 and 1500 m respectively. Competitive swimming requires high rates of energy turnover. Sprint events depend relatively more on anaerobic production of energy, while longer distances demand more aerobic use of muscle glycogen. High levels of blood lactate (12–20 mmol/L in elite males; lower levels in females) are often observed at the end of races, particularly 100 to 400 m events. In many events, the disturbance of acidity levels within the muscle cell places a likely limitation on performance.

The usual long-course program for key international meets runs over eight days with both morning and evening sessions. A total of 26 gold medals are available for swimmers at the Olympic Games and 32 at the Swimming World Championships. Typically, 400-m events and relays involve heats (morning) and finals (evening) on the same day, whereas events of 50 to 200 m are conducted as heats and semi-finals (same day) and finals (following evening). The 800-m and 1500-m distance freestyle races involve a morning heat and finals on the evening of the following day. It is becoming less common for an elite swimmer to compete in more than two events at any major championships.

Nevertheless, the race programs of exceptional swimmers such as Michael Phelps and Libby Trickett may require competition on six to seven days of the 8–day program, with two or three races on some evening sessions (semi-final of one event, final of another event, and a relay leg).

A unique aspect of the 2008 Beijing Olympics was that finals were swum in the morning to maximise television coverage where viewing audiences were largest.

Other high-level events such as World Cups and Grand Prix programs may be held over 1–3 days, sometimes using a timed final to decide the winner. At a lower level, carnivals can be held over 1–2 days, although age-group championships also have 4–5 day programs. A warm-up including some race-pace swimming is completed before each competition session, with the swim-down after each event being an important recovery strategy. Training is often scheduled on non-competition days.

Physical characteristics

Success in swimming is achieved by the production of high power outputs that are applied in a highly refined technique to move the swimmer against the resistance of water. To produce this power, swimmers must have good muscular development, especially in their upper bodies—back, chest, arms and shoulders. However, strong legs are also required for kicking and for generating speed in the dive start and turns. Swimmers are typically tall, since long bodies and long arms provide biomechanical advantages, but distance swimmers and breaststroke swimmers tend to be shorter and lighter than sprinters, butterfly and backstroke specialists. Swimmers specialising in distance events often have higher body-fat levels than sprinters do.

Swimming is a weight-supported sport, where the buoyancy of the body reduces the energy cost of moving it. Elite swimmers used to carry higher body-fat levels than elite endurance-trained athletes in other sports. However, in recent years there has been a trend to lower body-fat levels, and some of the standout swimmers look very lean as they step onto the blocks. There is no clear evidence that this leanness is the cause of their success—after all, it could simply be a by-product of the hard training and healthy eating that have been part of their winning plan. But it is worth considering whether and how leanness might benefit swimming performance.

Theoretically, any benefits of body fat in terms of greater buoyancy can be counteracted by the extra resistance or drag produced by the movement of a curvier body line through the water. This is one reason why swimmers often find that an increase in body fat is accompanied by a slowing of race times (although that could also be a side-effect of the poor training and badly chosen eating plans that have produced the gain in fat). It is also one explanation of the effects of the now-banned 'fast suits' on swimming performances. Although the materials in these suits do have special properties, their tightness and rigidity reduces the ripples produced when lumps and bumps (e.g. breasts, thighs) move through the water, thus reducing the drag.

Common nutritional issues

The overlay of adolescence

The high training volumes of many swimmers are undertaken in adolescence and early adulthood, a time with its own nutritional demands. Early-morning training sessions are a tradition in swimming—especially for school-age swimmers—and breakfast tends to be eaten on the run. At the other end of the day, the family dinner may be planned around the training and transport needs of school-age athletes. It is a busy schedule, often managed by parents. Many swimmers find it difficult to assume responsibility for their food intake as they move away from home to live alone or in a college or institute. This issue is covered in the chapter on Rugby League and Union. It is important that the adolescent swimmer eat nutritious food choices, since growth and development will increase their needs for protein and micronutrients such as iron and calcium. The guidelines for such sound eating are found in Chapters 1 and 2.

The physical changes of puberty may help to explain an interesting observation—that male swimmers are more likely to have trouble eating enough kilojoules to meet energy needs, while female swimmers struggle to lose body fat. This is because male adolescence is a period of skeletal growth and muscular development, requiring much energy, while females undergo hormonal changes that promote an increase in body fat. For young men, the addition of an intense training program means total energy needs can skyrocket to almost unbelievable levels, while young women, despite equally strenuous training, works uphill against the hormonal messages to lay down fat.

The developing swimmer often encounters conflict between meeting the nutritional demands of their sport and facing the many issues of adolescence and early adulthood. The long hours of training place heavy restrictions on a swimmer's lifestyle, keeping them away from many of the social and recreational activities typical of teenagers. This can either reduce the opportunities to eat in a busy daily schedule, or conversely, increase the inclination to eat for comfort or pure enjoyment. This is another reason why problems of both underweight and overweight are common in swimming.

High energy requirements

The energy demands of swimming training can be immense, particularly when they are added to the demands of adolescent growth. This issue is particularly acute for male swimmers, and getting enough quality kilojoules into them can be hard. During the coverage of Michael Phelps's astounding eight gold medals at the Beijing Olympics, the *New York Post* created a sensation when it reported that he fuelled his five hours of training by consuming 12,000 Cals (~50 megajoules) a day. According to Phelps, the sum of his daily activities was 'eat, sleep and swim'. His menu was full of high-energy sports drinks, multicourse meals and large serves of high-energy foods (French toast topped with sugar, choc-chip pancakes, whole pizzas, fried-egg sandwiches with mayo, etc.) There was some debate among nutrition experts about the accuracy of this report—the consensus was that it was likely either an exaggeration of his everyday diet or represented a single day's eating at the high end of his normal range. But it did show that meeting high energy needs can be a challenge. (Though in the case of an extraordinary athlete like Phelps, his success would allow him to have a team of people looking after his needs.)

There are a number of clever strategies that can be used by swimmers to achieve a high energy intake despite busy lifestyles. These include increasing the number of meals and snacks and making use of energy-dense foods. Planning ahead to have a portable and compact food supply can also be crucial. See Checklist 3.4, and Nick's story below, for more ideas.

Daily recovery

Strenuous daily training calls for a high-energy, fuel-providing diet. The American physiologist David Costill conducted a study on male members of a college swimming team who suddenly doubled their training load over a 10-day period. While some of the squad adapted to the increased workouts, the other swimmers experienced difficulty, complaining of fatigue and muscle soreness. Analysis of their diets showed that the first group had automatically increased their energy and carbohydrate intake to match the increased fuel cost of training, while the second group had not made this adaptation; their muscle glycogen levels were significantly lower as a result. It should be noted that the two groups of swimmers were equally able to perform a 25-yard sprint at the end of the period—at least, their times over this short race were not substantially different. However, the stroke efficiency of the under-fuelled group was reduced. Presumably, over a longer race, or after a longer period of poor training, the differences between fuelling well and poorly would become more evident.

Many of the sections in Part I provide information to prevent or unravel a situation like the one in Costill's study. You can read about the importance of matching carbohydrate and energy intake to actual needs in Chapters 1 and 2, with specific guidelines for achieving carbohydrate needs (Checklist 1.4) and for following a high-energy diet (Checklist 3.4). Chapter 5 provides specific hints on recovery after key workouts, and Checklist 5.1 covers issues related to the key pool workouts undertaken by swimmers. In the case of Nick below, help was needed to find compact vehicles for large amounts of carbohydrate and energy. A bulky diet requires more time to chew than most busy athletes can afford.

Fluid needs in training

Swimmers churn up and down the pool for hours—often in the steamy environment of a heated indoor pool, and occasionally outdoors in the late afternoon heat. However, they are generally able to drink during their workouts—as well as the accidental swallow of water from the pool. As long as they bring a bottle onto the pool deck, they usually have the opportunity to drink between sets. But how much do they need to drink? And how can you tell what your sweat losses are when you are already wet?

We would expect sweat losses during water-based training to be less than in sessions carried out on land. After all, the water is cooler than the body, so some, at least, of the heat produced during exercise can be dissipated without the need for sweating. Figure 2.3 provided a strategy for estimating fluid losses in a given workout. Doing this for water-based exercise is a little more difficult. You need to account for water taken up by your hair and swimsuit in the post-workout weigh-in. When we conduct sweat testing on swimmers at the Australian Institute of Sport, we get around this problem by having them dive in and get wet (and then towelled dry) for the pre-workout weigh-in. Of course we know that there will still be errors in our calculations if swimmers swallow pool water or wee in the pool without our knowledge. We try to be as meticulous as we can, but acknowledge that we need to interpret our results carefully. This is what we have found when we conducted sweat testing to the best of our ability:

- An average sweat rate is ~130 ml per km swum in the session, but there is considerable variation between swimmers and between sessions
- Males sweat at higher rates than females
- Workouts involving sustained high-intensity or race-pace efforts involve higher sweat rates than recovery sessions
- Afternoon workouts generally produce higher sweat rates than morning sessions—this could be a product of the type/intensity of the session, or it may happen because the swimmer has accumulated some heat before coming to the session so sweating is turned on earlier
- Pool sessions undertaken after another session (e.g. weight training or a run) will produce higher sweat rates because, again, the swimmer is hotter at the start.

Our studies have shown that some swimmers underhydrate in some sessions, but rarely enough to reach a fluid deficit of more than 2 per cent of body weight. On the other hand, some swimmers drink more than they sweat—which might explain the bathroom visits before the main set is attacked. A good reason to drink during the session is to consume a sports drink to provide carbohydrate support for key sessions. Of course sports gels, cereal bars and sports bars can also allow the athlete to refuel during fuel-intensive workouts, especially in a heavy training week. So it makes sense to consider good drinking and refuelling strategies during workouts, and to practise in workouts until you find a plan that is right for each session.

Weight control and the female swimmer

If you compare the photos of Dawn Fraser and Shane Gould from the 1960s and 1970s with images of Inge de Bruin and Libby Trickett from the last decade, you will notice a striking difference in the physiques of the two pairs of champions. Of course, many things have changed to explain the super-fast times of today's swimmers—goggles, fast swimsuits, biomechanical analyses and specially designed pools. But it would be easy to draw the conclusion that more muscular and lean physiques also play a role. As we outlined in the section on physique, it is hard to quantify the importance of low body-fat levels in swimming performance independently of the effects of hard training and good diet. Nonetheless, female swimmers today are under great pressure to be lean and to avoid gaining body fat when they go through puberty.

Female swimmers fight a notorious battle—with themselves and their coaches—to keep body-fat measurements to desired levels. Despite heavy training they often complain that they do not seem to burn as many kilojoules as they'd expected to. Not only can this become frustrating, but the constant focus on diet and weight loss can mean that thinking about food becomes almost an obsession. Everything starts to revolve around food—and it can paradoxically become more likely to be used as a source not just of energy but of entertainment, comfort, celebration or commiseration. It can become a vicious circle: You eat because you are upset, your skinfold measurements go up, making you more upset, so you have something to eat to make you feel better. And so on.

Coaches are now being taught not to insist on generic targets for weight and body fat for all members of their squad. It is also dangerous to conduct public weigh-ins and body-fat assessments in the absence of a structure that relates the results to individual goals and performance issues. Instead, each swimmer has a range of desirable physical characteristics within which she (and he) trains and performs well. The key is to allow swimmers to develop and find their ideal range over their lifetime as a swimmer. Female swimmers may need to accommodate growth and changes in body fat during adolescence, as well as a conditioning effect over years of committed training. As in all things, reaching your peak doesn't happen overnight. And there can be times—such as the return from a break or injury—when the swimmer has gained body fat and needs to follow a program to get back into the desired range. If this is the case, Chapter 3 provides a background for understanding about realistic body-fat targets and the need to commit to a long-term fat-loss program that also allows you to train well and stay healthy. The advice of a sports dietitian is very valuable in getting this balance right—especially in the case of young swimmers who are yet to develop good nutritional knowledge and practice, but are vulnerable to insecurities about their body image. The time to strike is before bad practice and poor self-esteem take hold.

Eating disorders and disordered eating

Some studies and recently publicised case histories have found that female swimmers are at high risk of developing eating disorders and disordered eating—resorting to unhealthy techniques such as self-induced vomiting (bulimia) and the use of laxatives to control their weight. Some of this can be traced to pressure within the swimming culture to stay lean, particularly at a time of life when it is normal for a girl to gain body fat. Experts note that the need to wear a revealing outfit can exacerbate poor body image among athletes. It's hard to hide any body fat when all you are wearing is a few centimetres of Lycra, and very tight swim suits can give even the leanest swimmers apparent 'muffin tops' at the intersection of suit and skin.

Most often, swimmers adopt disordered eating practices as a short-term solution to weight problems. Such practices, of course, do not solve or even properly address the real problem. And, in many cases, the 'problem' is exaggerated by excessive concern about body fat and a poor self-image. Read Chapter 3 for a sensible approach to goal-setting, with body-fat targets and a fat-loss program. For a swimmer flirting with an eating disorder, the best help may come from talking things over with professionals—a sports psychologist, who can help you to restore your self-confidence, and a sports dietitian, who can support you to get back into healthy training nutrition. Early intervention is important to prevent problems from developing.

Competition nutrition

Although pool swimmers train like endurance athletes, they compete like sprinters and middle-distance athletes. Preparation for competition generally involves a pronounced tapering-off of training. Depending on the event and beliefs of the coach, this may start 2–3 weeks before the competition, meaning that the swimmer will need to adjust her energy and fuel intake over a substantial period. Some swimmers gain weight in this lower-training period because they fail to respond to their new lower energy needs. This may result from a lack of knowledge, but it can often be caused by failure to adjust portion sizes or habitual eating practices. Making weight control all the more difficult, at the very time when fuel needs are lowest, that opportunities for eating over the day are increased—and the swimmer may also be exposed to an unfamiliar environment and new, tempting foods (see the comments on communal eating below).

Once the race program starts, swimmers should concentrate on making sure their energy budget provides adequate fuel for their targeted races. Generally, they should be able to fuel up for each session by focusing on carbohydrate-rich choices in the 1–2 meals beforehand and the recovery afterwards. This may be challenging for the Michael Phelpses who race in nearly every session of the meet—and sometimes more than once. The challenge comes not only from the fuel needs of so many races (17, in Phelps's Beijing campaign). At the elite level of competition, swimmers often have to accommodate many other commitments around their swimming program. In the typical race schedule involving morning heats and night-time finals, swimmers generally schedule their pre-event breakfast according to the time of their warm-up, then return to a carbohydrate-rich lunch after the heats. Many swimmers like to sleep after this meal, then consume a carbohydrate-rich afternoon snack before returning for the evening race session. Dinner is eaten as soon after this session as possible—however, in the case of elite swimmers, this may be delayed by medal ceremonies, drug testing, and press conferences. Sometimes, swimmers will have to choose between sleep and eating as they try to recover for another early start. Between events, and in the warm-ups and warm-downs surrounding races, swimmers have opportunities to fine-tune fluid and fuel levels and attend to stomach comfort.

It makes sense for all swimmers to examine their individual race schedules and plan their meal routine and pool needs carefully around it. On many occasions, the meet will be away from home base, and swimmers may be relying on hosts in a homestay program, a hotel or an institutional dining hall for their food. He may need to bring supplies from home to ensure that swimmers have a safe, suitable and familiar stock of foods and drinks available. They may also need to bring supplies to the pool so they can fuel, rehydrate and recover at the right time in relation to their events, or have a portable 'back-up' meal if their commitments prevent them going back to their accommodation. Sports drinks and gels are often used for a quick top-up before and after races. Carbohydrate-rich snacks such as yoghurt, fruit, cereal, sports bars, sandwiches or rice cakes can be brought to the pool—particularly in an Esky—and eaten in longer gaps between races or as a recovery snack at the end of a session. Don't forget fruit smoothies or commercial liquid meal supplements if your stomach or timetable calls for a 'lighter' recovery snack combining protein and carbohydrate.

Communal eating—the dining hall

A communal dining hall can be a culture shock for young swimmers, especially if they're on their first trip away from home. This situation may be encountered at swimming camps, at the dining hall in the Athletes' Village during big competitions, or during residence at the Australian Institute of Sport. It has many features in common with 'buffet dining' experiences in hotels. Although the challenges posed by a dining hall might be temporary, they often coincide with a crucial time in the swimmers' life and career. For many, the change from the family dinner table can bring anxiety, temptation and bad food choices. These can result in both short-term consequences (perhaps upsetting competition performance) and long-term problems (upsetting training nutrition goals). The experience of a swimmer we'll call Sara shows how these challenges can be overcome.

Profile: Nick

Chewing through the fuel and energy

Since he'd been invited to train with the elite swim squad in his home town, much of Nick's day was spent staring at the black line on the bottom of the pool. This new squad trained twice a day, so he was now doing twelve training sessions a week, twice as many as he had done at his previous club. At first he coped with the extra training load, but by the end of the second month he was feeling fatigued. Not only were his times beginning to drop off, but his schoolwork had started to get the better of him as well. He was anxious to please his new coach, but despite his efforts to show enthusiasm, his times and his lactate levels told a different story. To cap it all off, his weight was going down despite his introduction to a resistance-training program (three sessions a week in the gym) and the fact that he was outgrowing his shoes every couple of months. Nick could not really afford to lose any more body fat—his skinfold measurements were already the lowest in the squad. Nick's mother encouraged him to eat a larger serve of meat at the evening meal, but by that time of the night he was often too tired to do more than pick at it.

A sports dietitian listened to Nick's story and examined his diet. She told him he needed extra kilojoules to cover the increase in his training volume, and that a lot of these needed to come from carbohydrate-rich foods—an important source of the fuel burned in training. Chronic depletion of muscle glycogen stores was the likely cause of his fatigue problems and explained why he was unable to complete a test set of repeated high-intensity swims. It also explained his low blood lactate levels after trying to do these sets: glycogen provides the quickly turned-over source of fuel that leaves lactate as a by-product. At 70 kg, he should aim for a daily intake of 500–700 g of carbohydrate, but his present diet lagged considerably behind that. And given that Nick was still growing, he needed adequate energy and nutrients to allow him to reach his height potential as well as grow bigger and stronger muscles in response to the weight training program.

When the sports dietitian looked at Nick's schedule and habits, she found he was missing the opportunity to consume foods and fluids before, during and after each workout to enhance his performance and support recovery. He usually just drank water during the session, often even forgetting to bring a bottle and having to dash to the drink fountain outside the change rooms if he felt thirsty. The dietitian explained that replacing water with a carbohydrate source would translate not only into better training performance but also into less breakdown of muscle protein during prolonged high-intensity sessions. It was unproductive to spend time in the gym stimulating protein synthesis before his morning pool session, then sacrifice the results (and perhaps even encourage further protein breakdown) by being in a fuel and energy deficit throughout the subsequent workout. So a better response to the weight training could also be expected from the recommended changes. The final benefit of consuming energy and nutrients at these strategic times would be simply to fit more kilojoules into his busy day so he'd reach energy balance. Nick needed to consider every waking moment as a potential time to make energy deposits.

The sports dietitian showed Nick and his mother a list of carbohydrate-rich foods, and Nick was pleased to note that they were all foods he liked to eat—bread, breakfast cereals, fruit, potatoes, rice and pasta. They all considered partner foods that could add protein, the other important recovery nutrient to a meal or snack—for example, milk on the cereal, meat sauce on pasta, ham and cheese fillings in sandwiches, yoghurt on his fruit. However, it would be tricky to fit all these foods into Nick's day. He already left the table feeling too tired or too full to eat another mouthful. Listening to Nick's typical daily meal plan, the dietitian pointed out that he relied on only three meals per day—breakfast, hastily eaten in the car on the way from the pool to school, lunch, juggled between school activities, and a late evening meal at home. Possible solutions might be to increase the *number* of meals rather than their *size*, and to choose recovery foods that were portable and easy to eat. To enable Nick to graze throughout the day, he and his mother would need to do some planning to ensure the right supplies were on hand at the pool, at school and during travelling times.

Another clever strategy would be to make use of nutritious high-energy fluids, simultaneously replacing his fluid losses over the day and providing a source of energy that didn't need to be chewed. Sports drinks were a no-brainer for training sessions, and outside the pool, Nick learned that rather than filling up with water or cordial (even though that did contain some carbohydrate), he should choose more action-packed drinks such as fruit smoothies and milk shakes, flavoured milk, and commercial liquid meals such as PowerBar Proteinplus or Sustagen Sport. These could be drunk as a pre- or post-training snack, as an accompaniment to meals, or on grazing occasions between meals, without making him feel uncomfortably full. And when he did go out with friends on the weekend, Nick should order a fruit frappe or thick shake rather than developing a coffee habit.

Nick worked with the sports dietitian to remodel his daily eating program, with clever eating before, during and after sessions and between meals as the centrepiece of the new plan. This was topped off with some minor tweaking of his main meals. For example, adding an extra 'layer' to his normal choices—such as yoghurt on his cereal and milk, or an extra protein filling in his sandwich—increased his kilojoule intake a little without the appearance of making him eat more.

Nick's new intake was summarised in the following plan (Table 8.1):

TABLE 8.1
Sample high carbohydrate/high-energy eating plan for Nick (swimmer)

Occasion	Plan
On the way to the pool before morning workout	• Cereal bar • Tetra Pak orange juice
Workout	• Sports drink during pool session • Weights before workout: recovery drink made at pool by adding water to 100 g liquid meal (carbohydrate-protein) powder between sessions • Key pool workouts: 100 g liquid meal supplement after main set
Weekday breakfast (in car on the way to school)	• Ice-cream container full of mixed breakfast cereals plus milk + chopped banana or other fresh fruit • Juice

Occasion	Plan
Weekend breakfast	• 1 bowl cereal + milk + fruit yoghurt • Eggs—scrambled or omelette on thick bread toast • Juice
Morning recess at school	• Large Tetra Pak of flavoured milk • Large piece of muesli slice or fruit bun or 4–5 pikelets
Lunch	• 2 salad rolls or wraps with meat/egg/chicken/cheese + light serve salad • 2 cartons yoghurt or Frûche or rice pudding • Juice 'popper'
After school on way to training	• Cereal or sports bar • Juice 'popper' or flavoured milk depending on GI concerns at upcoming training
Workout	• Sports drink during pool session • Key pool workouts: 100 g liquid meal supplement (carbohydrate-protein) after main set
On way home from training	• 100 g packet of dried fruit/nut mix • Tetra Pak drink
Dinner (waiting at home)	• Large serve of rice/pasta/potatoes • Lean fish/meat/chichen • Vegetables or salad • Juice or milk
Before bed	• Smoothie made with skim milk, fruit (banana, berries, mango, etc.), ice-cream and extra skim-milk powder.
Other snacks if out and about on weekends	• Dried fruit/nut mix or apricot chews • Muffin • Boost juice or smoothie or thickshake

Occasion	Plan
Other snacks if home on weekends	• Crumpets, pancakes, muffins • Jaffles/toasted sandwiches with leftovers or canned tuna or ham/ cheese/tomato • Homemade smoothie

This proposed eating plan would increase Nick's intake to a maximum of ~800 g carbohydrate on a heavy training day and a total 21 000–23 000 kJ (5000–5500 Cal). Since many of the snacks were connected with a training session, the plan would adjust itself up or down according to his training load. It concentrated on everyday foods when possible, saving the more expensive sports foods for situations (such as at the pool) when it was hard to store other foods. Within three weeks Nick reported a new feeling of energy at training, and a weight gain of over a kilogram. His eating program certainly required some planning and organisation, such as packing a cooler bag the night before with food for school and arranging to have access to the staff-room fridge. But with his new lease of energy, Nick has plenty of enthusiasm to get it done!

Profile: Sara

Eating in a communal dining hall—special tactics for a special situation

By the time Sara returned from the Commonwealth Games, she had gained over 2 kg. Her coach at home was half expecting it. He had heard of other swimmers going to the Australian Institute of Sport and gaining 4 kg in the first six months, mostly from increased body fat. His own daughter was heading off to a university dorm life with trepidation. Thanks to her obsession with American teen soaps, she had heard all about the 'fresher 10'—the 10 lb that college students in the US allegedly gain in their first (freshman) year. His son, on the other hand, who'd gone off to university the previous year, came home at the end of each term complaining that there was never enough to eat in his college dining room.

Most people who eat in an institution, whether it's a boarding school, a hospital or the Olympic Athletes' Village, have definite views about the food there. Common complaints are: 'there's no variety', 'all the goodness is cooked out of it', 'it's fattening—you'll put on weight', and 'there's never enough to eat—weight just drops off'. Dining rooms specially set up for athletes, such as those at the Australian Institute of Sport or at big sports meets, or the 'training tables' for athletes at American universities are definitely not guilty of these charges. In addition to serving massive volumes of food, and staying open for long hours to cater for the varying schedules of the athletes, the cooks at these dining rooms pay particular attention to the nutritional needs of athletes. It is the athletes who are ultimately responsible for what goes into their mouth. In most cases, when a complaint about bad food is closely examined, the real problem is found to be the athlete's choices not the foods themselves.

Most people are accustomed to eating at home, where the cooking is done by them or a family member. They are used to having one or two items on the 'menu' at a time, and although they may think they eat a variety of dishes, they probably stick to a handful of favourite recipes with only an occasional change. In any case, it is all very familiar and under control. The sudden switch to a communal cafeteria-style dining hall brings:

- Great quantities and many different choices of food. You can serve yourself as much as you like from a neverending supply, and there are so many nice things to try. Many athletes find that they lose the plot in such circumstances—because it's so easy to eat more than usual, and more than they need.
- Limited access to food outside designated eating times. If the dining hall is only open at certain times, athletes with enormous energy needs may not be able to consume enough food at the customary three meals and may lose weight.
- Different and unusual foods. It can be challenging to find a counter laden with new foods and dishes. You may be reluctant to experiment when it comes to trying new foods, or maybe you are unsure of their nutritional value. This can lead to weight loss or failure to meet nutritional goals.
- Lack of supervision. Many athletes come unstuck when they first move to the dining hall and find that Mum is no longer around to make them eat their vegetables.

- Distraction from other athletes. Surrounded by the eating habits of a large group of people, you may find it hard to concentrate on your own nutritional goals. And, given the competitive nature of athletes, it isn't surprising that official and unofficial 'eating competitions' can take place.
- Eating for entertainment. An athlete may not have much time or scope for leisure activities during the day. If the dining hall becomes a substitute, he may demolish a lot of extra food in the name of relaxation and recreation.

Faced with these challenges, athletes must take special steps to use the dining hall to its optimum potential. Checklist 8.1 will help you make good decisions. Note that many of these ideas come in handy in any buffet dining situation.

Profile: Tom and Tammie

Old swimmers never die, they just become larger than life

During the 2008 Olympic Games, many past sporting champions appeared on TV as commentators. This brought together many veteran swimmers. It was a great time for reminiscing about the Good Old Days and trying to recognise friends who hadn't been seen in years.

Tom was a larger-than-life member of the swimming commentary panel. He had ballooned since his glory days. Once he had been a triple medallist. Now, triple referred to his XXXL shirt size—and a triple bypass might be somewhere in his future. It was hard to believe that he had been lean and trim only a decade before. But the old footage didn't lie—and his present waistline couldn't be hidden.

When Tom retired from swimming after the Athens Olympics, he had been keen to make up for the 'lost time' of his early adulthood. While his university friends had been out partying and having fun, he had spent his time eating sensibly under the watchful eye of his mother, going to bed early, and pounding up and down the pool. His coach had believed in high-volume training, and his program usually required 20–25 hours a week of high-intensity swimming and gym workouts.

After his last race, he'd vowed to limit his water exposure to baths and showers. He partied hard, laughing at how he now came home from a night on the town at the same time when he used to leave home for morning training. Beer became his new sports drink and he rehydrated strenuously. He moved out of home into an apartment with some friends. Their fridge provided liquid refreshments and on its door were the phone numbers of pizza places and fast-food restaurants. If it wasn't for the roast on his weekly family visit, Tom would have been lucky to meet a vegetable.

Tom's weight gain was quick. But he joked that he'd enjoyed every gram of it since it was achieved by a lifestyle that seemed like liberation from his years of regimented and disciplined existence. After two years, he was ready to settle down. He thought that one of the benefits of getting married would be having all his meals cooked for him. But even regular meals only seemed to make things worse, since he snacked a lot and piled his plates with favourite foods. In his new job as a swimming coach he did little exercise. It was back to 4.30 a.m. starts to supervise squad training, and staying on the pool deck until quite late at night. He periodically tried to start swimming or running at lunch times, but usually abandoned his good intentions after a week or so because of fatigue and lack of time.

Tammie also surprised her former team mates with her new look. People remembered her as a chubby but talented swimmer whose career had ended prematurely because of her gradual weight gain and the resulting battles with her coach. Looking back, it had involved more misery than enjoyment or success. After she retired she too vowed to step right away from the pool scene. Although she didn't party as hard as Tom did, she enjoyed the freedom of not having to train or watch what she was eating. Her coach and her mother had always been on her back about her diet. This had led to guilt, worry, secret eating, and at least 16 hours of the day spent thinking about food. Now she could enjoy what she wanted. After all, she wasn't planning to wear a swimsuit for quite some time.

In the first six months she gained a little weight. However, after a while Tammie began to lose her obsession with food and eating. As long as she knew that she could eat if she was hungry, she found that she could take food or leave it. She began to leave it, and settled into a healthy eating plan. She also took up playing basketball in a team with some friends. It wasn't a serious competition, and she enjoyed the novelty of team play and not having to be 'The Best'. She found herself going out for a run a few nights each week, just to keep fit for the game. And a swim or two each week kept her 'feel' for the water intact. Ten years on, trim and fit, she can hardly believe she struggled so hard with her weight in her competitive swimming days.

Tom and Tammie represent the opposite ends of the Life after Sport spectrum. Tammie's story shows that sometimes the pressures of elite-level sport create eating problems that have nothing to do with the nutritional demands of the sport in question. Away from the pressures, the problems can resolve themselves.

Tom's story is an all-too-common one. It doesn't occur only at the end of an illustrious swimming career. Sometimes a swimmer just gets sick of the discipline of training and reverts to a life of sloth—at least for the short term. Sometimes injury forces retirement. When swimming stops, that may be the end of all exercise. Other commitments take up time and energy and may introduce new sources of temptation like business lunches. Alcohol may also play a big new role in the ex-swimmer's life.

During elite sports careers, athletes are often required to eat more than their appetite ever suggested. It can be difficult to 'listen' to their appetite when massive kilojoule intakes are no longer needed, or to realise that the strategies that made kilojoules easy to eat before, such as high-energy fruit smoothies, are now counterproductive.

When a sports career is over, all athletes need to take stock of their eating and activity patterns and find a new balance. In some cases, a change in body physique is to be expected. However, this should be judged according to what is healthy rather than by the requirements of the (former) sport. Because they tend to retire young, swimmers may need extra help to find new dietary patterns and a new outlook on exercise. Given time and good management, a retired swimmer can move into a new, healthy and happy lifestyle.

CHECKLIST 8.1
Eating well in a cafeteria-style dining hall

- Develop the right attitude. The food is not 'fattening' or 'bad for you'. You can control your own nutritional destiny by the way you choose your foods.

- Have your goals clear, especially if you are at a time of altered energy needs or competition demands. Treat the dining room like a restaurant. If there is no written menu, survey the choices before you commit yourself to a queue. Look for nutrition cards that will tell you more about each dish. Decide what you will have, before you are served.
- Don't get into the line and keep piling more food on your plate as you pass each dish. We call this 'compost eating'. Apart from the likelihood that you will overeat, this style of dining minimises the sense of variety from night to night. You will quickly get bored with it.
- Be prepared to exercise restraint with portion sizes or menu choices, even if the menu is advertised as being athlete-focused.
- Don't be distracted by the other foods you have not chosen for this meal. There will be other opportunities to try the things you missed today.
- Ignore what other athletes eat. Stick to what is right for you and keep in mind that your nutritional needs and theirs may be very different.
- Allow yourself some flexibility for special treats—but choose them well, with your nutritional goals in mind.
- Leave the dining hall once you have finished eating. If you join those hanging out there beyond mealtimes, you will soon find yourself eating for entertainment rather than need.
- If you need more energy than the offered meals provide, take a snack for later on—a sandwich, some fruit or some flavoured yoghurt are good choices.
- Seek help if you need information or have special food requirements. There is often a dietitian or food-service expert who can help with any queries or problems.

Road Cycling

Road cycling enjoys a long history of organised competition: the Tour de France is more than 100 years old. Men's road cycling is a professional sport dominated by sponsored trade teams made up of cyclists from all over the world. Many of these cyclists are household names in Europe, the heart of the racing scene. The successes of Australian cyclists such as Cadel Evans, Mick Rogers, Robbie McEwan and Stuart O'Grady have helped to increase the profile of professional road cycling back home, and Adelaide's Tour Down Under is now first on the calendar of international ProTour races. Apart from the professional circuit, top cyclists also compete for their national teams at World Championships (annually) and the Olympic Games (every four years). Women too engage in the sport, though the professional circuit for female road cyclists is newer and less developed.

Training

World-class riders typically cycle 25 000 to 35 000 km a year. Training is done between events within the racing calendar or in the form of less important races. Most time is spent on the road, although wind-trainers and rollers allow some training to be done indoors. The focus in the pre-season and early season is often on riding 'into shape' to reduce body-mass and body-fat levels. Riders typically organise their training and competition program to allow them to peak for specific races or tours within the season. At the height of the season in Europe, cyclists may do little training because they are continually racing, thanks to a packed race calendar and a selection of longer stage races.

Specialised training techniques such as interval training and altitude training assist the performance of road cyclists. However, racing itself appears to be an important form of training. Tools such as SRM PowerMeter cranks have allowed us to examine the high power outputs achieved by elite cyclists during races, and it seems that these can be achieved only by racing. This helps to explain why professional cyclists improve their performance over the competitive season even against the background of such high-volume training. Spending so much time on the bike, elite cyclists rarely undertake any other type of training. One possible exception may be in the relatively short pre-season or while rehabilitating from injury, when an elite cyclist may engage in some weight training, flexibility work, or other forms of aerobic activity.

At the serious club level, cyclists generally do 300–600 km of training a week and may have more opportunity to undertake specific training programs between their weekly or seasonal racing commitments than the elite cyclist on the ProTour circuit. Such training is undertaken to improve the cyclist's aerobic base and capacity for high-intensity work, but also to improve riding technique and aerodynamic positioning.

Competition

Professional cyclists typically race about 100 days each year. Competitive road cycling offers a number of common race formats. The shortest races are the prologues, or brief time trials for individual riders, often held at the start of a stage race or tour. Such races can be completed in as little as 10 min. However, the duration of an individual time-trial event at the world championships or Olympic Games is typically around 40 km (~60 min) for men and 20 km (~30 min) for women. The world record for one hour of cycling is a well-recognised target for elite road cyclists, despite being completed on a cycling track or velodrome. The individual time trial represents a true test of the rider's cycling ability, requiring efficiency in technique and riding position and the ability to sustain high and relatively constant power outputs for the duration of the race. Analysis of the performance of elite time-trial specialists shows that they are able to sustain exercise intensities near, or even slightly above, their lactate threshold, the point at which lactate starts accumulating in the blood, for 30 to 60 min.

Mass-start road races, whether single events or stages within a tour, cover a range of distances and typically last 2–8 hr. Road races can be conducted on a loop course, but many courses cover the distance between two towns or landmarks. Criterium races, or crits, involving multiple laps of a small loop circuit, are popular with spectators. Mass-start road races are made up of lengthy periods of submaximal or aerobic work interspersed with periods of high-intensity activity. Cycling intensity is affected by features of the race course—climate, wind, hills, and road surface—but more particularly by race tactics. Drafting, or riding behind another cyclist or group of cyclists, reduces the drafter's energy cost by reducing his drag or aerodynamic resistance. As a result, the exercise intensities of cyclists riding within a large bunch (called a *péloton*) can be quite modest, around 150 watts. However, power-output data collected during actual races show multiple brief efforts at very high intensities along with sustained periods of hard effort as the cyclists climb a hill, break away from a pack or sprint to the finish line. A professional cycling team generally contains a range of cyclists who excel at different specialties (e.g. time trials, hill climbs, or sprints) or who are assigned different tasks within the race (e.g. *domestiques*, who ride to support the team leader). As a result, the overall race performance of a cyclist is affected by both the type of course and his designated role within a team.

Some mass-participation races allow professional riders and recreational cyclists to compete in the same field, in a similar mix as that in Big City Marathon events. Some of these bike races attract large fields—for example, the annual 105-km Cape Argus tour in Cape Town, South Africa, is limited to 35 000 competitors! Popular mass-participation rides in Australia include the Round the Bay in a Day and the multi-day Great Victorian Bike Ride.

Physical characteristics

A successful road cyclist can generate power to move efficiently against the rolling resistance of the road, wind resistance, and, in the case of uphill cycling, gravity. The striking characteristics of elite road cyclists are a high aerobic capacity and the ability to sustain power outputs at a high percentage of this capacity. Physical characteristics vary according to the specialisation of riders. All cyclists strive for low body-fat levels to increase their power-to-weight ratio. However, hill-riding specialists are smaller and lighter than other cyclists and thus less subject to gravity's pull. Level-ground time-trial specialists are typically larger and heavier than other cyclists because a higher muscle mass can generate more power. Furthermore, a low ratio of body surface area to body mass improves aerodynamic resistance. Although some genetically gifted athletes inherit these characteristics, most cyclists will strive through training and dietary manipulation to enhance muscle mass, body mass, and body-fat level according to the needs of their desired specialty or for all-around excellence.

Common nutritional issues

Training nutrition

Training for road cycling is time and energy consuming. The long kilometres and hours of training undertaken by elite cyclists call for a high-energy diet—high in protein, vitamins and minerals, and matching carbohydrate to muscle-fuel needs. (Chapters 1 and 2 provide a discussion of the optimum training diet.) Daily recovery between heavy training sessions may require extra energy and nutrients, but also clever timing of meals and snacks to enhance refuelling and repair/adaptation processes. As Chapter 5 explains, a carbohydrate-protein snack or meal immediately after a long training session will kick-start muscle glycogen synthesis to prepare fuel stores for the next day's training session and supply the building blocks for new muscle fibres. Also related to the timing of food intake is the idea of periodising the training diet—changing nutritional priorities according to the type of training that is being undertaken and the specific goals that are set. This is also discussed in Chapter 2.

As well as providing timely nutrient intake after training sessions, a pattern of frequent meals and snacks can help to ensure that energy and carbohydrate needs are met when requirements are high (Chapters 2.9 and 3.8). The sheer bulk of food needed to supply a high-energy diet may make it hard to pack enough into three meals a day. Some dietary studies of elite cyclists have estimated their average daily energy intake at over 20 MJ (~5000 Cal). Imagine trying to reduce this energy target to three 7000-kJ meals—it would be the equivalent of three Christmas dinners each day! Many cyclists who manage a high energy intake graze throughout the day as well as consuming substantial amounts of energy on the bike and immediately after training sessions.

Body-fat levels and body weight

Low body-fat levels are as much part of modern cycling as carbon fibre is of bikes! Cyclists specialising in hill climbing or preparing for a hilly race also want to reduce body mass, often at the expense of their muscle mass. (Note the relatively skinny upper bodies and arms of top cyclists.) Cycling culture is replete with tales of the sacrifices made by elite cyclists to become lighter and leaner—and the rewards they've reaped by doing so. Lance Armstrong is a notable example. In his book *It's Not About the Bike*, he explained that weight loss was an unexpected benefit of the chemotherapy he received for testicular cancer: 'There was one unforeseen benefit of cancer: it had completely reshaped my body . . . now I was almost gaunt . . . Eddy Merckx had been telling me to slim down for years, and now I understood why . . . I had lost 15 pounds. It was all I needed.'[1]

In the sequel, *Every Second Counts*, Armstrong described the effort it took to stay lean:

> You had to become a slave to data, to performance indicators like pedal cadence, and power output measured in watts. You had to measure literally every heartbeat, and every morsel you ate, down to each spoonful of cereal. You had to be willing to look like a vampire, your body-fat hovering around three to four per cent, if it made you faster. If you weighed too little, you wouldn't have the physical resources to generate enough speed. If you weighed too much, your body was a burden. It was a matter of power to weight.[2]

Many individual stories and some studies describe methods used by cyclists to reduce or maintain a low body weight and body-fat levels. They include deliberately undereating during high-volume training periods—which even includes stage races that the cyclist aims just to complete rather than perform well in. Cyclists may also restrict their fuel intake before or during training sessions to promote 'fat burning'. Of course, negative energy balance is not conducive to optimal performance, and if taken to extremes may cause the problems associated with low energy availability (see Chapter 3.5). Cycling with inadequate fuel intake is likely to impair performance and may increase the risk of illness and injury.

Mastering this topic involves making the correct choice of race weight and identifying the best way to achieve any weight/fat loss. It is likely that all cyclists will return after the off-season or a period of injury with body fat that needs to be shed. It's hard to argue against gravity, friction and wind resistance. However, as Lance Armstrong noted, it is a matter of 'power to weight' not weight alone! The successful cyclist will find a body weight and an eating plan that allow them to train hard so they'll be able to generate high power outputs and have adequate fuel in their muscles on race day. Sometimes, cyclists will allow their race weight to fluctuate over a season, achieving their lowest level as part of their peak for an important race or a race requiring special physique characteristics (e.g. a hilly course). But in all cases, they will need a careful eating plan to achieve the energy deficit required for weight loss without sacrificing key training targets or their own health. See Chapter 3.4 for ideas—and a note on the benefits of consulting with a sports dietitian.

Special needs for female riders

Female cyclists especially need to find a sensible approach to weight and body-fat loss. The casualties of excessive dieting can include a healthy menstrual cycle, strong bones and a comfortable feeling about food—for more information, read Chapters 2.6 and 3.5, and the story of Lola in the next chapter, on distance running. Although we need studies to investigate this, it's likely that the negative effects of low energy availability on bone are more pronounced in cyclists than on athletes in other 'thin-build sports', since cycling is a non-weight-bearing activity and does not have the same protective effect on bone as running or gymnastics do. Calcium intake is also important for building healthy bones (Chapter 2.6).

Some female cyclists contribute to their weight problems by overdoing pre-race fuelling and post-race recovery eating. This is especially true of young riders who are stepping up to a higher level of competitive racing. The race distances in women's cycling are usually much shorter than in men's racing, and it's easier to follow 'male models' and take in more energy than is actually needed. Many young riders also over-fuel for fear of 'bonking' or being dropped from a race. A sports dietitian can help you to understand the real fuel and nutritional needs of racing and develop a plan that hits your individual targets. Sometimes it takes a season or two of racing before young riders develop the strength, endurance and tactics to stay with the pack. Overeating will not only hinder this process, it will create another set of problems.

Inadequate iron intake may be an issue for all cyclists with a heavy race program, since the focus on carbohydrate for fuel needs can override concern about overall micronutrient intake. This may be especially true for female cyclists, who need more iron than males but less energy. Read Chapter 2.5 and see how adequate iron intake can be meshed with other nutritional goals, such as a high fuel intake or reducing body-fat levels.

Race preparation and the pre-race meal

Generally, exercise lasting longer than 90 min of continuous work saps an athlete's muscle glycogen stores. Fuel needs can be hard to judge in a road race, the intensity of the work may vary according to the tactics of the day and the terrain, but a good rule is to prepare for each individual race in which you wish to perform well by topping up muscle fuel stores during at least the 12 to 36 hr before the event. The longer and more important the race, the better the fuelling should be. Opportunities for fuelling will vary depending on your program and goals. They may be few in a race series or stage race where events are scheduled every day, or when you are is continuing high-volume training right up to a race. Even when you are watching energy intake for weight-loss purposes, you should consider the benefits of better fuelling just before a race. It also makes sense to make use of every hour between stages in a tour by starting to eat or drink carbohydrate as soon as is practical after the end of each stage. Chapters 4 and 5 provide strategies for fuelling up and refuelling.

Many cycling races start in mid-morning or afternoon, allowing riders time for a substantial carbohydrate-rich breakfast or brunch. Choose a pre-race meal based on your individual race nutrition plan, the practical opportunities provided by the schedule, and the lessons learned from previous races.

Food and fluid needs during long rides

Whether in training or racing, cyclists ride over distances that challenge their fluid and fuel levels. Sweat losses can be high in hot weather and when working hard, but you may not notice this if the sweat evaporates quickly in the wind. In a hot laboratory, a fluid deficit of as little as 2 per cent leads to measurable physiological impairments (heart function and temperature control) and reduced ability to cycle (perception of effort is increased and work output decreased). Some scientists argue that in real-life conditions, a fluid deficit has less impact. The cooling effects of wind and moving through the air are difficult to simulate with laboratory fans. In the field, they may provide extra assistance to keep body temperatures from overheating. Of course, if you are drafting or riding in the middle of a péloton, you are trying to avoid this movement of air over your body, so you may miss out on its cooling benefit.

Some cyclists feel that fluid lost through sweating is also a loss of weight to carry. There are reports that some top cyclists make a calculated decision to let themselves become dehydrated before hitting a mountain stage so the energy cost of riding uphill will be lower. A study organised by Tammie Ebert at the AIS compared full hydration with a 2 per cent fluid deficit, achieved by restricted drinking in the early part of a ride, when cyclists had to ride uphill in hot conditions. The 'uphill' effect was simulated by riding on a treadmill with a steep 8 per cent incline. When they were lighter, cyclists were able to do the hill climb at the same speed as when fully hydrated but with a lower power output (308 W vs. 313 W), showing that they were more efficient. However, their ability to continue riding at this speed was reduced by ~29 per cent. Therefore, the ill effects of dehydration appear to outweigh any physical advantages of weight loss, albeit under a laboratory simulation of race conditions. This finding needs to be tested in a race setting.

Chapters 2 and 4 describe strategies for monitoring fluid levels during training rides and races. These will help you to assess typical volumes of fluid lost via sweat and your success in replacing these. It is not necessary to replace them entirely during a workout or race, but the general aim should be to keep your fluid deficit low—below 2 per cent of body weight. On a training ride, drinks need to be carried on the bike or the rider. For longer training rides, it might make sense to stop to replenish these supplies. In races, feeding zones are set up where volunteer handlers or professional team *soigneurs* hand out drinks (and food) to their riders. In professional races, team cars also follow the riders, and it is the job of the team's *domestique* riders to ferry extra bottles to the designated leaders.

When should you add refuelling to your race tactics? Several laboratory-based studies suggest that benefits may be seen in races as short as ~40 km or 1 hr duration. Chapter 4 explains that in these brief but high-intensity events, even a small amount of carbohydrate may give your brain a buzz and make you feel like working harder. In longer races, especially when you haven't fuelled up fully beforehand, the benefits of carbohydrate intake come from providing a substantial fuel source for your muscles. The general target is 30–60 g/hr, although in stage races, where very high energy expenditures are maintained for a week or longer, cyclists often consume more than 1 g carbohydrate per hour. This generally comes from a mixture of sports drinks, sports gels and bars, and everyday foods. In longer races, too, cyclists like to have a range of choices to avoid flavour fatigue and the discomfort of an empty stomach. Popular everyday foods include bananas, cakes and bread rolls. A range of supplies is often packed into a *musette* bag and provided to cyclists at the race feeding zones.

Multi-stage races: the challenge of recovery

Whether in recreational bike tours like the Great Victorian Bike Ride or in important professional stage races, many cyclists ride day after day. In the Grand Tours—the Tour de France, the Giro D'Italia and the Spanish Vuelta—individual stages may be up to 200 km and the events may last up to three weeks. Such constant hard work places enormous stress on cyclists' fuel and fluid reserves, and if they are not topped up fully, the deficit carries over to the next day. Riders need to adopt special nutritional strategies to assist recovery overnight as well as meeting the needs of each stage. The main factor in success is not being the best on any one day but being able to do it again tomorrow. This was highlighted by the feat of Greg LeMond, who in winning the 1990 Tour de France became the first rider to gain overall honours without having won a single stage along the way.

Recovery nutrition is covered in Chapter 5. Particularly relevant to cyclists are the sections on fluid and carbohydrate replenishment and, in the case of long tours, maintaining adequate total nutrient intake. From a practical point of view, nutritional arrangements for multi-day events may be left up to individual competitors or teams, or they may be part of in the overall organisation of the event. Often, accommodation and meals are included in the race or tour package. These may vary from camp sites with army-style cooking to hotel hospitality.

The disadvantages of relying on the event organisation for food include unsuitable food, a need to follow their feeding timetable rather than one designed to meet your needs, and the need to compete with many other people for the same food. It may be safer to arrange part or all of your race diet and catering yourself—especially if the race organisation is unfamiliar to you or if your nutritional needs are crucial to good performance. It doesn't hurt to bring some of your own supplies, especially the specific foods and drinks that are part of your race and post-race eating strategies. Professional teams in important races will often come with a full back-up team and an aggressive nutrition plan.

Profile: Tour de France

Energy in/energy out

The Tour de France is no picnic—4000 km in 20-odd days over some of the most rugged terrain in Europe. Yet eating and drinking, especially on the bike, play a crucial role in getting competitors through this gruelling race. Several studies of the Tour de France and other long road races help us understand how. An extensive investigation was carried out on the 1988 race by some Dutch physiologists, led by Wim Saris. They followed the fortunes of five male cyclists from one of the leading professional teams. Daily energy expenditure was estimated, and the cost of each day's cycling was taken from the detailed descriptions of each stage. Body weight and body fat were checked over the course of the race, and cyclists kept a record of all food and fluid intake.

The most remarkable result was the estimate of energy expenditure for the race—an average 25 400 kilojoules (6060 Cal) a day. The heaviest day of exercise was estimated to cost 32 700kJ (7800 Cal), and on the sole rest day, energy expenditure was estimated to drop below 13 000kJ (3100

Cal). Despite this colossal energy output, only minor changes in body weight and body fat were noted over the three-week race. Indeed, the average estimated energy intake from food, drinks and supplements was 24 700kJ (5900 Cal) a day. The riders not only balanced their energy needs over the three weeks, but managed to balance intake and expenditure remarkably well on a daily basis. This was important, since with the large amounts needing to be eaten it would be hard to catch up from one day to the next if one's intake fell behind. There is only so much that a person can put into his stomach each day!

Carbohydrate was well looked after, making up over 60 per cent of total food intake. The cyclists churned through an average of nearly 850 g of carbohydrate each day—12–13 g per kg of body mass per day—further evidence of the remarkable fuel needs of the race. Protein intake, at around 220 g per day, was more than adequate, and supplied about 15 per cent of total energy during the period, or an intake of over 3 g per kg body mass per day. Fat intake, supplying about 23 per cent of energy intake, was well below levels seen in the typical Western diet. Vitamin and mineral intakes were above requirements, both on the basis of standard recommended dietary intake levels and from blood measurements of micronutrient status. These nutrients came not only from food but from fortified liquid formulas (such as high-carbohydrate and liquid meal supplements) and from additional vitamin supplements as well. As would be expected based on sweat loss, fluid intake was high—an average of 6.7 L per day per cyclist.

So what did the cyclists eat? The range of carbohydrate-rich foods listed included cakes, pasta, bread and breakfast cereals, while high-protein foods were dominated by meats, dairy products and eggs. An important contribution to both carbohydrate and energy intake was made by carbohydrate-rich drinks—soft drinks, and more particularly sports drinks, liquid meal supplements and high-carbohydrate formulas. About a third of total carbohydrate intake was provided by these drinks—which offer obvious advantages in terms of compact and digestible energy. It is also of interest to note that a substantial part of each day's intake was consumed on the bike. Nearly half the day's energy and nearly 60 per cent of total carbohydrate intake was consumed during the race at an average hourly rate of 94 g (~1.4–1.5.g of carbohydrate per kg body mass). Fluid intake while on the bike averaged 4 L per day.

Asker Jeukendrup, a Dutch exercise physiologist now working at the University of Birmingham, has described his experiences with the Rabobank cycling team at the Tour de France. He highlighted the practical challenges of trying to achieve extremely high energy intakes for weeks on end, explaining that cyclists are often exhausted, have lost their sense of hunger, have been eating the same foods every day for two weeks, and are suffering from gastrointestinal disturbances. He noted that they learn through experience how much they need to eat to prevent a major energy or fuel deficit—this is one of the advantages of racing 90–100 days a year.

Jeukendrup's description of a typical day in the life of a Tour de France cyclists starts with a substantial breakfast of bread, muesli, cornflakes, and some fruit, with coffee, milk, and orange juice. Sometimes when the stage ahead is very long, a plate of pasta or rice is added. On the bike, riders eat small cakes, white rolls with jam, energy bars and 2–8 per cent carbohydrate solutions, depending on the weather conditions. Water and cola drinks are also consumed. After each stage, they consume a carbohydrate-protein drink or drink a carbohydrate solution and eat a ham sandwich. They continue to snack on fruit, energy bars, and cakes until dinner. Dinner is usually the largest meal of the day—plates of pasta or rice, often accompanied by chicken, fish or meat. The quality of this meal is entirely dependent on what the hotels provide; sometimes the food is well prepared but often the meals are overcooked and not very tasty. In the evening there is still time to eat smaller amounts of sweets, cake, and fruit before the riders go to sleep.

Jeukendrup refers to this pattern as functional eating, since it has little to do with appetite, comfort or enjoyment. He also describes the importance of having new foods or 'treat' foods along the way to break food boredom and add a flavour fillip to fatigue. His recent scientific studies have looked at carbohydrate drinks that are better absorbed than the conventional sports drinks. Jeukendrup found that mixing a couple of different carbohydrate sources—specifically, a mixture of glucose and fructose in a ratio of 2:1—achieved better absorption than glucose alone. This occurred because the different carbohydrates were taken up from the gut via different transporters. The practical implications of his work included not only a better delivery of fuel to muscles, but reduced discomfort from undigested carbohydrate in the athlete's gut.

It is enormously challenging to maintain the large energy intakes required in a long and gruelling road race in the face of limited appetite or time available for eating. But with good planning and the support of science, it can be done.

Profile: Caffeine and the road cyclist

Is Coke the real thing?

If you've watched a road cycling race, triathlon or marathon in the last five years, you may have noticed a curious thing. After drinking a sports drink for most of the race, competitors suddenly switch to their 'secret weapon'—Coca-Cola! Feed zones and aid stations are awash in cans and bottles bearing the iconic red-and-white logo. The Coca-Cola company's marketing prowess is well known, but there is no advertising campaign telling athletes that 'things go better with Coke in the last third of an endurance event'. Nor does Coca-Cola mount sponsorship drives to put its products on bikes or in the hands of runners. Can experienced athletes really be turning their backs on sports drinks, supported by millions of dollars worth of research and hundreds of scientific publications, in favour of a beverage that's mostly sugar, caffeine and flavouring?

Caffeine . . . At marathons in the 1980s, it was common to see runners pouring cups of strong black coffee from thermoses as they finished their warm-ups and congregated at the race start. Cyclists are still connoisseurs of the pre-race coffee, and the coaches of many pro teams travel with coffee machines that would be at home in any Italian cafe. Caffeine has been known as a stimulant and used in sport for its ergogenic properties for at least a century. But relatively new scientific evidence both supports the competition caffeine hit and explains the recent sudden increase in its popularity. In the late 1970s, papers began to appear in the peer-reviewed literature ascribing metabolic and performance advantages to the consumption of caffeine in the hour before to endurance exercise. The first of these came from the Human Performance Laboratories of Ball State University in Indiana, under the leadership of Professor Dave Costill. Costill's reputation in running circles as a 'sports science guru' ensured that this information quickly spread, via articles in popular running magazines and word of mouth, to large groups of runners of varying abilities. Many studies published since

Costill's have confirmed the ergogenic effect of consuming moderate to large doses of caffeine (5–6 mg per kg of body mass) in the hour before a range of exercise activities.

The number of endurance athletes switching to Coca-Cola in the last part of a race intrigued us and our fellow sports scientists at the AIS. Although cyclists told us they drank Coke for the 'caffeine kick', we felt the dose (~1–1.5 mg per kg of body mass) and the timing (in the last 20–60 minutes of the race) would be unlikely to achieve the same effects as the standard caffeine protocol developed in the 1980s. We suspected that either the Coke was delivering a placebo effect or that other aspects of switching to it (such as its higher carbohydrate content compared to sports drinks, or the change in taste) were also involved in performance changes. In any case, enthusiastic testimonials from athletes prompted us to investigate the mysterious 'Coke effect'. Together with colleagues from RMIT University in Melbourne and the University of Canberra, we completed two studies based on the same protocol. Each study involved well-trained cyclists or triathletes, who undertook a 2.5-hour cycling task on four separate occasions, after 24 hours of controlled training and diet and abstinence from foods and drinks containing caffeine. The cycling task was divided into a two-hour segment completed at a steady aerobic workload followed by a 30-min time trial. This allowed us to monitor metabolism for the first part of the race, then measure performance. The athletes ate a carbohydrate-rich pre-race meal and drank sports drink (about 1 L per hour) throughout the task—in other words, they followed recommended race nutrition strategies.

In the first study, twelve athletes completed the trial. For each of their four cycling bouts they received one of the following treatments:

- A single caffeine dose of 6 mg/kg body weight consumed 1 hour before the 'race'
- Six 1 mg/kg caffeine doses consumed every 20 minutes during the 'race'
- A switch from sports drink to defizzed Coca-Cola for the last 40 minutes of the 'race'
- A placebo treatment of dummy capsules

Despite beliefs that caffeine increases the use of fat as an exercise fuel and spares precious glycogen stores, we found no differences in muscle fuel use among these four treatments. But in the time-trial (Figure 9.1), the cyclists rode ~3 per cent faster when they took caffeine or drank Coke than when they took the placebo pills. The size of the caffeine/Coke intake made no difference, nor did its timing. We were stunned! Of course, the cyclists knew when they were receiving Coke, so if they expected it to make them go faster, they may have talked themselves into a better time-trial through the powers of positive thinking.

Because of this, we did another study under a fully 'blinded' protocol—meaning that neither the subjects nor the key researchers knew which treatment was being received. Because the switch to Coke at the end of the race meant not only a caffeine boost but a change in flavour and an increase in carbohydrate intake over sports drink, we used similar drinks with different combinations of caffeine and carbohydrate. Eight athletes completed the same four bouts of cycling as in the first study, but this time they all had their sports drink switched at the end of the race to ~750 ml of a cola drink of the following formulas:

- 6 per cent carbohydrate, no caffeine (i.e. a cola-flavoured sports drink)
- 6 per cent carbohydrate, 13 mg/100 ml caffeine (sports-drink carb content; caffeine content of Coke)
- 11 per cent carbohydrate, no caffeine (a cola-flavoured drink with added carbohydrate)
- 11 per cent carbohydrate, 13 mg/100 ml caffeine (Coca-Cola)

Compared with the cola-tasting sports-drink placebo, Coca-Cola again provided a ~3 per cent boost in the time-trial, confirming the results of our first study were real. Our stats man helped us to tease out which components of Coke provided the benefits—a 2 per cent improvement came from the relatively small amount of caffeine (~1.5 mg/kg body mass) and a 1 per cent improvement from the drink's increased carbohydrate content over sports drink (Figure 9.2).

These studies are part of a new wave of caffeine research showing that even very small doses enhance performance, especially when they are consumed when the athlete is starting to become fatigued. In fact, the caffeine doses provided by the Coke treatment in our study are the smallest that have been shown to provide a performance advantage under sports-specific conditions. In addition, we confirmed that there is no extra benefit from consuming caffeine in larger amounts. This is good news for athletes who want to get a performance boost without the side-effects of large doses of caffeine, such as interference with sleep. We didn't find an explanation for caffeine's beneficial effect on sports performance in our study. However it is likely to be related to the drug's effects on the central nervous system—caffeine masks the perceptions of fatigue, allowing the athlete to keep exercising at optimal pace rather than slowing down. In fact, our study shows that caffeine's use in sport can be similar to its use in our everyday lives. Rather than maxing out on a single large dose of caffeine to supercharge the day, most people stop for a small shot of caffeine when they become tired—after which they feel refreshed and able to resume their activities.

In summary, we found that the athletes with their red cans were right—switching from sports drinks to Coke in the last part of an endurance race does give a worthwhile boost to performance. The fact that caffeine appears to have this effect at doses indistinguishable from those involved in normal eating and drinking also speaks in favour of the decision by the World Anti-Doping Agency to remove caffeine from the list of banned substances in sport. Future sports-specific studies should focus on identifying situations in which modest intakes of caffeine might be beneficial to sports performance, and on educating athletes that this approach is safer and more effective than the uncontrolled intake of large amounts of caffeine. Table 9.1 provides a summary of some common sources of caffeine in our everyday diet or for use in sport.

TABLE 9.1
Caffeine in common foods, drinks, sports foods and over-the-counter tablets

Food or drink	Serve	Caffeine (mg)*
Instant coffee	250 ml cup	60 (12–169)*
Brewed coffee	250 ml cup	80 (40–110) *
Short black coffee/espresso	1 shot	107 (25–214)*
Starbucks brewed coffee Venti size	600 ml	415 (300–564)*
Iced coffee—commercial brands	500 ml	30–200*

Food or drink	Serve	Caffeine (mg)*
Frappuccino	375 ml cup	90
Tea	250 ml cup	27 (9–51)*
Hot chocolate	250 ml cup	5–10
Chocolate	60 g bar	5–15
Coca-Cola	375 ml can	49
Pepsi Cola	375 ml can	40
Red Bull energy drink	250 ml can	80
V Energy drink	250 ml can	50
PowerBar caffeinated sports gel	1 sachet	25
PowerBar double caffeinated sports gel	1 sachet	50
Gu caffeinated sport gel	1 sachet	20
Carboshotz caffeinated sports gel	1 sachet	80
PB speed sports gels	1 sachet	40
PowerBar Acticaf performance bar	1 bar	42–50
NoDoz	1 tablet	100

* The caffeine content of tea and coffee varies widely, depending on the brand, the way the individual makes the beverage, and the size of their mug or cup. There is variability even between commercial serves of tea and coffee.

FIGURE 9.1
Different protocols of caffeine use and a cycling time trial

Placebo trial:
29:18 ± 0:44 min
6 mg/kg caffeine
1 h pre-race:
28:18 ± 0:40 min
Mean improvement
= 3.4%
Likely range
= 0.2 to 6.5%
6 × 1 mg/kg caffeine
During race:
28:24 ± 0:57 min
Mean improvement
= 3.1%
Likely range
= --0.1 to 6.5%
2 × ~350 ml Coca-Cola
Last third of race:
28:24 ± 0:30 min
Mean improvement
= 3.1%
Likely range
= −0.2 to 6.2%

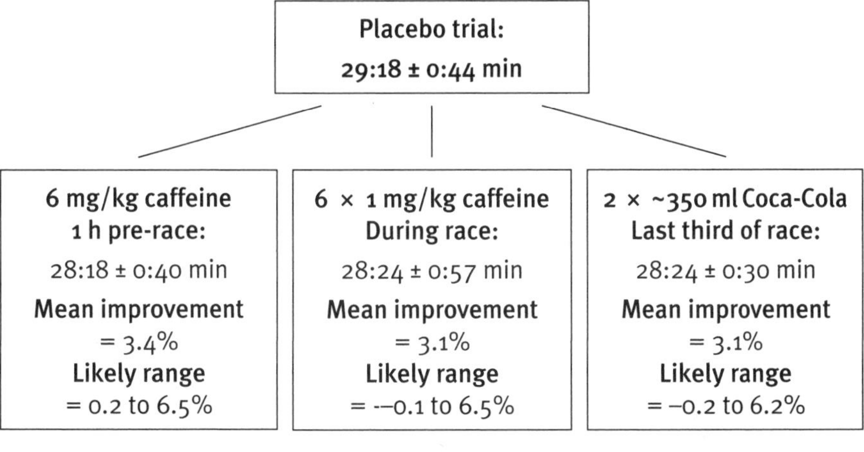

FIGURE 9.2
Teasing out the effects of switching to Coca-Cola on a cycling time trial

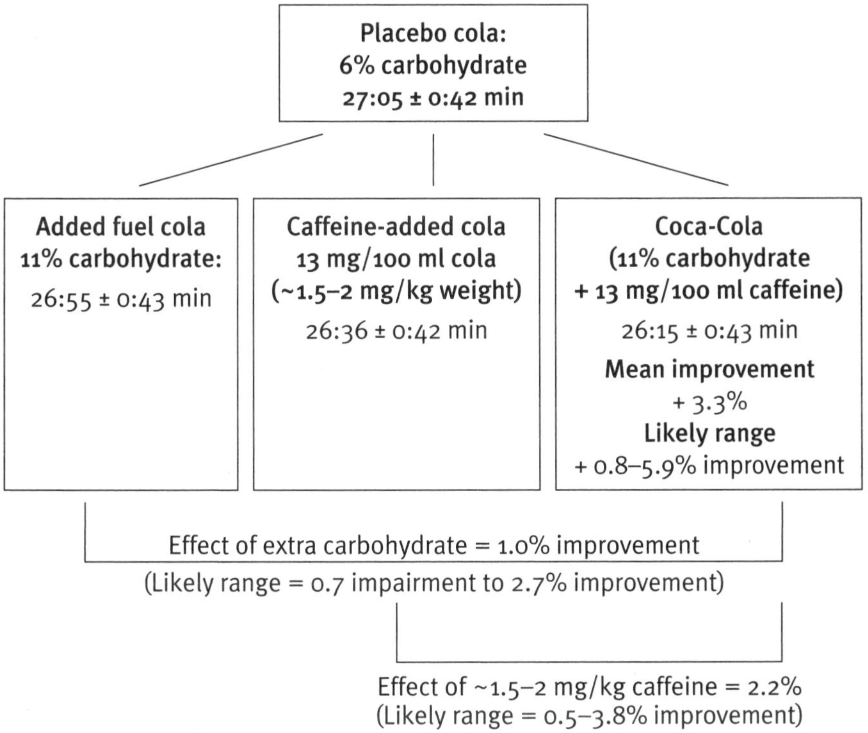

Placebo cola:
6% carbohydrate
27:05 ± 0:42 min
Added fuel cola
11% carbohydrate:
26:55 ± 0:43 min
Caffeine-added cola
13 mg/100 ml cola
(~1.5–2 mg/kg weight)
26:36 ± 0:42 min
Coca-Cola
(11% carbohydrate
+ 13 mg/100 ml caffeine)
26:15 ± 0:43 min
Mean improvement
+ 3.3%
Likely range
+ 0.8–5.9% improvement
Effect of extra carbohydrate = 1.0% improvement
(Likely range = 0.7 impairment to 2.7% improvement)
Effect of ~1.5–2 mg/kg caffeine = 2.2%
(Likely range = 0.5–3.8% improvement)

Distance running

Distance running covers races of greater than 5000 m; common events are 10 km, 15 km, half marathon (21.1 km) and the marathon (42.2 km). Although there is a 10 000 m event conducted on the track, most distance running involves road races or cross-country runs. The World Cross Country Championships include races over 8 km for females and 12 km for males, while the 10 000 m and marathon are included in both the world championship and Olympic track and field programs. 'Fun runs' of various lengths are a great leveller of age and ability, with participants from teenagers to 70-year-olds, and from recreational runners to elite athletes. Big City Marathons can also feature large and varied fields. The 10 000–40 000 entrants in each race include top runners vying for a world record time and considerable prize money, as well as community members, often running to raise money for charity as well as for personal pride. Ultradistance races such as 50-mile, 100-km and 100-mile events are not included in the Olympic Games or world championships and generally do not attract a large following, particularly at the recreational level. Exceptions to this are races such as South Africa's 90-km 'Comrades' run, which attracts a field of 12 000 competitors each year.

The elite level of distance running and cross-country racing, particularly in males, is dominated by runners from East Africa: Kenyans and Ethiopians. Distance runners typically mature with age, requiring years of base training to build up to an elite-level program. Consequently, most elite competitors reach their peak in their late 20s to 30s and remain competitive until about 40 years of age. New features of the marathon include the movement of elite middle-distance runners into the longer race and the specialisation of runners into marathon racing at an earlier age. These two features were demonstrated in the amazing marathon results of 2008: Ethiopian former track champion Haile Gebrselassie broke the world record in 2 hr 3 min 59 sec, while a 21-year-old Kenyan, Sammy Wanjiru, won the Beijing Olympic marathon in very hot conditions in an Olympic record time of 2:06:32.

Training

At the recreational level, many runners train primarily for fitness or health, and compete in a number of fun runs, and perhaps a marathon, each year. Daily training sessions might add up to a weekly distance of 50 km, perhaps peaking at 80–100 km before a marathon. Elite distance runners generally run up to 150–200 km a week in a highly periodised program. A typical training week involves two training sessions a day in a microcycle, following a hard-easy principle. Different types of sessions are undertaken, each with a specific physiological emphasis. These include longer slow runs for aerobic endurance, and intense continuous runs, *Fartlek* or 'speed play' sessions and track (interval) work, all undertaken to improve anaerobic capacity and speed. Some runners include water running and weight training in their programs, but this is the exception rather than the rule and is traditionally done for rehabilitation of injuries. Specialised training techniques such as altitude training and heat acclimatisation before competition in a hot environment may also be undertaken.

Competition

In general, the main competition for track and field occurs in summer, whereas cross-country has a winter season. Most mass-participation road races are scheduled from spring to late autumn. The schedule of Big City Marathons, which includes races in London, Paris, Berlin, Boston, Chicago and New York, extends from April to November.

The elite runner may compete in a number of races of varying distance each year, with a few key events being chosen for full preparation and peaking. Many will compete weekly or fortnightly over a season of races—including road races, cross-country runs or the track series of

World Cups, Grand Prix or Golden League—treating many of these as hard training sessions Marathon runners are unlikely to compete more than once or twice a year over this distance.

Events in hot weather are usually held in the early morning to avoid the heat, while cross-country events may be held on winter afternoons. Distance races are normally held as a once-off competition, i.e. without heats or qualifiers. However, the 10 000-m race at the Olympics or world championships usually involves a heat run several days before the final. In such international events, only exceptional runners will contest both the 10 000-m track event and the marathon, since the races are separated only by a number of days.

Distance running is predominantly an aerobic activity, with elite athletes running continuously from less than 30 min (10 km) to just over two hours (the marathon). Recreational runners can take twice as long as this (or more) to complete the same distance. Aerobic metabolism accounts for the great majority of the energy cost of these events, especially the half-marathon and marathon. However, there are critical times in these races which require anaerobic effort—for example, a surge, a hill, or a sprint finish—and which may ultimately determine the outcome of the race. The factors that limit performance vary between events, according to the duration and environment of the race. Because many of these factors—such as fluid balance, the availability of carbohydrate fuel, and even the disturbance to acid–base balance arising from the anaerobic breakdown of glycogen—can be manipulated by dietary strategies, nutrition is an important component of the athlete's preparation. Races longer than 30 km will probably challenge the usual carbohydrate-storage capacity of most runners, who will need to take steps to increase or supplement muscle glycogen stores.

Physical characteristics

Successful distance runners need a high maximal aerobic capacity, the ability to use a high fraction of this for long periods, and an economical running style. Their defining physical features are a light build, low muscularity in the upper body, and a low level of body fat. There is also some evidence that elite runners carry particularly low levels of body fat on their legs, and that the running efficiency of the East African runners is due to their very slight legs and heels and their more elastic Achilles tendons.

Although distance runners vary in size, many of the world's top competitors have a small and compact physique. Being small makes it easier for your body to regulate its temperature if you need to run in hot conditions. Typically, runners go more slowly in races run in heat and humidity because they need to reduce their accumulation of metabolic heat to compensate for their absorption of environmental heat. Small runners are protected from an excessive rise in body temperature because they produce a smaller absolute amount of heat (thanks to less muscle mass) and achieve a more efficient dissipation of heat generated by the body (higher ratio of body surface area to body volume). The significance of this factor is demonstrated by the results of the 2004 Olympic marathon for women in Athens, where the winner was a tiny Japanese runner, Mizuki Noguchi (~39 kg, 150 cm), while the world's best marathon runner, Paula Radcliffe (54 kg, 173 cm) was unable to finish the race.

Common nutritional issues

Recovery and carbohydrate: the amount and the timing

Daily and twice-daily training sessions call for recovery strategies, especially when two hard sessions are held back to back. Even recreational runners may find that their typical diet does not provide sufficient fuel for marathon training. In fact the first time many runners hit the wall is during their early weeks of big training mileage, as a result of a gradual falling-off of muscle glycogen levels. Recovery will be aided both by the right amount and timing of carbohydrate intake (see Chapter 5). Chapters 1.3 and 2.2 will help you estimate your daily carbohydrate requirements and build the dietary habits necessary to meet them.

After long, hard training sessions or races, not only are your muscles depleted of carbohydrate, but the running will have caused some damage to muscle fibres, which will delay glycogen recovery. Having some carbohydrate immediately after the session or the race will let the muscles take advantage of their most rapid recovery time.

Low body weight and body-fat levels

The low body-fat levels of elite distance runners are primarily a result of genetics and high-volume training. However, even elite runners—males and females, Caucasian and East African—eat carefully to ensure that they stay in shape. They may further fine-tune their body weight/body-fat levels as they peak for special races. Dedicated weight/fat loss may also be needed on an athlete's return after the off-season or after a period of injury. Many recreational runners also need to reduce body-fat levels—in fact, many people take up running in order to lose weight. Dietary measures can assist this process as well as improving running performance.

Regardless of the calibre of the athlete or the starting point for weight loss, the processes should be the same. The first step is to set a realistic target—a body-fat level that will support good health as well as good performance, and that can be achieved and maintained with a sound diet and a sensible workload. You can find more information about this in Chapter 3.

Fat phobias and the female athlete triad

For some runners, particularly females, setting and achieving a desirable body-fat level is difficult. Many female runners set unrealistic targets—either to get below their natural body-fat levels or to lose weight too fast. This can result in a cycle of frustration and further trouble. Remember that the female body is designed to carry a higher level of fat than the male body. An athlete can afford to create only a certain energy deficit before she runs into the problems of low energy availability. In studies, many female runners report a surprisingly low intake of kilojoules—less than you would expect for the training they do. It's not that they don't enjoy eating. In fact, many spend hours each day thinking about food. Sometimes the discrepancy occurs because they underreport or underestimate what they really eat. But often they do need to restrict energy intake far more than their male colleagues to keep their weight down to what they regard as appropriate levels. Often the situation becomes progressively worse—the more they restrict their intake, the less they need to eat. Chapter 3.5 explains the concept of restrained eating, and how the body adapts to low energy availability to reduce its energy requirements. Of course, not all situations of low energy availability result from deliberate choice. A runner may step up the volume and intensity of her training but because of lack of appetite or time be unable to consume enough food for their increased energy requirements.

Some runners complicate the situation further by adding weird and wonderful diets, excessive training, and problem eating behaviours to their weight-loss techniques. Not all runners who practise anorexic (food restriction) or bulimic (bingeing) behaviours have a true eating disorder—many are driven to these actions in a desperate attempt to hit their weight targets. However, many scientific studies as well as anecdotal reports suggest there is a high prevalence of eating disorders and disordered eating among female distance runners. If you are stressed or feel your eating or weight are out of control, then your ideal physique may not in fact be ideal for you. The penalties associated with chasing unrealistic goals are twofold—the problems that arise from pursuing such goals, and the problems that arise when your body is starved or overloaded—or both alternately.

The female athlete triad is a term coined more than a decade ago to describe a bunch of problems that were seen to coexist or cluster in female athletes—with runners being prime candidates. The syndrome was originally seen in black-and-white terms: to be diagnosed with it, the female athlete had to have an obvious eating disorder, loss of menstrual function and osteoporosis (low bone density). As explained in Chapters 2.6 and 3.5, these problems are interrelated and put women at risk of both short-term problems (career interrupted with stress fractures and bone injuries) and long-term ones (earlier onset of osteoporosis). However, in 2007 the American College of Sports Medicine updated its position to recognise that each corner of the triad—energy, menstrual function and bone health—was a separate area that existed on a spectrum (see Figure 10.1). The idea was to warn female athletes that moving down the spectrum on any of the three corners was undesirable, and warranted intervention as soon as possible. Part of the reason for this change was the recognition that all these issues are interrelated. Low energy availability, for example, affects bone mineral density directly by increasing the rate of bone breakdown and remodelling, and indirectly by impairing menstrual function, thus reducing the bone-protecting effects of the hormone oestrogen.

Chapters 1 and 2 explain why the key elements to a healthy diet are variety and an adequate kilojoule budget. If loss of body fat is a healthy option for you, then Chapter 3 will help you with a sensible plan of attack. If you feel caught in a cycle of frustration, a sports dietitian, together with a sports psychologist, can help you to break free. Any interruption to menstrual patterns should be considered a problem requiring the input of a sports physician. The case history of Lola provides an example of these problems.

Iron deficiency

Distance runners, particularly females, are at relatively high risk of low iron levels, perhaps even iron-deficiency anaemia. As discussed in Chapter 2.5, many iron-deficient athletes report feeling fatigued, and although anaemia clearly impairs endurance-sport performance, iron deficiency may also interfere with training adaptations and recovery. Experts still argue about the severity of iron losses from gastrointestinal bleeding, sweat and red-blood-cell damage, but it is probable that the iron requirements of runners are higher than those of sedentary people. The main culprit in iron deficits in females is a low intake of well-absorbed iron. Women not only need more iron than men (to cover menstrual blood loss), they also consume less iron (because of a smaller kilojoule budget, often further compromised by poor dietary choices). On paper, many runners look as if they get enough dietary iron, but on closer examination this may be mostly non-heme iron, from plant food sources, which is not always well absorbed. Male runners who are iron deficient should examine their iron intake but also consider the possibility of iron/blood losses. The story of Zac, below, shows what happens when a runner overlooks his iron needs.

Gastrointestinal problems

Many runners report gastrointestinal problems during hard runs, particularly races. It's hard to achieve a personal best when you are suffering from stomach cramps, diarrhoea or wind. Some runners experience problems at the top end, with burping and heartburn, and a few even find that they pass blood during races. The cause of these problems is unknown, but it seems to be related to the intensity of the running, the stress of competition and perhaps, dehydration. Some runners are able to pinpoint certain problem foods, but this is an individual matter. Probably the best general advice is to experiment with the type and timing of food you consume before running. Sometimes you will need to avoid certain problem foods or eat your pre-race or pre-workout meal well in advance. If problems persist, for important races you might need to empty your gut by switching to low-fibre foods and/or replacing meals with liquid meal supplements over the last 24 hours. A sports physician can advise you about suitable medications or provide a referral to a gastrointestinal specialist who can investigate any underlying gut problems or food intolerances. See Jason's story in the middle-distance running chapter.

Race preparation

Runners need to store sufficient muscle fuel to see out the event. A trained runner should not have too much difficulty preparing for events up to the half-marathon. In Chapter 4.2 you read that adequate muscle glycogen levels can be stored with a high-carbohydrate diet (daily intake of 7–12 g per kg of body weight) and 24–36 hours of taper or rest. For weekly events, such as a season of cross-country races, you may like to schedule training sessions to achieve an adequate taper at the end of the week.

Carbohydrate loading is almost synonymous with the marathon—and rightly so. Races of this length and longer will burn up as much muscle glycogen as you can store. But despite the hype—or perhaps because of it—many runners do not know how to carbohydrate load properly. In the case study reported below, some runners did a better job of 'garbo-loading' than 'carbo-loading'. Read Chapter 4.3 for the low-down on loading. Runners who like to race with a light stomach can modify the fibre and bulk in their diets over the 12–24 hours before the event to help clear out their gastrointestinal system.

The pre-race meal

With early-morning races, it is tempting to sleep in for as long as possible—thus skipping breakfast. Some runners worry that they will suffer from gastrointestinal upsets if they eat a big breakfast before a race. However, the pre-event meal is vital. It is the last opportunity to top up glycogen stores—particularly in the liver—and fluid levels. In many cases, a light snack, even a couple of pieces of toast and a drink, might be the best menu. If your race starts later in the day there might be time for a larger meal three to four hours beforehand. Don't forget fluids, especially if the day is hot. Liquid meal supplements provide a compact and quickly digested alternative to solid food in situations where time is scarce or pre-race nerves are a problem.

Race fluids and fuel

For events up to the half-marathon, you should have all your muscle-fuel needs on board, although it's possible that a carbohydrate boost might give your brain something to feel happy about. Race nutrition should also consider whether fluid is needed. In races of 10–15 km and even the half-marathon, the main threat of overheating comes from the pace at which you are running—the faster you run, the more metabolic heat you produce. But severe dehydration will add to the problem. So make sure you start the event at least in fluid balance. In races of less than 10–15 km in cool conditions, there may not be any need to drink during the event, and the top runners will not want to sacrifice any time. As the distance increases and/or the temperature rises, however, you will start to find aid stations along the route. Make use of these according to your sweat losses. If you are running for more than an hour, you should aim for a comfortable fluid intake—perhaps 500–600 ml, spread over the race. Water is the drink most likely to be supplied, but sports drinks are also suitable.

In the marathon and longer events, you'll enhance your performance by taking in carbohydrate during the run. This will be crucial for events of 50 miles or more. An intake of 30–60 g of carbohydrate per hour is a rough guide for events that outstrip the capacity of your muscle glycogen stores, although you may need to experiment to find what works for you.

For most runners, replacing about 80 per cent of sweat losses will mean a fluid intake of 500–700 ml/hr. With a sports drink that is 7–8 per cent carbohydrate, and an intake of about 200–250 ml at each 5-km aid station, fluid and carbohydrate needs are generally taken care of, though you may feel thirstier on a very hot day and want to drink more. The front runners may have difficulty swallowing this amount, but in the middle of the pack you should be able to spare a little more time at the aid station. Other in-race carbohydrate choices include gels, lollies and cola drinks. Even though cyclists may feel they championed the practice of drinking coke in the last phases of their races, it's interesting to note that Frank Shorter drank Coke during his win in the 1972 Olympic marathon in Munich! Many marathon runners like to vary their rate of carbohydrate intake at different points of the event. They may drink water or dilute carbohydrate drinks (2–4 per cent carbohydrate) in the first part of the race to attend to fluid needs, then shift to the higher carb levels of full-strength sports drinks or cola drinks, or add gels and lollies for a more substantial fuel boost. See Chapter 4.7 for more ideas.

In ultradistance races of 50 miles and more, runners even manage some solid food—but then they are usually running at a relatively slower pace. Even so, most runners are best served in mid-race by liquid forms of carbohydrate, including gels.

Travelling to races

Many athletes undertake their most important races away from the safety of home. At the elite level, runners may need to travel interstate and overseas to find suitable competition, or to race in major events. Even at the recreational level, runners may organise their holidays so they can participate in a well-known marathon or distance event. It can be challenging to achieve your special race nutrition strategies before and during races when you're travelling. You may need to decide whether you'll trust your special high-carbohydrate needs and pre-race timetable to restaurants, or whether you'd prefer accommodation that allows self-catering.

Be prepared and organise ahead. You may need to bring some of your favourite foods with you if they are not available in your new location. Be wary of carbohydrate-loading banquets and parties that may offer a menu higher in fat than in fuel. Think about fluid supplies—especially if you are going somewhere with an unsafe local water supply. It may be useful to carry a water bottle around with you over the last days before the race, particularly if you are in unfamiliar surroundings.

That way you can be sure of staying well hydrated even when taps and fridges are hard to find. However, it is usually unnecessary to overload on fluids, especially if you are a recreational runner who'll have adequate opportunities to drink during the event.

Profile: Lola

The bare bones of running

Lola couldn't believe her bad luck as she viewed the results of the CAT scan. The sports physician pointed out the 'hot spot' of weakened bone in her lower leg. All that hard work and dedication down the drain! The doctor agreed that it was unfortunate, but suggested that factors other than luck could be involved. He finished his clinical examination and concluded that Lola was a typical female distance runner—all legs and lungs. Then he questioned Lola about her training program and diet, and listened as she described the lifestyle of a committed long-distance runner.

Lola was midway through her fourth season of running seriously, but had been frustrated by disappointing results and a stop-start program of racing over the summer. She had missed the first three weeks after coming back from a leg niggle, and had to skip various races or run at less than full power owing to a series of colds. This wasn't what she'd expected in the early days of her running career, when everything had seemed easy. Three years before, when she'd joined her first running club after a successful few years in school sports, she had doubled her training volume and increased her intensity to match the other girls. Noticing how lean and light they all were, she put herself on a rigorous diet, cutting out all food with more than a couple of per cent fat content. The lighter and leaner she became, the faster she ran. Soon she dominated the inter-club under-age competitions over 1500 m and 5000 m.

At the end of her second season, Lola started making the transition to senior competition, picking up some places in distance events on the track in state championships. She also picked up hints from the runners around her. A taste of international competition on a University Games team increased the pool of people with whom she could trade ideas. She returned from this trip even more convinced that she needed to be light like the Kenyan girls. Despite being at the tall end of the range for a runner, she worked to whittle herself down to the magic 50 kg.

Lola was a surprise winner of the Sussan 10 km road race at the end of the summer, taking a large chunk off her PB. She even found herself on the cover of *Runners' World* magazine, with the headline: 'Could This Be Our New Lisa Ondieki?' After that, her running career hit a series of bumps, literally and figuratively. Her troubles began with a stress fracture during the cross-country season. She had to watch her diet even more closely and increase food restrictions to avoid gaining weight during enforced periods of reduced training. She limited dairy foods because she thought this might help to relieve her frequent sniffles and runny nose. When she was able to resume running, she added extra sessions of training, outside the program set by her coach, to try to increase her fitness and leanness. How else would she match the skinfold measurements of 31 mm that Lisa Ondieki achieved when she ran at her best?

The next year was a bleak one for Lola. Her training was sluggish, her mind was always on her weight and body-fat levels, and the harder she tried to stay lean, the harder it seemed to become. She performed credibly in a few races, then seemed to lose her spark. She set herself the goal of doing a hard winter of training and cross-country racing to try to find her lost promise. She had started the current cross-country season with a nagging pain in her shin. She tried to nurse it along until she just couldn't run any more.

The diagnosis of this stress fracture drew her attention to even more, hidden problems. When the doctor asked Lola if she had regular menstrual periods, she laughed. 'Of course not!' she said. 'I've heard that hardly any of the top girls do. It's one of the rewards of all the hard work. And who needs to spend a week every month off their game?' The doctor explained to Lola that amenorrhoea (lack of periods) in athletes was no longer considered harmless or a reward. As with menopause in older women, the loss of periods is associated with a drop in blood oestrogen levels—and he reminded her that an important function of this hormone was to maintain bone mass. Studies have shown, the doctor said, that athletes with amenorrhoea have lower density at some bone sites than normally menstruating athletes—and a higher incidence of stress fractures.

Stress fractures result from the failure of a bone to adapt to excessive trauma. They can occur whether bone density is low or normal, although a weakened bone is theoretically more likely to give way. The doctor sat down with Lola and her coach and discussed the potential causes of an excessive training load—too much too quickly, hard surfaces, inadequate shoes and poor running style. However, Lola's medical workup also needed to assess her menstrual function and hormone levels in case some non-sporting factor had caused her periods to stop just over a year ago. Being female, Caucasian and lightly framed made her more likely to have low bone density anyway, so a special bone scan was scheduled.

A key ingredient of a program to restore low oestrogen levels would be to resume a regular menstrual cycle. Since one of the likely causes of her menstrual problems—and an extra direct cause of bone loss—could be diet, Lola was also sent to see a sports dietitian. When she described her rigid dietary plan (see Table 10.1), it was easy to see that it was lacking in many nutrients. Her typical daily calcium intake of about 300–500 mg was below the Australian recommended intake of 1000 mg a day, and well below the 1300 mg recommended for postmenopausal (and presumably other low-oestrogen) women. Lola asked if she could remedy the situation with a calcium supplement. She had heard of other runners doing this to prevent stress fractures. The dietitian replied that many aspects of inadequate nutrition were contributing to the problem, so while an increase in calcium intake would help, total remodelling of her eating patterns was needed rather than a simple Band-aid approach.

The sports dietitian explained that her central concern was Lola's energy intake. After some quick calculations based on information that Lola provided about her training program and body composition, she offered the opinion that Lola was in a situation of low energy availability. Lola looked confused. 'But I'm not losing weight,' she said. Then she described some of her distance running friends, who she felt took risks with their nutrition but never seemed to suffer any problems. First there was Chloe, who was the leanest of all the girls in the squad. And then there was Hannah, who had come back from a year off and was steadily losing body fat. Weren't they low in energy too?

The sports dietitian sat Lola down and explained in detail (see Table 10.2).

'Assessing energy availability involves calculating how much energy the body has to carry out all the functions needed to stay healthy. Training consumes a certain amount of energy. Therefore, energy availability is the total daily energy intake from food minus the daily energy cost of exercise. The resulting number should be related to lean body mass, since this is the tissue that needs most of the support.

'Energy availability is different from energy *balance*, which involves a comparison between the total energy consumed in a day and the total energy expended (both in exercise and in other body activities).' As explained in Chapter 3.5, if energy consumed is greater than energy expended—yielding a positive energy balance—you would expect a gain in body fat/muscle. If it's less than energy expended—a negative energy balance—you would expect a loss of body fat/muscle.

'If we know your energy intake, the kilojoules you burn in training, your total energy expenditure for the day and your body-fat level (and have a calculator handy),' the dietitian went on, 'we can work out both energy balance and energy availability.

'The example of Chloe shows that a low body-fat level didn't necessarily cause any health problems for a runner. Chloe seems able to maintain low body weight and body fat while eating a relatively high-energy diet. Her energy availability is on target for a healthy person. It is likely that she is genetically suited to low body fat levels and she has achieved them gradually and safely. By contrast, Lola, you have a much lower energy intake, and because you're in approximate energy balance (not losing or gaining weight), your total daily energy expenditure is also apparently low. The energy cost of your training is probably similar to Chloe's, leaving you with an unusually low energy expenditure for the rest of your body functions. Perhaps some contributors to energy expenditure, such as resting metabolic rate, have gradually reduced over time as a way of trying to cope with your extreme energy restriction. This scenario explains impaired body activities such as hormone and menstrual function. And in your case, Lola, it can occur without a very low body-fat level or weight loss being present.'

The dietitian then considered Lola's friend Hannah. 'She is in a negative energy balance—in the process of losing body fat. However, she has been careful enough to reduce her total energy intake just enough to create an energy deficit but without dramatically reducing energy availability. According to studies by Anne Loucks, the body is robust enough to cope when energy availability is reduced by approximately a third. Hannah has the best of both worlds, achieving her weight-loss goals with her health intact.'

Clearly, it was Lola who deserved the attention of the sports dietitian. Her low energy intake was probably behind her loss of menstruation, and therefore affecting her bone health because of the altered oestrogen environment. Low energy availability was also probably directly affecting bone turnover, and low energy intake meant Lola wasn't consuming enough of the nutrients needed for bone formation, body adaptations to stress, and training fuel. Since it was hard to imagine the situation getting worse, Lola agreed to try increasing her energy intake and the variety of foods in her diet. Both factors would allow her to boost her intake of protein, carbohydrate, calcium and iron. She used the liberalisation of her diet to ensure that each meal provided some quality protein, and that snacks—particularly after training—could kick-start refuelling and adaptation with some well-chosen protein–carbohydrate partners.

Lola found her more liberal diet was more enjoyable and gave her the flexibility for more social eating. She was glad to swap her watery fake-chocolate drinks for a mug of delicious milk-based cocoa at home or a steaming hot chocolate at her favourite café. In summer, this could be reconstructed as a frappe made with ice, skim milk and a chocolate carbohydrate–protein liquid meal powder. Lola found that her fears about milk were unfounded. There was no runny noses or mucus to worry about after her dairy serves. In fact, she had fewer colds over the next months than during any of the previous three winters. But the milk went a long way towards achieving a dietary calcium intake of ~1000 mg a day (see Chapter 2.6 for more ideas.) Lola was advised to add a calcium supplement to this mix.

Although her new food plans gradually added 2000 kJ to her daily intake, Lola found that her weight and body-fat levels stayed surprisingly stable. And she seemed to easily accommodate the small gain—she had plenty of energy for her cycling rehab and resumed her running without mishap once the stress fracture had healed. Perhaps it was because all her mental energy could now go into enjoying training rather than thinking about her next meal or next weigh-in. After five months, Lola's menstrual cycle resumed. It will take some years of monitoring to see how her bones fare. However, Lola's running program has had no further hiccups to date. Her revised training program now includes less total mileage and some ongoing water running sessions—she became expert at this while the stress fracture healed. And she frequently lectures her running friends about seeing a sports physician at the first sign of disruption to their periods.

TABLE 10.1
Lola's diet before and after counselling

Before	
Before morning run	1 toast + Vegemite
Breakfast	Bowl of wholegrain cereal Small amount of soy milk Black tea 200 ml orange juice
Lunch	Roll or sandwich with lots of salad and occasionally chicken breast or tuna Piece of fruit Diet Coke
Afternoon tea (before training)	Muesli bar or rice crackers
Dinner	Small serve chicken breast or fish Big salad or vegetables Low-joule jelly + large fruit salad
Supper	Large low-fat muffin Cup of light 'chocolate' drink made with powder and hot water
After	
Before morning run:	Toast and vegemite
Breakfast:	Bowl of wholegrain cereal Good serve of calcium-boosted milk or carton of yoghurt Fruit or juice
Mid-morning snack	

Later lunch:	Roll or sandwich Lean meat/chicken breast/salmon with bones/ egg/reduced-fat cheese Piece of fruit
Afternoon tea (straight after training)	Carton of yoghurt and piece of fruit OR Summer smoothie (milk, ice, fruit, carbohydrate-protein powder)
Dinner	Small serve lean meat, chicken or fish Big salad or vegetables Custard or low-fat yoghurt and fresh or baked fruit
Supper	Cup of hot chocolate or cocoa made with calcium-boosted milk Small muffin or toast with grilled (reduced-fat) cheese

FIGURE 10.1
***The female athlete triad*: The issues of energy availability, bone health and menstrual function vary along a spectrum from healthy to impaired (thin arrows), while each of the issues affects the others (thick arrows).**

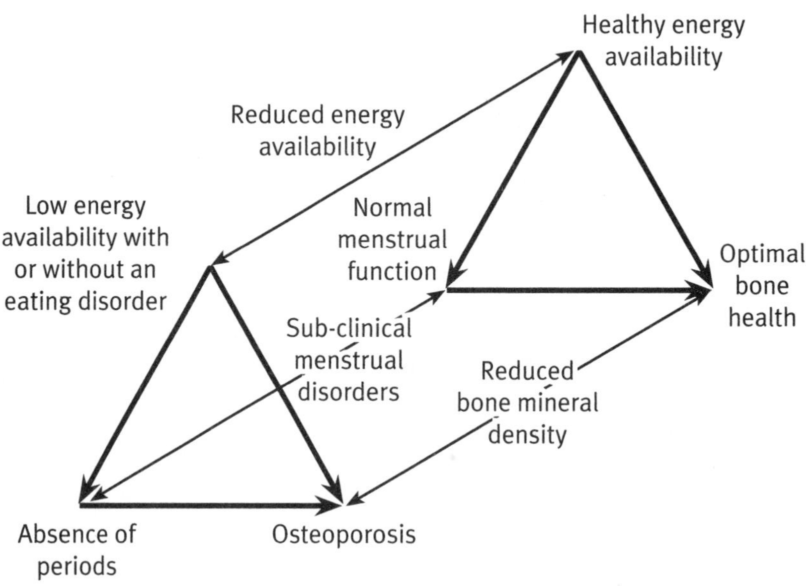

TABLE 10.2
Energy balance and energy availability calculations for Lola and her teammates

	Energy balance (EA)	Energy availability (EB)
	= Energy intake – energy expenditure This sets the potential for weight loss (if negative) or weight gain (if positive)	= energy intake – energy cost of training Generally: daily energy availability for a healthy person in energy balance = ~ 190 kJ/kg lean body mass (45 Cal/kg/d)
Chloe—female runner • 48 kg runner • 12% body fat • Weekly training: 100 km = 21 MJ (5000 Cal) per week = 3 MJ/d • Actual daily energy intake = 11 MJ (2620 Cal) • Actual energy expenditure = 11 MJ (2620 Cal)	= 11 – 11 MJ/d = 0 Chloe is in energy balance and should be weight stable	= 11 – 3 MJ/d = 8 MJ Lean body mass = 42 kg Energy availability = 190 kJ/kg/d (45 Cal/kg/d) Chloe has good energy availability
Hannah—female runner • 55 kg runner • 20% body fat • Weekly training: 100 km = 25.2 MJ (6000 Cal) per week = 3.6 MJ/d • Actual daily energy intake = 10.6 MJ (2520 Cal) • Actual energy expenditure = 13 MJ (3100 Cal)	= 10.6 – 13 MJ/d = –2.4 MJ/d (–570 Cal/d) Hannah is in negative energy balance and should be losing weight	= 10.6 – 3.6 MJ/d = 7 MJ/d Lean body mass = 44 kg Energy availability = 159 kJ/kg/d (38 Cal/kg/d) Hannah has reduced her energy availability but it remains in a healthy range

	Energy balance (EA)	Energy availability (EB)
Lola—female runner • 52 kg runner • 15% body fat • Weekly training: 100 km = 23 MJ (5500 Cal) per week = 3.3 MJ/d • Actual daily energy intake = 8.3 MJ (1980 Cal) • Actual energy expenditure = 8.3 MJ (1980 Cal)	= 8.3 – 8.3 MJ/d = 0 Lola is in energy balance and should be weight stable You would expect Lola to have a greater energy requirement for her weight and body mass	= 8.3 – 3.3 MJ/d = 5.3 MJ/d Lean body mass = 44 kg Energy availability = 120 kJ/kg/d (28 Cal/kg/d) Even though Lola isn't losing weight, she has low energy availability and is at risk of health problems

Profile: Zac

Feeling ironed out?

Zac hadn't been training well for the last month. He felt tired all the time, despite plenty of sleep, and didn't seem to recover fully between training sessions. After getting used to lunch-time runs to keep fit for a weekly squash game, he had decided six months ago to try a marathon. He joined a running group and had been doing things by the book, gradually stepping up his program. Strangely, he had coped better with the greater mileage at the beginning. Now, when he had expected to be right on top of it, little problems were emerging. His knees niggled a bit, but one of his training partners kept him well supplied with anti-inflammatory drugs, and these seemed to keep it under control. Thinking that perhaps he wasn't eating enough fuel for training, he decided to see a sports dietitian.

The dietitian questioned him about his symptoms, his training and his diet. Zac described his daily meal routine, pointing out that he had put it together himself from a running magazine article. Not being a terrific chef, he had kept things simple—such as alternating between rice and pasta most nights. The dietitian questioned him further about specific foods and found that he didn't often eat meat. He liked the simplicity of boiling up his fuel food, opening a jar of pasta sauce and throwing some cheese on top. Variety meant adding a tin of tuna or chopping some lean ham into the sauce. When he was out at a restaurant he ordered fish (he didn't know how to cook it himself). In fact, the only meat he ate these days was on the monthly visit to his Mum, when she'd serve a roast leg of lamb. However, since he ate the lion's share of this meal he thought that should tick the red-meat box for a while.

On the checklist of other regular sources of dietary iron, he didn't go too well. He didn't eat packaged breakfast cereals, but made his own muesli from rolled oats and added bran. He didn't eat eggs—his father had a cholesterol problem. He rarely ate legumes or green leafy veggies—unless they were in the frozen-vegetable mix. Dried fruit and nuts? A little in his muesli. He didn't take any vitamin or mineral supplements, or use any fortified sports products.

The dietitian suggested that inadequate iron, rather than inadequate muscle fuel, might be at the root of his fatigue problem. He was eating plenty of wholegrain bread, rice, pasta and oats for carbohydrate—and these were also his major source of dietary iron. Although his estimated iron intake appeared to be well above the Australian RDI for a male (8 mg a day), almost all of his dietary iron was in the non-heme form that is least likely to be absorbed. And his meal mixtures hardly enhanced iron absorption. Additionally, it was likely that Zac's iron requirements were higher than the typical sedentary male. The increased training mileage, all run on hard surfaces wearing his favourite well-worn shoes, could be causing additional damage to red blood cells. And it was possible that his chronic use of anti-inflammatory drugs was causing a small but consistent loss of blood through gastrointestinal bleeding.

The dietitian arranged for Zac to see a sports physician, who would take a full medical history and order a blood test to determine his iron status. The results came back a few days later: his haemoglobin level was at the low end of the range, and his ferritin concentration (a storage form of iron) was at a low level of 12 nanograms/ml. While these tests are often hard to interpret, it was likely that Zac was in the first stages of iron deficiency. The sports physician excluded other medical causes of iron loss that might need treatment. Then he discussed Zac's training and the appropriate use of anti-inflammatory drugs. Finally, it was time to discuss strategies to reverse Zac's low iron status and prevent it from recurring.

The doctor passed Zac back to the sports dietitian to implement a dietary plan that included 12 weeks of therapy with an over-the-counter iron supplement.

The sports dietitian explained to Zac that he needed to take the iron supplement on an empty stomach each day, along with orange juice to assist the absorption of the elemental iron. This would boost his iron stores while he reorganised his diet to meet his iron needs. The dietitian gave Zac the following nutrition plan:

- Continue with fuel-rich foods at the evening meals following your major training sessions for the week, but learn ways to add a small portion of lean red meat, chicken, liver pâté or shellfish to the menu.
- Focus on quick-cooking red-meat meals on nights when refuelling needs are less important. (Zac liked to cook a steak or beef kebab on the barbecue on his patio during summer, but hadn't realised that this could be part of a runner's dining repertoire.)
- Add some iron-fortified breakfast cereal, such as Sustain or Sports Plus, to your home-made muesli mix.
- Expand food choices by trying legumes, green leafy vegetables and egg dishes.
- Add some vitamin C foods, such as orange juice or fresh berries/citrus/tropical fruits, to any meal in which plant foods are the dominant source of iron.

The dietitian gave Zac some simple recipes for dishes like stir-fries, risottos and lasagnes. He especially enjoyed the Popeye lasagne, which added a spinach layer to the lean beef mince. (Of course, he realised that it was a myth that spinach increased your strength—or even that it was a particularly good source of available iron. But it tasted good!) But he found that many of these recipes were quick and within his abilities. He could afford to buy diced or stir-fry cuts of lean beef and lamb, and it didn't take long to make a pasta sauce or stir-fry with them. Besides, he found that cooking more substantial meals created leftovers for other meals—further spreading the iron as well as saving time. He was glad to hear that it was a better plan to spread a small amount of red meat or shellfish across a number of meals than to try to eat half a cow in one go.

Other ways to spread the well-absorbed iron were to order a roast beef and salad sandwich at the lunch shop rather than his usual ham, cheese and tomato.

The other major change in Zac's eating habits was to increase the variety of foods at each meal or snack. When you are an unadventurous and time-poor cook, it is easy to stick to as few ingredients as possible. However, there are benefits to mixing different food types at the same sitting—matching meat or vitamin C–rich foods with plant sources of iron (breakfast cereal, wholegrain bread, green leafy vegetables, legumes etc.) is one example of how this enhances the overall nutritional quality of the meal. Making this change required new recipes, more organised shopping, and experimentation with new foods. For example, Zac discovered frozen vegetable medleys, which let him not only increase his range of veggies in general but have many of them on his plate at once. Shopping at a market allowed him to buy a range of seasonal fruits to spread around his meals rather than sticking to the safety of an apple on the way to a training session.

At the end of three months, Zac reported feeling more energetic and more adept in the kitchen. His ferritin levels had increased to more than 60 nanograms/ml, so it was agreed to stop the supplement and retest him in another six months. Pleased with this success, Zac asked if he should recommend an iron supplement to his training partners if they also felt tired. The dietitian said many runners considered iron supplements a quick 'pick-me-up' for fatigue or used them 'just in case of a deficiency'. It was true, she said, that iron supplements could be bought over the counter at pharmacies. However, self-prescription and casual use of these supplements often lead to an unnecessarily high intake of iron, which can interfere with the absorption of other minerals such as zinc.

However, the real problem with Zac's 'iron for all' idea lay in seeking a simple solution for a complex problem. For a start, fatigue could be caused by a number of things, including lack of sleep, overtraining and inadequate fuelling. These would not be rectified with an iron supplement. Zac was reminded that his own iron problem had been carefully assessed and comprehensively treated. His friends who self-diagnosed and self-treated would miss out on such expert advice. They might never discover or treat the underlying causes of the iron deficiency, nor benefit from counselling on all aspects of training nutrition. For example, they might easily have a medical condition causing the iron loss, such as an ulcer. Self-diagnosis and treatment could mean missing the chance for an early diagnosis. The dietitian reminded Zac that he had added plenty of good ideas to his new eating patterns, including clever timing of meals and snacks after training sessions to promote recovery. That kind of smart eating can't be found in a bottle of supplements.

Zac went back to his squad with renewed vigour and steadily continued his marathon training program. At last report, he was confidently counting the days until the big event.

Profile

Carbohydrate loading—a load of?

The issue of carbohydrate loading hit scientific journals in the late 1960s, and the first study on it of practical importance to sport showed that runners raced faster over a 30-km event after loading than if they followed their usual diet. If you were trying to pick an event that was ideally suited to carbohydrate loading, it would be hard to go past the marathon. After all, a 42.195-km run is a predictable drain on glycogen stores, and any way to get over the dreaded 'wall' seems well worth trying. The publicity created by the British distance runner Ron Hill was another factor in making the marathon and carbohydrate loading inseparable partners. As far as we know, Ron was the first notable adopter of this nutrition strategy, using it at the European Championship marathon in Athens in 1969. The race was memorable because it featured a spectacular reversal of performance by Hill, who was well behind the race leader, Gaston Roelants of Belgium, at 20 miles, but ran strongly in the later stages of the race to win comfortably in a time of 2 hr 16 min 48 sec.

In a curious turn of events, Hill's carbohydrate loading preparation at the 1972 Olympic Games in Munich was disrupted by the infamous terrorist hostage-taking. Hill followed a strict form of carbohydrate loading, starting with an extreme depletion phase that was almost carbohydrate-free. He had already started this regimen when the massacre occurred and caused the marathon to be rescheduled. He was a highly favoured starter in the race, and it is sometimes suggested that having to alter the timetable of his carbohydrate loading made him underperform and finish sixth. His experience suggests that getting carbo-loading right can be tricky.

Picture the scene. You have been training hard for six months for the marathon, and there are only three days until the gun sounds. Now for the real fun! Good-bye careful eating for the next couple of days while you create new records in pizza and chocolate munching. On the final evening, you organise a carbo-loading function with your training buddies, and fill your stomach to within an inch of bursting. Looking at the caramel mousse, you wish you hadn't eaten so much lasagne. However, you find room on the way home for a couple of doughnuts, convincing yourself that this will come in handy over the last ten kilometres. This carbohydrate loading is great stuff, right?

Wrong. Runners who practise this version of carbo-loading do themselves a double disservice—an uncomfortably full stomach and a questionable intake of carbohydrate for muscle glycogen storage. In a study of the carbohydrate-loading techniques used by 76 runners competing in the 1983 Nike marathon in Canberra, we questioned runners about their training and dietary program over the final week before the race. The results showed a variety of practices: some depleted their glycogen stores in the early part of the week, some tapered their training over the last three days, and others continued their normal training right up to race day. Chapter 4.3 explains the modified loading technique that is now recommended.

Of most interest to us were the high-carbohydrate diets eaten over the last three days before the event. A summary of the results shows the average daily intake was ~470 g—just under 7 g per kg body weight. This would sit at the low end of the recommended range for optimal muscle glycogen storage. Some of the runners in the group achieved levels of 600–800 g per day—probably maxing out their fuel-storage capacity. But at the other end of the scale, some runners managed only 200 g or so of carbohydrate a day, and targeted only 30 per cent of their total energy intake to this fuel source. These results showed that some runners did not understand carbohydrate-rich foods and high-carbohydrate eating. So where did they go wrong?

If you read the sample diet for carbohydrate-loading in Table 4.1, and the suggestions for carbohydrate-rich eating in Checklist 1.4, you will be able to identify correct eating strategies. Instead of this, the runners in our study showed evidence of the following classic mistakes:

- They continued to eat large amounts of non-carbohydrate foods at meals, such as protein foods and low-carbohydrate salads. Although these are part of a nutritious diet, the main goal of carbo-loading days is to meet carbohydrate intake goals. You can afford to sacrifice some of these other foods (and their nutrients) to make more room on your plate and in your stomach for the carbs.
- The runners fell for the idea that 'junk foods' are good carbohydrate sources. Many ate large amounts of foods they considered to be low in nutritional value—take-aways, chocolate, cream cakes and rich desserts. Most of these foods contributed more fat than carbohydrate to the diet.
- While many food ingredients are correctly identified as carbohydrate-rich, people don't often understand how they are assembled into a dish or menu. For example, few runners wouldn't recognise that pasta is a good source of carbohydrate. However, many do not realise that a typical lasagne recipe may contain only a few sheets of pasta and a lot of meat, oil and cheese. The overall effect can be relatively low in carbohydrate and high in fat kilojoules.
- The runners continued their healthy habits of eating 'no added sugar' and artificially sweetened foods. While these might assist with the health-based strategy of moderating sugar intake in the everyday diet, during the three days of carbo-loading before an event, it is OK to stray outside the usual dietary 'rules'. Canned fruit and juices with added sugar, confectionery, soft drinks and sports drinks are easy and compact ways to boost carbohydrate intake.
- Few runners made use of high-carbohydrate fluids—including fruit smoothies, soft drinks and fruit juices, as well as special supplements like sports drinks, gels, bars and liquid meal supplements. Don't overlook these as other compact sources of carbohydrate.

In this study, the group of runners who finished the marathon in less than three hours reported significantly greater training mileage and more carbohydrate in their loading diets than the runners who took more than 3.5 hours. This is, of course, only an observation and does not prove that the extra carbs improved performance. It is just as likely that the best runners knew more about what they were doing as that a good loading diet improved race times.

The moral of the story is that carbohydrate loading might be on the tip of every runner's tongue, but to get it right you need to carefully consider which foods go into your mouth. This study is more than 25 years old, and we hope that the top athletes these days see sports dietitians to make sure that they get their event eating right. It would be interesting to check whether this is the case, and also to see what recreational runners do. If you have been in a Big City venue in the days before a marathon is held, you will have seen the buzz of excitement. Regardless of the calibre of the athlete, glycogen stores will be crucial to success. Just as all modern runners have access to top technology in cushioned running shoes and sweat-wicking T-shirts, they should have the best science and practice in nutrition on their side.

Middle-distance running

Middle-distance running is generally considered to cover events ranging from 800 m to 5000 m, the common link being that each is run as a track race, and each requires the development of both aerobic and anaerobic energy supply systems. Although championship races are often tactical and physical, world records are heavily reliant on speed endurance. Like distance running, the elite level of middle-distance running in males is dominated by African-born runners: while Kenyans and Ethiopians dominate the longer events, athletes from North Africa have been outstanding competitors in the shorter events.

The mile (1.6 km) race has a special mystique in middle-distance running, and remains the only non-metric distance for which the International Association of Athletics Federations (IAAF) continues to keep world records. The breaking of the 4-minute mile by Roger Bannister in 1954 was a landmark event in sport itself, as well as in middle-distance running, since it involved a huge psychological and physiological barrier. Today, the record for the mile is 3 min 43.13 sec, held by Moroccan Hicham El Gerrouj. The women's record, held by Russian Svetlana Masterkova, is 4 min 12.56 sec. Progress can also be measured by the observation that high-school athletes and runners over 40 years old now run the mile in under 4 min, and exceptional runners such as John Walker and Jason Scott broke the 4-min mark more than 120 times each.

Training

Training for middle-distance events is highly periodised and combines characteristics of both distance running and sprint training to prepare all energy systems to handle the diverse metabolic demands of training and racing. Middle-distance runners often train similarly to their long-distance counterparts in the winter off-season, although total weekly mileage and the distance of their 'long runs' may be slightly less. Training is undertaken twice a day, with a mixture of continuous runs and track interval work (see Distance running, previous chapter). Weight training and plyometric training are included when time and facilities permit, and the middle-distance runner may also consider altitude training and heat acclimatisation work.

As the competition season approaches, greater emphasis is placed on track work and improvements in speed. There is usually a drop in mileage as the quality of the sessions increases. Training is normally reduced over the days leading up to the race, depending on the importance of the event.

Competition

Competition begins with school athletics and continues through club level to the international scene. In addition to the Olympic Games and world championships every two years for both the regular and indoor program, the IAAF now champions a World Athletics Tour, consisting of 25 international meets (Grand Prix, Super Grand Prix and Golden League meets) in which athletes accumulate points to qualify for the World Athletics Finals. In addition, there are a variety of major competitions at continental and regional level.

Middle-distance athletes normally specialise in one or two distances, such as the combination of 800 m and 1500 m races. At national and international level, a runner will rarely compete in more than two races on the program, although at the inter-club level some athletes will try themselves over a variety of distances. At specialised meets, such as the Grand Prix circuit, the restricted program will usually offer only one event suited to each runner. For example, in one year's program a 1500 m race may be offered, while the previous year the 800 m race was featured.

The competitive season is traditionally summer. Elite Australian athletes competing in the northern hemisphere summer have to organise their training to extend their competition peak, or to peak out of time from their own domestic season. Inter-club meets are held over a day, usually in the afternoon, with some athletes competing in a couple of different races. Some national and international track meets are held over a number of days, often with heats and semifinals (if needed) on the same day, and the final on the following day. Events at such meets are generally held in the afternoons or evenings, although heats may be scheduled for mornings. The Olympic program is run over 10 days, with 1–2 days separating the rounds of the shorter middle-distance events and up to 3 days between the heats and finals of the 5000-m race. Other European and international meets on the World Athletics Tour involve a single evening's program of selected events with a straight final held between invited runners.

The middle distance runner is a hybrid athlete, combining the distance runner's excellent aerobic capacity with the sprinter's ability to maintain a finishing kick that can be as long as a lap of the track. Championship races are usually highlighted by tactical running at varying speeds and physical jostling. Of all runners, middle-distance specialists require the greatest degree of tactical intelligence and instantaneous decision-making as they consider their position in the pack and the length and timing of an accelerating burst. However, best times are produced by more consistent pacing over a race. Middle-distance events are not long enough to challenge the normal glycogen stores of a well-trained athlete. However, with athletes competing up to 15 to 20 times over a season, especially on the European and international circuits, where mid-week competitions can entice runners to compete three times in a fortnight, recovery of glycogen stores between races becomes an important issue.

Middle-distance running requires a high rate of energy turnover from all energy systems; for example, at the extreme of middle distances, elite 5000-m runners run at a pace close to their maximum aerobic capacity for ~13 min, while a 1500-m runner will work at more than 110 per cent of that capacity for ~4 min. In general, the limiting factors during middle-distance events arise from the body's system for anaerobic breakdown of glycogen, which leads to the build-up of blood-acidifying hydrogen ions and other metabolic products. Training and nutritional strategies can help athletes increase their capacity to buffer this acidity.

Physical characteristics

The physical characteristics of a middle-distance runner are similar to those of a long-distance runner—indeed, many of the top distance runners are former middle-distance runners who increased their competition distance. Low body weight and low body-fat levels help the economy of movement. However, because middle-distance runners are not required to transport their body weight so far, being slightly heavier, particularly in terms of height, carries less of a penalty. In fact, middle-distance runners tend to be taller than their long-distance counterparts—longer legs assist with the stride length needed for speed.

Common nutritional issues

Many of the nutritional issues of middle distance running are similar to those of long-distance running, and only the differences will be discussed in this chapter. You should read the previous chapter carefully, and note especially the first seven sections, on training diet and race preparation, as well as the first two profiles. The nutritional concerns peculiar to middle-distance runners are summarised below. The profile of Jason below explores the issue of gastrointestinal upsets during running—a common concern in both middle- and long-distance running.

Periodisation of eating

The training programs undertaken by serious middle-distance runners need to develop all muscle energy systems to a high level. Therefore, training is highly periodised, and includes sessions and cycles that range between a distance runner's training and the preparation of a sprinter. The energy and fuel requirements of these different phases and sessions of a training program are quite varied. Ultimately, the runner needs to treat these differently in terms of dietary practices. This means increasing total carbohydrate and energy intake during times of high-volume training, and decreasing intake when volume and intensity are reduced.

Specific training phases or sessions that are focused on enhancing anaerobic power and capacity are reliant on carbohydrate, and may call for a focused intake of fuel foods, particularly to prepare for, and recover from, a session. Total energy requirements might be reduced during such phases. The bottom line is that middle-distance runners need to have a flexible eating plan that is in tune with their training and their competition goals. This is often a good reason to seek the advice of a sports dietitian.

Race preparation

Middle-distance runners do not need to carbohydrate-load for competition, since their normal glycogen stores will be more than adequate to see them through a single race. With a sensible focus on carbohydrate foods in combination with rest or tapered training over the final 24–36 hours, a middle-distance runner should be sufficiently fuelled for the event. However, there may be situations in which post-race recovery will overlap with preparation for the next event. Young athletes in particular who have several races over a 1–2-day program may need to increase their carbohydrate intake above normal during this period and make an extra effort to fuel up in advance. Similarly, athletes who have spread-out heats (and semis) over a longer program, or who are racing on a circuit every couple of days, will need to be organised with post-race refuelling and recovery. Chapter 5 discusses the benefits of speedy intake of carbohydrate and protein after a hard session such as a middle-distance race.

Since races can be run at various times of the day, pre-race plans will vary. A breakfast or brunch-type meal will be suitable for events held early in the day. If you are running in an evening race, you might like to continue your normal meal plans until lunch and then finish with a light pre-race meal or snack. See Chapter 4 for more details.

Buffering for race performance

Racing over middle distances hurts in a special way. Although runners think of lactate build-up as the 'bad guy' behind the pain and the fatigue, these are more likely to be caused by the excessive acidity that is a by-product of anaerobic carbohydrate burning. Theoretically, high-intensity exercise could continue for longer if there were some way to neutralise this acid build-up. Training itself tunes up your muscles' own buffering system and increases your tolerance for high-intensity work. But as explained in Chapter 6, there are several ways in which you can help this process along.

In other conditions when we produce too much acid in a part of our bodies—for example, heartburn or urinary-tract infections—consuming a source of bicarbonate or citrate is able to neutralise the acid and its associated pain. These well-known buffers work by temporarily increasing the blood's capacity to neutralise acid. After high-intensity exercise, though, the acidity produced inside the muscle has to move outside it, into the bloodstream, before it can be mopped up. Nevertheless, there is reasonable evidence that taking 'bicarb' or citrate might enhance performance in an 800–1500-m race, or help with the fast last lap of a 5000-m race. Table 6.2 explains two different protocols that might be used. The most common one is the 'acute' protocol undertaken for a single race, and involves consuming a large dose of buffer in the hours leading into the event. The second, more experimental protocol, is to spread some doses of bicarbonate over a couple of days to build up blood bicarbonate levels. There is some evidence that these levels are sustained for a day or so after the last dose, thus giving the athlete more flexibility in timing bicarb consumption before a race.

The downside to bicarbonate loading is that it can be rough on your gut. Many people experience bloating and diarrhoea from a single large bicarb dose. This is probably exacerbated by running's high-intensity jogging motion. The multi-dose protocol, if it can be proven to effectively maintain blood bicarbonate levels, could offer the advantage of putting distance between the last dose and the race. It could also be handy for athletes who plan to compete more than once in a day or days. Trying to load twice in a short time (before heats and then the final) is likely to increase the risk of side-effects. Spreading the dose out might reduce this risk. However, all use of bicarbonate needs to be trialled to find evidence of benefits along with absence of side-effects.

Another new idea for buffering comes from the use of B-alanine supplements (see Table 6.2). This amino acid, found normally in fast-twitch muscle-based foods such as chicken breast and fish, is able to build up levels of carnosine, which is a buffer inside the muscle cell. Unlike bicarbonate, this build-up apparently takes months rather than hours and is maintained for a similar period. It is too early to know how well it works, but it offers potential as a buffering agent in its own right as well as a two-pronged solution when combined with bicarbonate. Perhaps boosting buffers both inside and outside muscle cells is the best way to tackle the acidifying effect of sustained high-intensity exercise head on.

Post-race recovery

Hard running causes damage to muscle fibres and impairs the replenishing of muscle glycogen stores. Muscle glycogen storage is aided by providing a rapid supply of carbohydrate to the muscle following exercise. The first few hours after exercise are an important recovery period for a depleted muscle, and a damaged muscle will also make better use of carbohydrate during the first 6–24 hours than over the next 24–48 hours. Repair and adaptation also requires protein for the building blocks of muscle, and an early supply helps kick-start these processes. Make use of the post-race window of opportunity to maximise your recovery, especially if you have a busy competition or training schedule. Don't presume that race organisers will look after your needs. Bring your own supplies of fluids and foods providing good carbohydrate and protein combinations—see Chapter 5 for ideas.

Travelling on the circuit

For those who compete on an international circuit there are many challenges. Some of these relate to being on the road, living out of suitcases and eating at restaurants. Another challenge comes from the compact competition schedule, which can mean ten big races in as many weeks. This timetable requires quick recovery and preparation between events, over and over again. Juggling training and racing, not to mention transport schedules, accommodation details and money, can be exhausting. It is often hard to stay at your peak both physically and mentally.

The travelling athlete needs to plan well in advance and to be aggressive about meeting nutritional goals on the road. An efficient preparation and recovery plan requires identifying suitable alternatives to the foods regularly consumed at home, and carefully scheduling training between events. See to immediate post-race recovery by consuming adequate fluid and carbohydrate straight away. Again, it may be wise to have your own recovery food supply—don't rely on the post-race party or a late-night meal in a foreign town. Get recovery on the road, and then take part in post-race celebrations—sensibly, of course!

Profile: Jason

Runner's trots

At the finish of his last 5000-m race, Jason doubled over with stomach cramps. It happened quite often at big events—pain, wind and the threat of diarrhoea. Frequent pit stops once interrupted his evening training, but he had gradually learned to control this need by cutting out afternoon snacks. However, the competition situation was still 'out of hand', and Jason feared that he might become another statistic in his running club—joining the group who usually had to respond to an urgent call of nature during a race.

His sports doctor organised a series of tests of his gastrointestinal function, which found no obvious abnormalities. He had no family history of gut problems. The doctor suggested that an anti-diarrhoeal drug might help in important events, but also recommended a session with the clinic's sports dietitian. The dietitian put a checklist in front of Jason and invited him to compare it with his own experiences (see Checklist 11.1).

Jason considered this list carefully. There was no doubt that nerves played a role—he was often agitated before important races and could almost feel his stomach tie itself in knots. He also remembered how anxious he had been before hard track sessions in his early days at the running club. There had been plenty of gut problems in those days—just as there had been last year around tax time, when work had been extremely busy and stressful. It didn't seem to matter how fast Jason ran—it was how much he worried about how fast he ran.

Looking further down the list, Jason decided dehydration wasn't contributing to his problems, since he was careful to keep his fluid levels topped up and his races really didn't last long enough for much of a fluid deficit to occur. At work Jason had several coffees as part of his daily routine in meetings with colleagues and clients. He typically grabbed a double espresso from the coffee shop next to his office as he left work, about an hour before afternoon training. The espresso kick was also part of his pre-race routine on weekends. He'd started it after seeing footage of a Tour de France cyclist showing off a *barista*-quality coffee machine in the team bus. He needed a double issue of his sugar-free gum to get rid of the coffee breath before training, of course. Now he listened with surprise as the dietitian told him caffeine was a gastric irritant and might be contributing to his stomach upsets. As for the chewing gum—he'd started using it as a way to clean his teeth after lunch but soon found that he was getting through several packets a day, overdoing the sorbitol. That was one habit that would be easy to break, something he couldn't say of his daily coffee fix!

Jason described his usual diet, which he thought was a varied and nourishing one. The dietitian asked about Jason's intake of milk and milk-based products (yoghurt, ice-cream, custard, etc.) and concluded that he was probably not intolerant of lactose (the sugar in milk). Jason could remember a couple of bad experiences before races—one after a big bowl of untoasted muesli and another after a generous intake of plums and apricots straight from the orchard. He'd learnt that too much dried fruit and raw oats didn't agree with him, at least not on the day of a race. However, fresh fruit and high-fibre foods were usually OK.

It seemed that the main cause of Jason's stomach problems was pre-race nerves. The dietitian suggested that he try reducing his stomach contents before less important races in combination with moderating his caffeine intake. It would be hard to simulate race stress in training, so Jason prepared to experiment with some of the early races in the competition calendar.

The dietitian suggested he change the timing and amount of food eaten close to the start of a race so his stomach would have time to empty. He couldn't give up eating altogether, though, and he worried about fuelling up before important races. For the 24–36 hours pre-race he would eat only low-fibre foods, and on the day of the race he would consume a liquid meal supplement such as PowerBar Proteinplus or Sustagen Sport as his pre-race meal. He also agreed to limit his coffee intake to two cups in the morning and avoid caffeine close to exercise. By race time—late afternoon—he should be feeling light and untroubled, the dietitian said. The chewing gum could go also.

Jason tried this a couple of times and reported an improvement, not just in his gut symptoms but in his pre-race anxiety levels. Worry about his gut problem, it seemed, had been adding to the problem. The thought that medication provided still another potential solution was comforting, but for the moment Jason decided to keep it as something to fall back on. A stress-management course offered at work has since taken his fancy, and he has decided to learn and practise relaxation techniques for pre-race as well as everyday stress relief.

CHECKLIST 11.1
Factors possibly associated with runner's diarrhoea

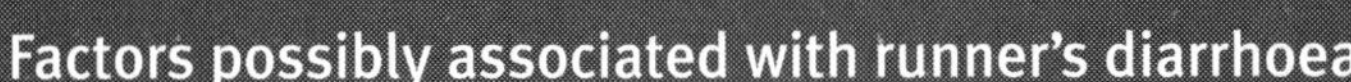

- Stress and nerves: Do your symptoms get worse when you are nervous or stressed?
- Intensity of running: Are symptoms worse during intense running—e.g. competing and training at or above race pace?
- Are there any underlying gut problems? Do you or members of your family have a history of irritable bowel syndrome, coeliac disease/gluten intolerance, Crohn's disease?
- Foods in your everyday diet: Have you identified whether certain foods, or large quantities of these foods, cause gut problems that become worse when you run?
  - Examples:

    too much fibre

    too much lactose (milk, ice cream and milk-based products)

    too much fructose that is not accompanied by a good ratio of glucose (dried fruit, fruit juices, certain fruits such as apples, pears, melons and grapes)

    too much sorbitol (e.g. sugar-free chewing gum)

    too many stone fruits (plums and apricots, etc.)

- Caffeine as a gastric irritant: How many serves of concentrated caffeine do you have each day, and when are they consumed in relation to training?
- Dehydration: Some studies have shown that dehydration increases the incidence of gastrointestinal complaints. Could this be adding to your problem—especially if you are limiting fluid intake in the belief that it could be the cause of your distress?
- Timing of pre-exercise meal: Have you experimented with changing the time of your last food intake before training or racing?
- Size of pre-exercise meal: Have you experimented with changing the amount of food eaten in the pre-exercise meal?
- Type of food in pre-exercise meal: Do your pre-workout menus provide significant amounts of protein, fat or fibre? Do they provide lactose or fructose? Have you experimented with changing the foods in these meals?
- Intake during exercise: Do you consume carbohydrate-containing drinks or solid foods during exercise? What are the types and concentrations of carbohydrate in these fuel sources, and have you experimented with changing them? If you are eating solid foods, do they contain significant amounts of fat, protein or fibre?

Jumps, sprints and hurdles

Track-and-field competition includes a number of events of short duration that rely primarily on the development of power through anaerobic energy. Some can be traced back to the ancient Olympics, and the idea of being the 'swiftest or highest' has always commanded great interest. The 100-m sprint is generally considered the blue-ribbon event of track and field, with all eyes focused on the 'fastest man on earth'. Other sprint events at Olympic-level competition are the 200-m and 400-m, as well as 4 × 100-m and 4 × 400-m relay events. Hurdles events are contested over 100 m (women), 110 m (men) and 400 m. The jumps consist of high jump, long jump, triple jump and pole vault. Some talented athletes compete in more than one event, combining, say, the 100-m, 200-m and relays on the same program, or entering special 'combined events'—a two-day program featuring seven track-and-field events for females (the heptathlon) or 10 for males (the decathlon). These combined events truly identify the all-round athlete, since competitors must master a range of often diametrically different athletic skills. Versatility is the key to success: dominating in a single event can actually be detrimental to overall performance.

Competition begins with Little Athletics and school athletics, with careers carrying through club competition to international events. The International Association of Athletics Federations provides a wide range of competition opportunities for high-level athletes. In addition to the Olympic Games and world championships every two years for both the regular and indoor program, sprinters and jumpers can compete in the World Athletics Tour, consisting of 25 international meets (Grand

Prix, Super Grand Prix and Golden League meets) in which athletes accumulate points to compete in the World Athletics Finals. In addition, there are a variety of major competitions at continental and regional level. While a full program of events is included at major competitions spanning a couple of days, there is a selected program at the specialised meets on the Athletics Tour.

Training

At school and club level, many athletes will not train specifically during the off-season. Many sprinters and jumpers are involved with other sports or study, and turn their attention to athletics only a month before the start of the inter-club season. During the competition season they may train three or four evenings a week and compete on the weekend.

At the elite level, training is a year-round pursuit of speed, speed endurance, power, technique, and flexibility. According to the phase of training and type of event, jumpers and sprinters undertake one or two workouts a day, including high-intensity intervals on the track, resistance training, flexibility work, technical drills, and plyometrics. To develop the ability to generate power relative to body weight, off-season training usually involves a considerable commitment to weight training, with about one-third of the total training load being carried in the gym. The other emphasis in off-season training is on the refinement of technique. In addition to running sessions on the track, drill sessions are conducted, for example to improve leg speed or knee lift. As the competitive season approaches, track work increases to include more intervals and sprints, although technical work and weight training are still maintained. Plyometric training, which involves drills of bounding, jumping, and hopping, is undertaken to develop the elastic properties of the muscle, increasing explosive power and the stiffness of the muscle, for example to speed start times and improve the ability to store and reuse the elastic energy from running and jumping.

The pre-competition training taper does not need to be as great as that practised by middle- and long-distance runners, since sprinters are already training for quality rather than quantity.

Competition

The competitive season usually spans five to six months over the summer. Sprinters and jumpers can compete regularly at weekend or mid-week inter-club meets during the season but usually target three to six special events. Elite athletes who wish to compete at home as well as overseas must be ready for an additional season and the need to work towards double or even triple peaks in their preparation.

At the inter-club level, athletes often compete in a number of events conducted on the same day of a competition—for example, a couple of sprints of different lengths, a jumping event and a relay race. At national and international level, most athletes qualify to compete only in their major event and perhaps a relay. However, highly talented athletes may dominate in multiple events, such as 100-m and 200-m sprints, the 4 × 100-m and 4 × 400-m relays and even the long jump—as did Usain Bolt at the Beijing Olympic Games or Carl Lewis at the Barcelona Olympic Games.

Some events involve a one-off race or straight final over a single day or night meet—for example, the Golden League and Grand Prix meets. By contrast, victory in the sprints and jump events at world championships and Olympic Games is decided by a multi-day program involving a series of heats, semi-finals, and finals. The winners of the sprint events must sustain their performance for three or four races over three to seven days. Within this program, the athlete must sometimes compete twice within the same session—for example, semi-finals and finals of the 100-m sprint. This is a particular feature of the combined events, in which the athlete undertakes three to five events on a single day. The men's decathlon program consists of 100 m, long jump, shot put, high jump and 400 m on Day 1, and 110-m hurdles, discus, pole vault, javelin and 1500 m on Day 2. The women's heptathlon program is Day 1: 100-m hurdles, high jump and shot put; Day 2: 200 m, long jump, javelin, and 800 m. Jumping events usually involve a qualifying round and final or a straight final program. However, within each session, each competitor must undertake several jumps, either doing a set number to determine the winner of the long jump and triple jump or following an elimination protocol to decide the winner of the high jump and pole vault.

Even though the event itself involves a brief explosion of energy, a jumping competition may drag out for many hours while all competitors take their turn. The athlete's fuel stores are not a limiting factor here. Muscle adenosine triphosphate (ATP) and creatine-phosphate systems are the most important energy source for events lasting seconds and are quickly regenerated between repeated bouts. Anaerobic metabolism of carbohydrate plays a greater role during events lasting up to a minute, but muscle glycogen stores should not be a limiting factor in events so brief.

Physical characteristics

Typically, sprinters carry a large lean body mass, with sufficient muscularity in both their upper and lower bodies to produce explosive power over short distances. The weight side of the power-to-weight ratio is also important, with elite sprinters showing off their leanness and muscular definition. Low levels of body fat and concern for total body mass become more important in longer sprints or where the athlete moves against gravity—for example, in the high jumps, hurdles, and pole vault.

Height and leg length play a role in sprint performance by influencing stride length. Hurdlers need to be tall, or at least have relatively long legs, to clear the hurdles well. Height provides an important advantage in high jump because it means that the jumper's centre of gravity, which must be raised above the bar to successfully complete a jump, is already high. Heptathletes and decathletes must achieve a physique that suits a range of sports with different biomechanical and physiological characteristics.

Common nutritional issues

Low body-fat levels

Although many elite sprinters and jumpers achieve their leanness and preferred racing weight as a natural consequence of genetics and training, others undertake deliberate weight-loss programs or at least make this a focus of their eating plans. Club-level athletes of both sexes who reduce or cease training over the off-season may need to lose body fat at the beginning of the next competition season. Where help is needed in this regard, read Chapter 3 for sensible and successful methods.

Increasing muscle mass and strength

Off-season may be the time for sprinters and other track athletes to hit the weights room and increase muscle strength and power. Chapter 3 deals with the questions about protein and energy needs, while Chapter 5 deals with the smart recovery strategies that allow the athlete to gain the most from these sessions.

Training nutrition

The goals of training nutrition are discussed in Chapters 1 and 2. Matching carbohydrate intake to the needs of training sessions is still a priority for sprinters and similar athletes, although understandably, their carbohydrate requirements do not reach the levels of endurance-type athletes. In many cases, there is a need to periodise food intake—over the week to accommodate different types of training sessions, and over the season to accommodate different emphases on building fitness and honing physique versus fine-tuning competition performance. It makes sense to ensure that carbohydrate stores are primed for key sessions of repeated sprints and speed endurance work. These sessions—and resistance workouts—should also benefit from well-timed meals or snacks that can help refuel muscles after the session (carbohydrate) and supply the building blocks (protein) the body needs for recovery and adaptation.

If you are unsure whether your eating plans meet your nutritional goals, a sports dietitian can assess your diet and guide you. Even if you think you are eating well, you may learn new ways to expand and enjoy your nutritional horizons—and getting a stamp of approval can be a great confidence boost, as it is in Michael's story below.

Preparation for competition

Since single jumps and sprints will not deplete muscle glycogen stores, there is no need to carbo-load before a competition. The gain in body weight arising from additional glycogen and water in the muscle—or simply from overeating—merely means extra weight to carry. This can impede performance, especially in jumps and hurdles, where you must lift yourself off the ground as well as propel yourself forward. Nevertheless, fuel stores must be primed for a meet, especially in competitions that involve multiple events or rounds.

The day of competition is best tackled with glycogen stores topped up to their typical resting levels. You should already be periodising your diet to fuel up for key training sessions. Competition is another time for a light but strategic carbohydrate top-up.

Competition-day food and fluid

Although your sport technically lasts only seconds or a minute, competition can be a variable affair. Competition-day nutrition needs can range from a pre-event meal before a single effort to a grazing picnic stretched over a drawn-out day of competition and balanced between warm-ups, events and warm-downs. Chapter 4.4 outlines the goals of the pre-event meal—fluid and fuel checks, comfort and confidence boosts. You will need to choose the foods and drinks that suit the needs of your events, and a plan that fits the day's schedule and your personal preferences. Experiment in training if an important competition is coming up and you are programmed to compete at an unaccustomed time of the day.

How should you handle a busy program, consisting of a number of all-out efforts interspersed with variable amounts of waiting around in between? What should you eat and drink between events, or during events that sprawl out over hours? Your nutritional goals are to keep hydrated, to maintain blood-sugar levels and to feel comfortable—avoiding hunger but not risking the discomfort of a full stomach. How you will do this largely depends on the time interval between events or efforts. Fluid and food intake must be matched with the general considerations for hydration, gastrointestinal comfort and fuel requirements over the hours of a competition session as well as the specific needs incurred by warm-up, events, and cool-down activities. See Grace's account below for ideas and, like her, be organised to look after your own needs.

Travelling to competition

Track and field athletes, like other athletes, frequently find their competition opportunities interstate or overseas. It requires forward thinking to ensure that competition eating goals can be achieved while away from home—particularly if you are eating at restaurants or hotels. The challenge is considerably greater if you are travelling on a Grand Prix circuit and away from a home base for a long time. It may be appropriate to bring some of your own supplies, particularly if you know that important foods will be missing, or that catering arrangements at the competition venue will not be ideal. The Tennis chapter provides some ideas for frequent travellers. Otherwise, think ahead to arrange appropriate food and be assertive in restaurants and hotels when ordering meals (see Golf chapter).

Supplements

Track-and-field athletes, particularly sprinters, are an enthusiastic audience for supplements and sports foods. Sports foods can provide a useful source of nutrition for special occasions, such as travel and competition—Chapter 6 summarises the types of products that are commonly available and their valuable uses. However, there is also plenty of interest in the range of alleged ergogenic supplements that promise to enhance strength, power, recovery and leanness. Despite the hype and interest, most of these are unproven. Read Chapter 6 to find the few supplements that have proven ability to support a strength or interval-based training program. But also weigh up the various costs of using such supplements.

Profile: Grace

A long day on the track

Despite being the most promising sprinter in the region, at last year's interschool athletics carnival, Grace could manage only one bronze medal. Her program had been busy—heats of the 100 m at 9.45 a.m., long jump at 12.30, final of the 100 m at 2.30 p.m. and the 4 × 100-m relay at 4.15 p.m. The morning of the meet was rushed. The sports ground of the host school was a long drive away, so she had to set off early. Grace had forced herself to swallow a mouthful of toast as she raced out the door. She consoled herself that she was too nervous to eat anyway.

By mid-morning, with the 100-m heats out of the way, Grace was ravenous. She eagerly scoured the sports-ground kiosk for something light to eat—after all, the long jump was not far off. The offerings were limited to pies, hot dogs, soft drinks and chocolate bars. She chose the chocolate, 'for energy', and made her way to the jump pit. With so many competitors, the long jump stretched out for well over an hour and as she sat out on the oval awaiting her next jump, Grace felt herself getting hot, thirsty and sunburnt. It was hard to concentrate, and she jumped badly.

There was barely time to warm up for the 100-m final, let alone get to the amenities block on the other side of the sports ground to find a tap. She ran, feeling tired and with a dull headache. She finished the day with a third place in the relay event—small comfort for the hours of training she had completed over the past three months.

This year the story was quite different, although her training hadn't changed and the meet program was almost the same as the previous year's. The difference was a careful plan for competition day, organised in collaboration with the school's new athletics coach.

Grace got up earlier than usual to allow herself to have a light but relaxed breakfast of cereal and fruit juice before leaving for the sports ground. Not willing to rely on the ground catering, she took along a picnic basket of provisions for the day—foods she had tested in training over the previous month. Once the 100-m heats were over, Grace had a small meal of ham sandwiches and juice, knowing that this would be comfortably 'digested' before the jumps started in two hours' time. Once they called for competitors in this event, she set up 'camp' on the oval near the jump pit, bringing with her a drink bottle full of cold sports drink and a small beach umbrella for shade. Some of the other competitors laughed at the sight, but they were soon feeling the heat of the midday sun and saying they wished they had done the same.

With a win and a personal best in the long jump under her belt, Grace started her warm-up for the 100-m final and followed up soon after with her second gold medal for the day. With just over an hour before the relay event, there was little time to eat solid food. Feeling a little empty, Grace was glad she had a 'ready-to-go' liquid meal supplement on ice in her picnic basket. Refreshed and revitalised, she prepared for the last event and helped her team win a silver medal.

While Grace knows that her medals were not just the result of particular food or drinks, her careful organisation did allow her to do justice to her talent and training rather than see it wasted by race-day mistakes. Some of her successful strategies are summarised in Table 12.1.

Profile: Michael

How do you assess dietary practices?

Michael, a 400-m hurdler, was aiming for selection in next year's University Games athletics team. He had been interested in sports nutrition for the past two years, gleaning information from his coach, from articles in *Runner's World* and from the occasional sports-medicine seminar. He'd tried to incorporate these ideas into his diet, although he was not always sure which foods were best. Wanting to leave nothing to chance in his running career, Michael decided to get a professional's opinion on his diet. He made an appointment to see the sports dietitian at the sports medicine clinic near his home, and his first question was: 'How will you tell if I'm eating well? Will you do a hair analysis or something?'

The dietitian explained that hair analysis, along with practices such as live-cell microscopy and iridology (eye examination), fall into the category of alternative therapies and are not regarded by scientists as valid ways to assess nutritional status.

A dietitian's major assessment tools are information about physique (see Chapter 3), lifestyle, exercise patterns, and a careful assessment of dietary intake. Medical examinations may be needed, including signs and symptoms of various nutritional conditions. Sometimes the dietitian will also have biochemical tests done to establish whether a nutritional deficiency exists.

Since biochemical tests are expensive and occasionally a nuisance they are best undertaken only when the other information points to a possible problem. For example, it is not necessary for athletes to have hundreds of tests to see which vitamins or minerals they might be lacking. However, if signs of a particular deficiency are apparent, and the athlete's usual eating patterns suggest he is falling short of estimated requirements for this nutrient, it is useful to do the appropriate blood tests to confirm this.

Michael's nutritional assessment began with a discussion about his sporting commitment—his goals, training and immediate competition plans. The dietitian then asked about his interest in nutrition and any special dietary principles he was already following. Did he live at home with his family, in an institution, alone, or in a shared house? Who did the shopping and cooking? What else did he have to fit into his day apart from training—university, full-time or part-time work?

The discussion turned to weight and body fat, and Michael said his weight never varied by more than one or two kilograms during the season. He showed the dietitian the results of a recent body-fat check by an exercise physiologist accredited in skinfold measurement procedures. Michael's score for the sum of seven skinfold sites was 32 mm, which made him very lean.

Next, the dietitian asked Michael to recount a typical day's eating. She led him through the day, noting his activities—particularly training—and eating habits. This gentle but thorough interrogation yielded a detailed account of the types, timing and quantities of foods and drinks Michael consumed, noting how they were cooked or prepared and why they were chosen. Special attention was focused on his intake before, during and after workouts. Weekends were described separately, with attention to any changes to his weekday pattern. The dietitian also asked about eating out, take-aways, and other variations in Michael's routines, such as differences between summer and winter eating. Competition nutrition was then explored, looking at dietary preparation, pre-race meals and tactics for race-day food and fluids.

'What can you learn from this?' Michael asked. The dietitian explained that, providing Michael had described his usual eating patterns accurately, this profile could provide a good general assessment of his success in meeting his nutritional needs. It not only covered what he consumed and when in relation to workouts, it also helped to explain some of the reasons why he chose particular food. This was important to know, especially when improvements were advised. For example, if availability or cost stood in the way of a better food choice, that would call for different tactics than if lack of nutrition knowledge was the only problem.

To complete the picture, Michael was invited to keep a food diary.

The dietitian explained that this was like having a video made of his running technique. Recording his food intake over a period of time would allow Michael to compare *actual* intake with what he *thought* he was eating, and also with what he *should* be eating for optimal performance. The diary would also help him track the timing of nutrition in relation to training and racing. A computerised dietary analysis could also be undertaken, estimating daily intake of kilojoules and nutrients based on Michael's diary records.

To make the most of the exercise, Michael was shown exactly how to keep a good food record. He needed to make sure that he kept it for long enough to reflect his usual eating patterns, and to accurately describe the type and amount of food and drink he consumed. He was happy to use paper and pen for the diary, though the dietitian told him that new techniques were being developed making use of mobile phones, digital photos and the Internet. Michael carefully kept a diary for seven days, which covered a full week of training and an inter-club meet.

The dietitian then studied Michael's diary, assessing the information quantitatively and qualitatively. She entered his food and fluid intakes into a computerised dietary analysis program to estimate Michael's daily tally of energy and nutrients and how this varied according to his training program. The results are presented in Table 12.2, along with typical meal plans from Michael's diary.

To evaluate Michael's diet, the dietitian worked through a checklist of goals for training and competition nutrition:

- Suitability of weight and body-fat levels: Michael's daily kilojoule intake is appropriate, maintaining his body fat at a low level to suit his sport.
- Nutrition knowledge and practical skills: Michael is motivated and is generally good at the time management and skills needed for planning, shopping and cooking good meals. He and his housemates might benefit from some cooking classes to widen his recipe range; learning to cook fish would be especially useful. A house roster will ensure that chores are all done and that Michael can contribute to the cooking on lighter training days and come home to a hot meal after his heavy workouts.

- Training support: Michael's estimated average daily carbohydrate and protein intakes look appropriate. However, they are not necessarily well spread over the day or week to give maximum support to his training. Michael could benefit from adjusting his carbohydrate intake from day to day to more closely track his fuel needs. A pre-planned weekly menu would schedule carbohydrate-rich dinners on the night before speed endurance sessions and other key workouts and focus on fuel intake at breakfast and lunch before these sessions. In longer sessions, he might benefit from some sports drink. He doesn't yet know how to monitor his hydration status from day to day or over long sessions. It would be valuable to monitor his morning urine output and fluid balance, particularly in summer.
- Recovery: Michael is doing a good job of scheduling a well-chosen breakfast after his morning workout to help with refuelling and repair/adaptation. However, his evening session is not as well supported. Even though Michael takes a snack to the session to eat on the way home, his choices have been carbohydrate-centred rather than carbohydrate–protein combinations. So although his average protein intake for a day is well above suggested requirements for an athlete, it is not necessarily targeting his real needs. Including protein in recovery snacks after key workouts and weights sessions would help a great deal by promoting adaptation and recovery, especially if the snack is eaten immediately after the session. The dietitian provided suggestions of other items to add to his post-session menu such as a liquid meal supplement (PowerBar Proteinplus or Sustagen Sport) or fruit-flavoured yoghurt.
- Adequacy of vitamin and mineral intake: Michael's intake of key nutrients is well in excess of the recommended daily allowances and provides a generous margin for when requirements are increased by heavy exercise. High nutrient intake is partly a result of Michael's generous energy intake, but also comes from his careful choice of a wide variety of nutritious foods. Although we don't have quantitative

information for all micronutrients and important food chemicals, if Michael is meeting his needs for key nutrients from a variety of foods, then he is probably getting a plentiful supply of other nutrients as well.

- Long-term nutritional issues: Michael's diet meets the guidelines for good health, with moderate fat and salt levels, and a variety of wholesome foods. As well as supporting his immediate athletic goals, this diet should lessen his risk of nutrition-related diseases in later life. He has no known family history of cardiovascular or lifestyle diseases that might require a special diet.
- Competition nutrition: Michael uses inter-club meets to practise the eating tactics he will use in more important competitions. He has fine-tuned his preparation and pre-race meal and takes his own food when he travels to an interstate meet. He has kept good records of all his competition outings over the past two years and has adjusted his nutrition on the day of an event to bring out the best in his performance.
- Social and enjoyment eating: Although Michael chooses wholesome foods and meals most of the time, he enjoys eating out with friends and occasionally scans the dessert menu for his all-time favourite—sticky date pudding with ice-cream. Careful but not fanatical, he feels happy with his menu.

The dietitian congratulated Michael, assuring him that his current diet met many of his nutritional goals as a hurdler, and that a little tinkering would further improve the interaction between his eating and training. All that remained to make his diet ideal was the confidence that he was eating well. Such a diet not only met his physiological needs—knowing that it did so would give him a psychological edge, a major advantage in top-level competition.

TABLE 12.1
Successful strategies for organising a competition-day nutrition plan for a track and field athlete

Strategy	Comments
Obtain the competition timetable and plan ahead • Pencil in a likely schedule of activities for warm-ups, events and cool-downs. • Work around this timetable to plan some times for eating and drinking	• Be aware of the potential for the timetable to change • Be aware of gut concerns—whether you are likely to be uncomfortable during exercise or get hungry with your plan
Investigate food supplies and food storage opportunities at competition venue	• Be prepared to take your own supplies and be self-sufficient if you can't rely on the competition venue — Portable and relatively non-perishable choices include sports foods—bars, sports drinks, gels and liquid meals — With your own Esky or access to a fridge you may be able to add a range of everyday foods to the menu—sandwiches, milk drinks, yoghurt, etc.
Use training sessions to gauge real fuel and fluid needs for your sport and event challenges • Monitor body mass changes and fluid intakes over a session to see what your typical sweat losses are, and how well you usually replace these (see Figure 2.3) • Think through the real fuel demands of your event and preparation/cool-down	• Be aware that it can be easy to overhydrate, as well as underhydrate—both can be unnecessary and undesirable. A moderate–large fluid deficit may reduce your concentration and performance. However, gaining weight because of overhydration can detract from performance and excessive fluid intake may also cause gut discomfort.

Strategy	Comments
activities. Monitor 'energy levels' over periods of training or low-level competitions	
Use training sessions or lower-level competitions to practise and fine-tune your plans	• You may not be able to replicate competition nerves, but most other aspects of competition day may be able to be practised
Monitor and debrief after every competition so that you learn what really works for you and how to achieve it • Note your performance • Where applicable monitor hydration status and energy levels over the day • Rate gastrointestinal comfort • Note the logistical challenges in carrying out your plan	• Record your competition plan for each occasion • Debrief as soon as you can after the competition to note what you actually did, and how well it worked. Memories aren't always a reliable source of information, so make your notes while it is fresh in your mind • Sometimes you won't see patterns until you have a series of debriefs to look at objectively

TABLE 12.2
An analysis of a typical day's eating for Michael

Typical food patterns from dietary history	
Early morning training before university classes	Water
Breakfast: eaten at home within 20–30 min of training	Wholegrain or light 'muesli flake' cereal—large bowl (100–150 g) + low-fat milk + sliced or canned fruit 2 slices of wholemeal toast + scrape margarine + jam Glass fruit juice and extra water 2–3 times a week: fruit added to cereal

During morning	Water, particularly if warm day
Lunch: at university on weekdays. Home or competing at meets at weekends	Summer—2 wholemeal rolls with scrape of marg OR mayonnaise, lean protein filling (chicken, salmon, egg or roast beef) and salad Winter—Thick vegetable soup + 2 rounds toasted sandwiches (fillings: baked beans, ham/cheese/tomato or 'leftovers') Scone or muffin, unbuttered Flavoured milk Piece of fruit
Gym training or second track workout after classes	Water or tries to have sports drink for quality session
On way home from training	Banana or plain bagel. Occasionally PowerBar
Dinner: home, later in evening when ready to cook Shares cooking with 2 housemates—occasionally comes home too tired to cook on heavy training day	Large serve (250–350 g) of lean meat or chicken. Likes fish but no one knows how to cook it Large serve of potatoes; rice/pasta: 1–2 times per week (2–3 cups) 3–4 other vegetables or salad All cooking is low-fat and dressings involve monounsaturated fats Juice
Before bed—dessert or snack	Fruit or fruit salad with low-fat yoghurt or ice-cream 1–2 times a week, pudding or cooked dessert If no dessert: bowl of cereal and yoghurt
Weekends	Eats out one night a week—likes Thai and Mexican foods Alcohol—rarely

Average nutrient analysis from 7-day food diary					
Nutrient	Intake/d	Target	Nutrient	Intake	Target
Energy	15.15 MJ (3606 Cal)		Vit A/ Beta-carotene	2675 μg	750 μg
Carbohydrate	525 g (6.7 g/kg, 58% of energy	5–8 g/kg	B1 thiamin	3.5 mg	1.2 mg
Protein	165 g (2.1 g/kg = 18% of energy)	1.2–1.5 g/kg	B2 riboflavin	4.3 mg	1.3 mg
Fat	94 g (24% of energy)		B3 niacin	69 mg	16 mg
Alcohol	Nil		Folate		
Iron	33 mg	8–17 mg	Vitamin C	525 mg	45 mg
Calcium	1120 mg	1000 mg			
Zinc	23 mg	14 mg			

*Targets include RDIs and general guidelines for athletes; see Chapter 2

Olympic weightlifting, powerlifting and throwing

Lifting and throwing require a combination of power, technique and flexibility. Performance is based on the generation of explosive power for a couple of seconds, relying almost completely on anaerobic energy. Muscle stores of adenosine triphosphate (ATP) and phosphocreatine are used to supply the energy for a single effort and are quickly regenerated afterwards. In the throwing events of javelin, shot put, discus, and hammer, athletes compete against each other in open competition. By contrast, in powerlifting and weightlifting (an Olympic sport), athletes are grouped into weight divisions and, in sub-elite competition, according to age.

In each of the lifting sports, athletes complete a number of separate lifts—the snatch and the clean-and-jerk in Olympic weightlifting, and the bench press, squat, and dead lift in power lifting. In weightlifting there is often an outcome for each lift category as well as the total of both lifts, whereas powerlifting recognises the total of all lifts. Depending on the event within lifting and throwing sports, the interplay of technique and skill involved ranges from small to complex. Whereas the lifts in powerlifting involve simple movements, Olympic weightlifting and the throwing sports are more technical, requiring greater flexibility and control. Although women compete in all lifting and throwing events, powerlifting and weightlifting competition is dominated by men.

Training

At school or club level, lifters and throwers may not train all year round. However, as the level of competition increases, so does the training commitment—both over the year and through each week. The focus of training varies with the demands of the event and the time of year. Lifters concentrate on weight training and—in the case of Olympic weightlifting, which involves more refined technique—flexibility. Throwers divide their training time between weight training, running and speed work, flexibility work and technical training. Specific training is done with free weights and resistance machines and often plyometrics and speed loading.

In the off-season or in base training, the main focus is on increasing muscle bulk and strength through general weight training. The number of sets and repetitions undertaken in a weight-training session is larger at this time of the season, boosting strength and stimulating muscle growth. As the competition season approaches, the repetitions are reduced and the weights increased to increase power output. More time is spent fine-tuning technique for specific events. Athletes who compete internationally may have to peak for two or three competition seasons each year.

Competition

During competition, the athlete is given a set number of opportunities to achieve a maximum weight or distance. Typically, throwing events allow three throws per competitor, and the leading eight athletes have another three throws to decide the final placings. The competition is usually conducted without a break and may take a couple of hours to complete. In large international competitions, a qualifying round may be held the day before the final, with the qualifying throw distance pre-set.

In the lifting events, each type of lift is undertaken separately. Within each category, athletes try to lift a series of gradually increasing weights. Each competitor can nominate the mass of the weight at which he wishes to enter the competition; he then has three attempts to lift each weight until he is eliminated. There is a weigh-in a couple of hours before the competition and a short break between lifting categories. Should two lifters achieve the same final weight, the one with the lowest body mass is designated the winner on a count-back. The weight divisions for Olympic weightlifting were reorganised in 2000; there are currently eight weight divisions for men (from <56 kg to >105 kg) and seven for women (<48 kg to >75 kg). There is a break between each section of lifts. Weigh-in starts two hours before the competition and lasts for one hour.

Typically, competitions in the lifting sports are conducted in an air-conditioned arena. The throwing events are generally conducted as outdoor field events and may expose competitors to a range of environmental conditions.

Physical characteristics

Since strength is related to muscle mass, the typical thrower or lifter has a large body weight and muscle mass. In the throwing events, where there are no body-weight limits, body-fat levels can also be high—even by community standards. Unless they are carrying so much fat that it interferes with their technique or puts their general health at risk, excess weight imposes less of a penalty on throwers than on other athletes. The exception is javelin throwers, who have a longer run-up before throwing and need to generate as much speed as possible over this distance. Javelin throwers would be expected to have the lowest body-fat levels among throwers.

Lifters, being classified into weight divisions, show a great variety of body weights and body-fat levels. Within any given division, we might expect lifters to try to maximise their strength by achieving maximal lean body mass and minimal body-fat levels. This seems to be the case in the lower-weight divisions of lifting sports. However, as the weight class increases, we see an increase in relative body-fat levels as well as muscle mass. Lifters seem less concerned than other athletes in weight-division sports about keeping body fat levels down. Heavyweight and super-heavyweight lifters may be justified in being concerned with absolute power rather than power-to-weight ratios.

Common nutritional issues

Bulking up: how much protein do you need?

In Chapter 3.7, we defined the necessary ingredients for successful gain of muscle mass and strength:

- the right parents
- the right training load
- the right diet—amounts and timing of nutrients

Hopefully, you have taken care of the first two, and all that stands between you and success is your diet. What constitutes the right diet is a point of some contention between strength-training athletes and most sports scientists. The folklore in strength sports is that a high protein intake is required—up to 3 g per kg of body weight, or up to 20 per cent of total energy intake. However, as we saw in Chapter 2.3, the consensus of most sports scientists is that while strength-training athletes do need relatively more protein than others, such high levels are unnecessary. Around 1.2–1.6 g of protein per kilogram of body mass is recommended during times of muscle growth, although adolescents may require 2 g per kg during growth spurts. Dietary surveys of strength-training athletes generally report that these protein intake levels are easily reached.

Chapters 2 and 3.4 also look at other dietary strategies that support the goals of resistance training. The first is adequate energy intake. As the story of Joey below illustrates, some athletes still find it difficult to pack enough kilojoules into their daily menu. They can address this problem by being more organised, and planning frequent compact meals and high-energy drinks.

The other important dietary strategy is eating to maximise recovery from training sessions. Chapter 5 summarises the value of consuming the building blocks for the synthesis of new protein—around 20–25 g of high-quality protein—soon after, the weights workout.

If you adopt both of these strategies—ensuring a high total energy intake and consuming a reasonably modest amount of protein around each training session—you are likely to exceed your protein targets. But you are also more likely to achieve your athletic goals.

Carbohydrate: a forgotten nutrient

Many strength athletes do not see a role for carbohydrate in their training diets. However, carbohydrate intake can optimise the gains achieved by a resistance-training program in three ways. Nutritional strategies for resistance-training should both assist the athlete to train hard (optimising the training stimulus) and provide the right environment for the synthesis and retention of muscle (optimising adaptation to training). Although the fuel for a single lift or throw is provided by the ATP and phosphocreatine systems, the repetition of these efforts draws quite heavily on muscle glycogen. Some studies show that specific muscle fibres can have no glycogen left after such a session, and that more work can be completed if resistance training is done in a 'carbohydrate-available' state (with adequate glycogen levels and carbohydrate intake during the session). Theoretically, at least, ensuring an adequate fuel supply for each session should allow the strength or power athlete to train harder and maintain optimal technique throughout the session.

The second advantage of eating enough carbs is that it provides a hormonal environment that reduces protein breakdown. Insulin is an anabolic (synthesis) hormone, while cortisol is a catabolic (breakdown) hormone. Consuming carbohydrate during and after an exercise session promotes an anabolic environment by increasing insulin concentrations and reducing cortisol.

Finally, recent studies have looked at the 'signalling' activities that occur in the muscle to promote adaptive changes after exercise. In Chapter 2.10, we discussed new theories that muscles respond better to the stimulus of endurance exercise when they are in a low-glycogen state. On this basis, some sports scientists say endurance athletes should do some of their training sessions in a low glycogen/carbohydrate state to 'train smarter'. However, it appears that at least one of the important pathways by which resistance training signals the body to synthesise more protein and muscle works best in the presence of high glycogen levels. Studies also show that adding carbohydrate to protein eaten after a workout produces a small increase in rates of protein synthesis.

It is difficult to turn all this information into definite carbohydrate guidelines for strength-training athletes, but two ideas make sense. While strength-training athletes may not chalk up the carbohydrate needs of endurance athletes, neither are they likely to get optimal returns from an eating plan that focuses on protein and ignores carbohydrate or from the low-carbohydrate diets that are touted from time to time in body-building magazines (see Body-building chapter). Such athletes may also benefit from increasing their carbohydrate intake around key training sessions.

Dietary supplements and sports foods

Another area of folklore in strength sports is the need for supplements to achieve optimal gain of muscle mass and strength. Many studies of strength athletes have reported heavy use of various products. The pages of body-building magazines and websites are filled with stories, advertisements and testimonials for products that make astounding promises. Chapter 6 provides a summary of the scientific basis for various sports foods and supplements.

Products such as sport drinks, sport bars, and liquid meal supplements may be used by strength and power athletes before, during or after a workout to meet needs for key nutrients. This may enhance performance and recovery—and help lifters and throwers to achieve better results from their training programs. These products may also increase energy intake and thus help optimise muscle mass and strength gains from resistance training. Creatine is one of the few claimed ergogenic supplements that enjoy strong scientific support for their claimed beneficial effect on resistance training. Other products also show promise—including caffeine or beta-alanine, said to help athletes train harder—but these have not been conclusively shown to produce overall gains in muscle mass and strength. Many of the 'space age' products discussed in body-building magazines and websites have simply not been tested in scientific studies. Whatever products lifters and throwers consider taking, they should weigh the potential side-effects, including the issue of contamination. The case study below illustrates how this hazard can have serious consequences for athletes who compete in sports with anti-doping codes.

Body fat: optimising power-to-weight ratios

Although in some lifting and throwing events a high body-fat level is not a great disadvantage, there are some instances in which athletes would be better off with less body fat. The best example of this is in the low and middle weight divisions of weightlifting and powerlifting, where competitors gain an advantage over their opponents by having the greatest muscle mass (and therefore lowest body-fat level) possible for their weight limit—a higher power-to-weight ratio.

Many lifters do not seem to appreciate this. It is almost a universal practice to compete in a lower weight division than one's usual training weight, theoretically so as to compete against smaller and weaker opponents. Like wrestlers and boxers, most lifters lose weight just before competition through dehydration and fasting. However, unlike wrestlers, studies of lifters report that many have higher body-fat levels than necessary and could profitably shed this weight by losing body fat. This could provide a long-term and safer way of making weight than is customary, as well as ensuring that lifters are in their most competitive weight division. Read Chapters 3.1–3.4 to learn about setting and achieving your ideal weight and body-fat level.

Making weight

Since weightlifting and powerlifting involve weight categories competitors face the issues of making weight. Chapter 3.5 and the chapter on boxing and judo below discuss the disadvantages of the dehydration and severe food-restriction practices that are usually involved. Unlike wrestlers, most lifters may need to use such drastic measures at only three or four major competitions a year. Many compete in higher weight divisions, or not at all, outside these occasions. And unlike wrestlers and boxers, they compete in events that are brief and power-related, so they're less likely to be impaired by dehydration and carbohydrate depletion. Nevertheless, there is a healthier and safer way to tackle the problem of making weight. As explained in Chapter 3.5, you should keep within reach of your competition weight while in training by using sensible weight-control techniques. The final kilo(s) can be shed easily in the later stages of preparation.

Blood lipids

Several studies of blood lipids in throwers and lifters have reported high levels of cholesterol and triglycerides, and low levels of HDL cholesterol (the protective form of cholesterol). This pattern has been linked with an increased risk of coronary disease. By contrast, endurance athletes generally have quite low-risk lipid profiles. There are a number of possible explanations for the poor profiles of strength athletes. First, some are overweight, with body-fat levels that make them obese even by community standards. Many athletes, trying to consume maximal protein in bulking-up diets, end up taking in large amounts of fat. And finally, the use of anabolic steroids is known to disrupt lipid levels.

If you share any of these characteristics, and particularly if you have a family history of heart disease, then you should have a blood lipid screening. Even if the results are OK, you would be better off switching to a healthier nutritional plan. Following the dietary principles outlined in Chapters 1, 2 and 3 will yield numerous benefits. Be at your ideal body weight and body-fat level, and eat a high-energy diet that is adequate in carbohydrate and moderate in fat. High protein levels can easily be achieved with such a plan.

Profile: Joey

Get massive? Get organised!

Joey weighed six kilograms less than the shot putter he wanted to be. At the end of the previous season he had resolved to be 100 kg by his next competition, but his efforts over the following four months produced a gain of 1 kg. For someone with his dedication this was frustratingly slow progress. He trained hard in the gym, ate constantly and until he was uncomfortably full, and supplemented his diet with the latest generation of weight-gain supplements and weight-gain powder. Finally, in desperation, he consulted a sports dietitian who specialised in strength sports.

The dietitian began by reviewing his goals. Had he set himself a realistic target? Had he allowed himself sufficient time to achieve it? Although a shot putter pays a lower penalty for extra body fat than other athletes do, Joey's target was to gain muscle (and strength) rather than weight *per se*. His coach assured him that his body characteristics and training program should enable him to bulk up well. It was theoretically possible for him to gain 1–2 kg of lean body mass a month under these conditions. Could the weak link be his diet?

Joey described a typical day of eating to the dietitian. A late but hearty breakfast of cereal, toast and eggs was followed by a session in the gym. Then it was home for a cooked lunch and off to afternoon lectures at the technical school. After a quick dash to training, and the evening workout, he returned home to an evening of eating. His mother would have dinner No. 1 ready when he walked in the door, and before he went to bed he would sit down to another meal of leftovers and a weight-gain milkshake. His family marvelled that at each of his evening meals he ate more than his mother, father and young sister combined. On weekends, Joey's routine changed because of his job as a bouncer at a nightclub. Working from 9 p.m. to 4 a.m. on Friday and Saturday nights meant having naps on Friday afternoon and between training sessions on Saturday. Sunday, a non-training day, was spent catching up on lost sleep. But lately he had been taking on some Sunday shifts at the nightclub. The extra money would come in handy for some new supplements.

The dietitian suggested that Joey keep a food diary during a typical week. The results came as a surprise to him, but it was easy to see his problem when it was written in black and white. Although he spent some parts of his day eating a lot, there were many long stretches when he ate nothing at all. Joey fitted many activities into his day—school, training, work and sleep. All these turned his attention away from food. Weekends were a complete upheaval, breaking up any eating routine that he might have developed during the week. Not only did he waste good 'eating time' during the day catching up on rest, but he took only a couple of sandwiches to work to eat on his short rest break. The result was almost eight hours of wasted energy-intake opportunities.

The dietitian concluded that Joey's problem was simply insufficient kilojoules to support the maximum gain of muscle mass. She explained that consuming more energy overall would increase his intakes of protein and all the other nutrients needed to build new muscle. He needed to find more efficient (and nutritious) ways to get kilojoules into his mouth. The keys to this were planning and timing.

Planning meant having foods on hand—for example, taking a

supply to eat on the way to the gym and while at work. Instead of taking a couple of rounds of sandwiches to the nightclub, Joey might take a couple of French sticks made up into giant meat, cheese and salad rolls. He could work his way through these over the course of the night.

In reviewing Joey's supplement program, the sports dietitian tried to take a pragmatic approach. She acknowledged the hype and buzz about 'volumising', 'super-bulking' and 'third-generation delivery systems' in the products Joey bought online or from the gym. She agreed that the lack of studies of most of these products means there is no scientific proof that they *don't* work, just as there is no scientific proof that they do. However, she suggested that Joey rationalise his spending on supplements, concentrating on those most likely to support his goals and provide value for money. As an example, she showed him a report in a study of his expensive 'serum creatine' product, which found that it contained very little creatine. In fact, creatine breaks down quite quickly and irreversibly when dissolved in liquid. If there were scientific proof that creatine might help Joey train harder in the gym and get better results, it would be worth continuing with this supplement. But even then he would be better off buying a simple and much cheaper creatine monohydrate powder from a reputable company and dissolving it in a drink just before consuming it. An immediate benefit of the money saved by such tactics would be that Joey could cut back on his extra shifts at work. Better eating and more sleep are definite performance enhancers.

High-energy drinks would also be part of the plan. The dietitian explained that there was nothing magical about the weight-gain powder Joey had bought online, despite a price that sucked up most of his wages. The trick was to use the principle of 'low bulk, no chew' nutrition more frequently, even three times a day, between meals. The dietitian showed him several cheaper options in the form of homemade thickshakes and smoothies, using a less expensive protein–carbohydrate powder or skim milk powder to boost their nutritional value. These drinks would be a mainstay on weekends, when Joey was trying to catch up on sleep. A snack and a drink could add up to plenty of kilojoules, yet be quickly consumed and easily digested.

Joey and the dietitian worked out a plan of six meals a day: breakfast as soon as he woke up; a mid-morning shake before he left for training; lunch as before; a couple of rolls and two Tetra Paks of a liquid meal for a snack between classes at school; the family dinner; and finally a lighter snack and a high-energy fruit smoothie. That plan would ensure that he went to bed feeling less bloated and was ready for breakfast as soon as he woke up. A different routine was planned for weekends.

With his energy intake spread more evenly throughout the day, Joey was able to increase his total intake by almost 30 per cent. This kick-started his muscle-gain program within a fortnight, and Joey achieved his target weight within six months. And that was without most of the expensive supplements on which he had previously spent so much.

Joey found that maintaining his new weight required dedicated adherence to his meal routine. After the annual school exams were over, he led a rather nomadic life for a fortnight, going out with friends at night and sleeping in later in the mornings. The scales showed a 2-kg loss and reinforced the lesson that gains are made through a carefully planned diet rather than haphazard eating. Joey now appreciates that for as long as he continues his shot put career, he will need to approach his diet with the same rigour and application that he shows in his training sessions.

Profile

Contaminated supplements: The end of a career?

In April 2008, four months before the Beijing Olympic Games, 11 lifters from the 14-member Greek national weightlifting team tested positive for a banned steroid. The coach blamed the results on contaminated dietary supplements from a Chinese manufacturer. There is evidence (see Chapter 6) that a large proportion of sports supplements contain products, including banned ingredients, which are not declared on the label. Many of these banned ingredients are stimulants or compounds like anabolic steroids which can be legally sold over the counter in some countries but are banned by sports' anti-doping codes. In some cases, the contaminant is a drug that would normally require a prescription. The contamination can arise from even a small crossover of ingredients during manufacturing—for example, a small coating of powder left on a machine used to make a steroid-containing supplement could find its way into the sports product made later in the day. However, in some cases, the amount of the banned product in a supplement is so large as to suggest that the ingredient was included deliberately, just not declared. The regulation of supplement manufacture in many countries is not strict enough to prevent such problems. So there are some reasons to believe athletes when they say a positive drug test must have resulted from accidental consumption of a banned substance 'hidden' in a supplement. Unfortunately, this has also become a convenient excuse used by cheats to cover up deliberate drug-taking.

The anti-doping codes of most sporting organisations insist on strict liability, so even if athletes can show that the banned substance ended up in their system by accident, they must still pay the penalty. How this penalty is applied can depend on the sport in question and the legal procedures open to them. Here are just some of the stories of athletes who appear to have been caught up in the crossfire of contaminated supplements.

- Rebekah Keat, a former junior world champion in Olympic-distance triathlon and winner of many half-Ironman triathlons, won the 2004 Busselton Ironman race in Western Australia but was disqualified after testing positive for a banned steroid similar to Nandrolone. She denied that she had knowingly taken a prohibited substance and attributed the result to her use of an electrolyte supplement called endurolyte. This product was manufactured and provided to her by her sponsor, the American company Hammer Nutrition. It had been designed specifically to address the nutritional needs of an ultra-endurance event, and came with a guarantee that it contained no banned ingredients. She received a two-year ban from sport. During this time, an accredited laboratory tested a previously unopened container of Endurolyte and found it to be contaminated with norandrostenedione. An appeal to the Court of Arbitration of Sport accepted that Keat's positive test was attributable to the use of a contaminated supplement, but upheld the ban. Keat was able to resume her triathlon career in 2007, and now lectures on behalf of the Australian Sports Anti-Doping Authority on the risks of taking supplements. In 2008 she joined in a lawsuit against Hammer Nutrition by two other high-profile athletes who had had a similar experience—US cyclist Amber Neben and Canadian off-road triathlete Mike Vine. This case had yet to reach trial at the time this book was published.

- A player from a third-league club in the German Soccer Federation tested positive for substances related to Nandrolone at a cup match. The player was suspended for doping, but this ban was lifted by the sports tribunal after seven weeks, when it was found that a creatine supplement given to the player by the team medical staff was contaminated with the banned products. The soccer club sued the supplement manufacturer and settled out of court.
- Hans Knauss, an Austrian downhill skier and silver medallist from the 1998 Winter Olympic Games, tested positive for Nandrolone in 2004. He was aware of the risks of supplement contamination and had therefore sought assurances from Ultimate Nutrition, the American manufacturer of Super Complete supplements, that they were neither contaminated nor contained listed ingredients that were banned. The supplier of the supplements gave him a written guarantee of this. After his test, he had the supplements examined, and they were found to be the source of his positive result. The Court of Arbitration in Sport rejected Knauss's plea of no fault or negligence, noting that since WADA and other sports federations had repeatedly warned of the risks of taking supplements, he could not be said to be free of fault or negligence. The tribunal accepted that he had taken significant steps to protect against the risk of contamination, but noted that he could have done more, including simply not taking the supplements. As a result, it ruled that his degree of fault justified reducing his original two-year ban by only six months. Knauss was banned from skiing for a total of 18 months. The Austrian hero—a former winner of a famous downhill race—retired from sport because of the difficulty of coming back into a competitive Austrian team and because he would now miss the 2006 Winter Olympics.
- American national team swimmer Kicker Vencill won a $500,000 lawsuit against the Ultimate Nutrition company when he was able to show that their steroid-contaminated supplement

was the cause of his positive drug test in 2003. As a result of this finding, his four-year suspension from his sport was reduced to two years. Although Vencill was pleased to win the court case, he said in an interview: 'Nothing can ever rewind the clock and give me back what I lost . . . what that whole situation equals is, this guy disrespected his sport, himself, his family, his team, his team-mates, the whole swimming community and athletics in general by testing positive on a drug test. And for someone who came from a small town in the middle of nowhere in Kentucky where swimming doesn't mean anything, and worked my way to a national and international level, only to be called a cheater when I knew it came from hard work, sacrifice and dedication . . . my family sacrificed, that's the hardest part about it.'

- Seventeen-year-old rugby player Adam Deane had scored a try in his debut game as an international player for England's under-18 team before testing positive for a Nandrolone-like substance in 2005. Barred from all rugby contact, he went from playing and training five days a week to not even being able to walk through the door of his club. Following the pressure to be 'bigger, faster and stronger', Deane had joined a 'hard-core' gym and begun taking muscle-gain supplements. Despite being educated about the risks of supplement taking, he had placed his trust in a product that listed no prohibited substances on the label and made claims of being 'suitable for drug tested athletes'.
- The Argentinian tennis player Guillermo Coria was ranked 30th in the world when he tested positive for a Nandrolone-related substance in 2001. His two-year suspension was reduced to seven months when he was able to prove that the multivitamin tablets that he had been taking (made by the US company Universal Nutrition) were contaminated with steroids. He returned to tennis and peaked at No. 3 before gradually dropping below 300th in the world in 2007 as a result of injury. In 2007 his lawsuit against the supplement company was finally settled for an undisclosed sum. His lawyer argued that Coria had lost two professional seasons, leading to losses in

> prize money, endorsements and appearance fees, and asked for more than $10 million in damages. However, Coria also said the injury to his reputation had been more painful than his loss of income.

These and other stories show how severe the consequences of a failed drug test due to supplement use can be. Several important questions deserve answers:

1. If the situation is so bad—in one survey, 15 per cent of supplements studied were found to be contaminated with steroid-like ingredients—why aren't we inundated with daily reports of positive drugs tests arising from supplement use?

- Only a niche group of athletes compete in sports under drug codes, so not all athletes may encounter the problems.
- The serving size of the supplement may influence the risk—for example, a protein powder that is consumed in 60–100-g serves may expose the athlete to a greater risk than a product that is consumed in 1 g capsules.
- Most athletes are not drug tested very often.
- It may all be in the timing—drug testing protocols may generally allow sufficient time after an athlete has consumed a contaminated supplement for it to be cleared from the body.

2. Why don't governments or the supplement industry fix the problem so that contamination—from impure raw ingredients or from mixing of products during the manufacturing process—don't occur? Why is the supplement industry so poorly regulated?

- The risk to public safety from contaminated supplements is generally low, so it isn't a huge priority for health authorities.
- Only a small number of athletes are concerned with anti-doping issues; some are actually happy with the idea that prohibited substances might be available in supplements. Therefore, even within sport, there isn't a huge push for a solution to the problem.
- Citizen free will is a hugely emotive issue: many people are against greater regulation of the industry because they feel

governments shouldn't interfere with their decision or ability to take supplements, or with the pricing of those supplements.
- Billions of dollars are involved—the supplement industry is a powerful political and business lobby.

3. What can an athlete do to eliminate the risk of testing positive because of supplement use (apart from not using supplements)?

- Recognise that the risk is real but can be minimised by careful decision-making.
- Weigh the likely benefit of using a supplement against risks such as contamination. Limit the use of supplements and choose products and manufacturers carefully.
- Make use of the risk-minimisation programs of various countries and sporting organisations, which give transparent information to athletes about supplement products.
- Get the input of a sports dietitian or a sports scientist who is an expert in this area to help with the steps above.

Body-building

Body-builders sculpt their own bodies to challenge the limits of muscularity and definition. Although the goal for most body-builders is simply to achieve their desired physique, some devotees compete in posing contests and for titles. The International Federation of Body-building and Fitness, which runs the top end of professional body-building has awarded the coveted Mr Olympia prize since 1965. Competitors such as Arnold Schwarzenegger and Lou Ferrigno have translated their body-building success into movie careers. Women also participate in body-building activities and competition, and the Miss Olympia title was created in 1980. Many women prefer to focus on Fitness and Figure competitions, which highlight muscle tone rather than size.

The body-building community is a flamboyant and close-knit one that can only be fully understood from within. Nutrition and training fads change regularly and often dramatically. Ideas come from hyped claims and testimonials spread through word of mouth in gyms, articles in muscle magazines and discussion online. It is hard to bridge the gap between the beliefs and practices of hard-core body-builders and conventional sports science. Although this chapter will try to bridge that gap, we will be realistic in stating that it's a wide one.

Training

The year of a competitive body-builder is divided into three phases. In the off-season, training is aimed at bulking up, or increasing overall muscle size. The result is that most body-builders are well over competition weight, and body-fat levels can be relatively high. As the competition season approaches, body-builders begin to 'cut up'—aiming to lose body fat so as to increase muscle definition without losing muscle mass or size. Finally, in the days or week before competition, body-builders take special steps to achieve cosmetic changes that will make their bodies appear 'pumped', with clearly defined muscularity and veining, or vascularity. Bodybuilders who do not take part in competitions may train simply to bulk up.

The training methods used by body-builders are diverse and often dramatic, and there are as many enthusiastically recommended programs as there are articles in body-building magazines. In general, both elite and recreational body-builders can spend many hours in the gym each day, usually following 'split routines' in which different parts of the body are trained at different sessions. Training typically involves three to five exercises for each of the six major muscle groups (chest, back, arms, legs, shoulders and abdomen). Each exercise normally comprises three to six sets of lifts or repetitions. Body-builders usually perform a greater number of repetitions per set (6–15) than do powerlifters or weightlifters (1–5), since this leads to bigger, more visible muscles. In the cutting-up phase, many body-builders incorporate more aerobic exercise into their programs to help reduce body-fat levels.

Competition

Body-builders may take part in contests sanctioned by a large number of organisations, ranging from professional associations to 'natural body-building' groups, which follow an anti-doping code and include drug testing during competition. Competitions are usually arranged into weight divisions, and there may also be divisions by age or experience—for example, a novice class. Ultimately, a body-building contest involves posing before a panel of judges. Typically, there are three stages of judging involved in body-building contests. In the symmetry round, all competitors appear on the stage together and gradually rotate their bodies while maintaining a single 'tensed' pose that allows all sides of their body to be scrutinised for symmetry and proportion. In the compulsory posing round, all competitors are again judged comparatively, and are required to undertake a series of set poses so judges can further scrutinise their physique. The individual posing round allows competitors to perform their own routine of poses to music; this lasts 1–2 minutes. The routine in this case is chosen to highlight the performer's strengths and downplay his weaknesses.

Competitions may involve a pre-judging round, in which contestants carry out these routines in a morning session attended by the judges. These rounds are repeated at the evening session in front of a larger audience. The final activity is a 'pose down', in which the top competitors again take the stage and spontaneously pose against each other. The judges' decision is announced after this, and is based on muscle size, shape, symmetry, vascularity and leanness. In preparing for a contest, body-builders attempt to minimise body fat so their muscles will look as 'cut' as possible. Removal of body hair and the addition of a tan and a sheen of oil during posing are all part of body-building's aesthetics.

Physical characteristics

The physical characteristics of body-builders are well known—and need little elaboration. Body-builders have a large total body weight owing to their large muscles. Depending on the time of year, body-fat levels may vary, from normal to high during the bulking-up phase, to minimal during the competition phase.

Common nutritional issues

Body-building vs traditional sports nutrition

Body building, more than any other sport, has placed nutrition on a pedestal. Body-builders are unsurpassed in their fastidious attention to diet. However, not all the nutritional philosophies of body-building agree with established scientific views. In fact, there is a huge gulf between body-builders and conventional sports nutrition.

For a sports dietitian, competing against the typical body-builder's nutritional beliefs and practices can be a losing game. For a start, it is hard to compete against the powerful communication and merchandising networks in body-building. Googling 'body-building or body-building supplements' yielded some 5 million links. That's a lot of 'free' information—although, of course, most of it comes from people with something to sell. Many of the nutrition experts within body-building have mainstream qualifications such as masters degrees and doctorates in sports science or sports nutrition. However, not all share mainstream views. And of course there are other 'experts' who have neither mainstream qualifications nor mainstream views. It can be hard to push the latter against ideas that have the triple advantage of being exciting, (allegedly) science-based and eagerly touted within a close-knit community. Finally, and sadly, it is sometimes hard for healthy dietary practices to match the undeniable results that can be gained through the use of drugs such as anabolic steroids and other unsafe practices.

From the perspective of the body-builder, conventional sports nutrition can seem frustratingly conservative. It's easy to conclude that its practitioners just don't understand the needs and proactive practices of the body-building lifestyle. Body-builders and the scientists who work in their corner are excited about new ideas, and find the practices of successful competitors compelling. They are not worried that few of these practices or the supplements hyped on the Internet have received scientific scrutiny. In fact, they may even be scornful of the system of peer review—scientists scrutinising each other's work—that decides what gets published in the scientific journals. It is true that there is some subjectivity in this process. Most scientists know of good studies that have been rejected by scientific journals and of poorly conducted studies that have been accepted and have thus become 'the truth'. Even the process of analysing the results of studies deserves criticism, because traditional statistics usually fail to detect small changes or differences that may have important effects on sporting outcomes. However, there are new ways to interpret the results of studies so that the real-life significance can be understood.

We hope that with time and communication, some of the gaps between body-builders and conventional sports scientists can be bridged. However, it seems likely that there will always be issues on which the two groups agree to disagree.

How can you evaluate nutritional advice?

Almost every body-building magazine or website carries articles in which top competitors or body-building scientists share the secrets of their training, diet and supplement programs (see the profile below). If you're a body-builder and feel overwhelmed with the volume and diversity of ideas that are thrust at you, you're not alone. Even sports dietitians find it hard to keep pace with the range and turnover of advice promoted to body-builders and other strength athletes.

The sheer numbers of products and dietary ideas are matched by the aggressive marketing campaigns prepared by supplement companies. Marketing tactics include testimonials from satisfied consumers, including impressive before-and-after photos and detailed accounts of the improvements credited to the product. Sometimes these anecdotes are accompanied by disclaimers that the results are not necessarily representative of typical or that the participants were paid for their stories. Other times the advertisements include statements required by the laws of various countries along the lines of 'these claims haven't been evaluated' or 'these claims are not intended as therapeutic (medical) advice'. However, these disclaimers are usually displayed in fine print and seldom understood or even noticed alongside the exciting information in bigger, bolder type.

Endorsements and testimonials from famous or successful competitors have a powerful influence on a lay audience. Luckily, most sport dietitians are aware of their limitations and can educate athletes about them. The tricky part is dealing with claims that a product or dietary strategy has been 'scientifically proven' to achieve various benefits. This may come in the form of endorsements from people who are said to be medical and scientific experts, or it may be accompanied by information and graphs from studies, or quotes from papers in scientific journals.

Unlike pharmaceutical companies, the makers of supplements are under no legal obligation to have their products rigorously tested before they hit the market. Nevertheless, some companies have realised that supportive research findings can enhance their products' credibility and sales. Many supplement makers employ exercise scientists and sports nutrition professionals to conduct or arrange scientific trials or write up the results. Unfortunately, however, some simply set up a smokescreen to make it look as if such research exists, using a 'scientist for hire' to add credibility to information that's been twisted to suit their story.

So how can you tell science from marketing, anecdote from truth, credibility from creative writing? Who should you listen to? How do you know who the real experts are? Checklist 14.1 provides some simple ways to answer some of these questions for yourself. The profile below illustrates the way in which marketing can twist or exaggerate science. If you have concerns about any nutritional information, seek the guidance of an expert like a sports dietitian. If he can't answer your question immediately, he will certainly know how to get the information needed to do so.

Nutrition for training and bulking up

During the training phase or off-season, a body-builders' main goal is to gain muscle size. This is achieved by consuming large amounts of energy and protein, with a pattern of multiple meals and snacks over a day. Even during this hypertrophy phase, body-builders typically show a rigid attitude to diet. Examples include scheduling meals every two to three hours (even setting the alarm to get up at night) and limiting food choices to a small range. Typically, meals are based on protein-rich, low-fat foods, and although attitudes to carbohydrate-rich foods appear to change from time to time, there is a general focus on 'healthy carbs'—foods with a low Glycemic Index that are also low in fat and high in fibre and micronutrients. Although these food choices were outlined in Chapter 1 as the backbone of healthy eating and sports nutrition guidelines, many body-builders take their focus on them to an extreme. They may follow the same food plan, involving a small rotation of foods, for months on end. A simple example of a day's eating in such a plan is provided in Table 14.1. You can often tell a body-builder simply by the large volume and narrow variety of foods that are in their shopping trolley!

Even though their meals and snacks are already focused on protein-rich foods, body-builders generally believe that protein supplements, including powders, bars, and free-form amino acids, are also necessary. Total protein intakes of body-builders from foods and supplements during this phase typically exceed 2 to 3 g per kg of body weight each day. You can see how quickly this adds up by looking at Table 2.9, which lists the protein content of various foods. This is well above the levels of less than 2 g per kg supported by scientific evidence. Though the multi-meal body-building diet is not always based on a correct understanding of the science, it is likely to provide protein at the right time in relation to workouts to maximise muscle growth.

Is there anything wrong with eating too much protein? This is a hotly debated topic. A few people with poor kidney function may have problems excreting the waste products of protein metabolism. A high protein intake may also interfere with calcium balance. The expense of eating lots of high-quality protein—especially when it comes in bars and powders priced for a spellbound audience—is probably the most obvious issue. But we should not neglect the knowledge that eating excessive amounts of protein increases the use of protein as an energy source rather than promoting protein storage. This is likely to be a problem if someone suddenly switches from a high-protein diet to a lower-protein one—as happens when a body-builder switches from a weight-gain diet to a strict pre-contest 'cutting up' plan. Having adapted his body to a high protein intake and got it used to using protein for fuel, the body-builder may end up unnecessarily sacrificing some of the muscle mass he has strived so hard to gain as he tries to adapt to the new dietary balance.

Although the dietary advice provided in Chapters 1, 2 and 3 of this book isn't as exciting or as regimented as the programs practised by body-builders or espoused on body-building websites, it provides an evidence-based approach to supporting training (Chapter 2), gaining lean body mass (Chapter 3.7 and 3.8) and losing body fat (Chapter 3.4).

The carbohydrate needs of body-builders are harder to pinpoint. There is currently no targeted research that identifies how much carbohydrate is needed to promote optimal muscle gain. But it is counterintuitive to severely restrict the amount and variety of carbohydrate-rich foods in a bulking-up plan. As explained in the Lifting and throwing chapter, it makes sense to have sufficient muscle fuel to train hard, and to help the body respond to that training. Base your plans on your sport's real needs rather than folklore.

Competition eating

Preparation for a body-building contest typically begins 6 to 16 weeks out from the show and involves cutting energy intake by as much as a half to reduce body-fat levels and increase muscular definition. In some cases, there is a severe restriction of carbohydrate intake or a cycling between minimal and moderate amounts (see the profile below). The characteristics of the body-building diet—restricted food variety and heavy supplement use—usually become even more pronounced at this time.

The week of peaking for a show is accompanied by further bizarre practices aimed at a final loss of body fat and the achievement of skin dehydration, muscle 'pump' and a flat stomach. These changes all help to produce the desired muscularity, vascularity and definition. Some body-builders drastically deplete their glycogen stores, then carbohydrate load to expand muscle volume, although one study has reported that this practice fails to measurably increase muscle girth. Other typical practices include drastic alterations to fluid and electrolyte intake, and dehydrating techniques involving diuretics and other drugs. There have been documented reports of body-builders restricting daily fluid intake to one to two cups of distilled water for a week before a contest, or not drinking at all for three days while taking other measures to induce further dehydration. (The body-builder who followed this last routine died of a heart attack shortly after winning the contest.) Some body-building websites promote drinking large volumes of water for a period—for example, 10 L a day—then drastically limiting or cutting out water in the 12–36 hours before the show. These practices are in clear contrast to the approach to fluid needs in Chapter 2. Other folklore-based practices for achieving a muscle that is 'volumised' and 'shredded' rather than looking 'flat' or 'soft' include drinking red wine (diuretic, vasodilator) the night before, and in the warm-up to, a show.

Again, it is hard to compete with the exotic but extreme competition practices that are romanticised in body-building circles. However, body-builders are encouraged to carry out their final preparation with more moderate methods that can achieve a pleasing appearance with fewer side-effects.

Post-competition blow-out

Not surprisingly, after a period of extremely restricted and disciplined eating, most body-builders enjoy a dietary splurge after the contest. Post-contest eating may double or triple usual energy intake, and increase fat intake tenfold. It may range from a welcome meal of previously denied foods to binge eating lasting weeks. Table 14.2 provides an example of a day of post-contest eating reported in a descriptive study of female body-builders by American nutritionist Janet Walberg-Rankin. Not surprisingly, weight gains of 5–10 kg are quickly achieved.

Some experts feel that the cycle of severely restrained eating followed by binges is a form of disordered eating. Indeed, some studies have reported that body-builders score highly on eating-disorder questionnaires. Whether these practices are simply part of the culture of the sport or represent behaviours that the body-builder can't escape from, they pose a threat to physical and mental health.

Supplements and sports foods

Body-builders are probably the largest consumers of sports foods and supplements of any groups of athletes. They provide an enthusiastic market for products claiming to enhance capacity to train, increase muscle size, promote fat loss, promote a muscle 'pump', change the body's water balance and maintain health. Products include powders, shakes, bars, pills, liquids and drops placed under the tongue. Many body-builders consume a large number of products each day and 'stack' and cycle supplements—strategies that mirror those of drug users in sport.

Even body-builders who do not use drugs may be avid consumers of supplements that are closely related to anabolic steroids (the so-called prohormones such as norandrostenedione and DHEA). In fact, many of the supplements produced for the body-building market bear names resembling those of anabolic drugs, and their makers heavily promote their (alleged) drug-like outcomes. Though these supplements may not be legally sold in many countries, athletes can purchase supplies from websites and by mail order. Typically, these compounds and supplements are also banned by anti-doping codes in sport. However, most body-builders pay no heed to these codes—many body-building competitions do not involve drug testing, and in any case many body-builders simply train rather than take part in contests. Nevertheless, these supplement compounds carry health risks—from both their primary ingredients and contaminants. The problem of contamination of supplements was covered in Chapter 6 and the Lifting and throwing sports chapter.

Chapter 6 gives the lowdown on the supplements and sports foods shown by scientific testing to benefit sports performance. This information is admittedly tame and unexciting compared to the material that fills muscle magazines and body-building websites, but it can help you achieve good results without damage to your health or bank account (see the Rugby chapter for ways to keep supplement costs down).

Profile

Understanding body-building literature

Body-builders are avid sharers and consumers of information about the latest 'best' practices. Before the Internet became a major venue for the exchange, we did a brief survey of the main muscle magazines to see what they were offering.

Muscle magazines are often published by companies that manufacture or market supplements, own gym franchises or organise body-building competitions. Depending on your perspective, these magazines either shape or report the beliefs and practices of strength and power athletes. At one end of what is a large and diverse range are the publications like *Muscle and Fitness*, which take a relatively science-based approach to body-building. The target market for *M&F* is presumably more mainstream or well-educated strength-training athletes. Magazines such as this feature an editorial advisory board of exercise scientists and qualified sports nutritionists. These scientists often have a track record in research, and may be consultants or direct employees of supplement companies. They contribute articles on training programs, nutrition and supplements which are usually written at a high level of 'lay science'. The articles are typically punchy, using a blend of scientific language and body-building jargon. Popular features include 'Top 10' lists of the best foods, supplements or diet and training approaches. The magazines promise, and often deliver, state-of-the-art information. For example, they often contain columns that summarise the abstracts of papers in peer-reviewed scientific journals and comment on how the findings can be applied to strength training or body-building. They may also offer Q&A columns where readers' questions are addressed by a scientist.

All this sounds good, and it mostly is. However, there are some caveats. In our opinion, some of the nutrition articles in the 'science-based' muscle magazines stretch information beyond the scientifically defensible. Sometimes, ideas from preliminary findings are presented like the Ten Commandments. Information from studies of animals, untrained people, or people with diseases may not be relevant to body-builders, but it is often treated as the last word in scientific truth. When we counted the advertisements and advertorials for supplements and sports foods in issues of *Muscle & Fitness*, we found that they took up more than one-third of the total space in the magazine. Many lay athletes can't tell the difference between sound science and something that simply sounds scientific—especially when both are presented in the same format, with sophisticated discussions of biochemistry and exercise metabolism, and lists of scientific citations. The authors of these features may be ahead of their time in predicting the next 'big thing' in sports nutrition. On the other hand, they may simply be contributing to a short-lived interest in something that will ultimately disappear as a fad.

At the other end of the spectrum are magazines like *Flex*. Although it's from the same publishing stable as *M&F*, *Flex* describes its audience as 'hard-core body-builders'. The space devoted to supplements in both magazines is about the same, but the products are often different—in *Flex* they are more likely to be promoted as having drug-like attributes. The language of the advertisements and the articles is 'in your face', using the popular language of body-building rather than the vocabulary of science. The articles are mostly written by body-builders, and as well as covering topics of diet and training, they also cover the outcomes of contests. The perspective is more likely to be, 'Copy my practices because I am a successful body-builder' than, 'This is underpinned by scientific evidence'.

How has the Internet changed body-building? First of all, it has exponentially increased the volume and accessibility of information. Countless sites devoted to body-building interests, including online versions of body-building magazines, are only a click away. The Web has also changed body-building practices, making supplements far more accessible—they can be bought from around the world, whether or not they are available or authorised in your own country—and increasing the amount of audible 'chatter' on how to eat and train, via blogs and forums.

Table 14.3 provides an example of the advice on diet, supplement and workouts that can be found on such sites. Many of the novice body-builders or other strength-trained athletes who read such advice may be caught up by the enthusiasm of the author, the muscularity shown in his pictures, and the mystique involved in following a puritanical eating pattern and exotic supplement program. Many will seek to emulate this regime, despite the expense, the boredom, the fatigue—and perhaps the absence of factors such as genetics, training and drug use that might be the real basis of Joe's achievements. Any sports dietitian will face formidable difficulties in helping body-builders find middle ground between these ideas and scientifically supported nutrition practices.

Profile

Sound science or scientific-sounding?

Many of the articles and advertisements in muscle magazines (and websites) wax lyrical about the 'scientific proof' that a particular supplement or diet aids the achievement of some body-building goal. An example of such information is provided in a fictional advertisement in Figure 14.1. There are many features that make these claims look impressive:

- Emotive body-building argot and technical language, which may impress or confuse the audience.
- A scientist who enthusiastically endorses the product and the science behind it.
- The endorsement of a top body-builder and testimonials from other body-builders about amazing achievements with the product.
- Patents
- Secret ingredients
- Ingredients that lend a scientific rationale to claims that the product works wonders.
- A study that shows fantastic results.
- References from scientific journals

FIGURE 14.1
Fictional advertisement for a body-building supplement

Are you prepared for a new and extremely powerful growth-enhancing hyper-dilation product?

Silvers Monsta Pump™

The ingredient profile of this scientific breakthrough is mind-blowing. Many of the ingredients in Monsta Pump™ are completely unique and relatively unheard of. The technology behind its state-of-the-art delivery system is patented.

Dr Cal Dugmann, research coordinator of the Silver Metabolic Laboratory says:

> *If you think there is something out there, or something that will come along, to outperform this product—think again! Simply, no product can come close to producing the growth, pump, mental focus, and performance factors that Monsta Pump™ does. Monsta Pump™ is an amazing accomplishment in the history of supplementation. But let the results speak for themselves.*

Clinical trials in our laboratory[1] yielded the following incredible outcomes:

- Five body-builders randomly selected from a local gym were allocated to a 12-week program of supervised workouts and twice-daily application of Monsta Pump™ in an intention to treat statistical design
- We monitored training load, recovery profiling and anthropometry
- After the program, subjects achieved a significant increase in weight and muscle girth ($P<0.001$), and a loss in waist circumference ($P<0.05$).
- Results for Subject A are demonstrated in the photo below (weight gain of 7.5 kg, increase in chest girth of 14 cm, 10 cm loss of waist circumference)
- Subjects recorded a mean increase in training load of 10.5 per cent, and reported a whopping 40 per cent improvement in recovery after each session. All reported a marked increase in workout pump which lasted 24 per cent longer than pre-trial

While we can't tell you all of our patented secret ingredients, we can let you know that they work in synergy with the highly popular arginine alpha-ketoglutarate (A-AKG). AAKG has the unique ability to perpetually sustain the flow of muscle-building agents to skeletal muscle by increasing the nitric oxide levels in your body.[2] Explode your muscles with Monsta Pump™! You'll understand why the reigning Mr Stratosphere, Joe Biceps, counts it as his favourite product!

References:

1. Dugmann C. New NO delivery supplement enhances body-building outcomes (abst). Bogus Assoc of Sports Science conference, 2009, p. 31
2. Hawley J.B., Hawley J. A. Effects of vasodilatory agent on cardiac muscle patency in transgenic MURF-I-resistant Mice. Journal of Nobel-winning Research 2009; 52: 2–5.

But appearances can be deceiving. In the case of the ad for Monsta Pump:

- Both lay and scientific language can be used to lend false credibility.
- A secret ingredient might sound cool and mysterious, but consuming it is diametrically opposed to the principle that athletes should only consume products known to be safe, legal and effective.
- Anyone can apply for a patent or trademark for a product or idea—this is not a measure of its real worth.
- Sometimes the scientists who provide scientific testimonials for a product are employed by, or directors of, the company that makes it. This does not necessarily invalidate their scientific opinion, but it does need to be taken into account.
- Many athletes, too, are paid for their comments. And nobody can say how much their success might owe to the use of a given product.
- Scientific studies require some basic design characteristics to be credible. In the Monsta Pump case:
    - There was no control group or control treatment—no

similar subjects undergoing the same training but not taking Monsta Pump. In a well-designed study, the control group would take a placebo—a product believed to be Monsta Pump—so they would be similarly motivated to feel special and train hard.

- Ideally, the only difference between the group receiving treatment and the control group would be Monsta Pump. The subjects in this case reported an 'increased training load'. So how does the study differentiate between the effects of this harder training and the effects of Monsta Pump? In addition, although the training was standardised, other factors that might affect the success of a training program, such as diet, were not controlled.
- The study sample was small (making it unlikely to be able to detect real changes from just one intervention). No information is given about the participants in the study, so we can't be sure that any results they experienced are applicable to the people who want to buy the product
- The measurements taken to record changes are poorly described. What do the authors mean by measuring 'recovery' or 'muscle pump'?
- Simply providing us a 'change' score, or an example based on a single study participant, gives us no point of reference, so we don't know the true size of the response. Sometimes the 'change' can simply be an error in measurement. If there can be a 20 per cent difference in a measurement taken on two occasions just from day-to-day variability, does it really matter if subjects on the Monsta Pump study were 10.5 per cent better at the end of the trial?

- Scientists make their arguments by compiling a list of studies that speak for and against their ideas. However, not all references provide the same quality or support when you are trying to make a case. The Monsta Pump advertisement takes two liberties that most scientists wouldn't accept.
  - The first 'reference' terms the summary of a conference presentation as a 'scientific publication'. Information about the Monsta Pump study may have been presented

at a conference, but that does not mean it was exposed to the peer-review process—evaluated by other scientists, or even that the study was well received. For all we know, the scientists to whom the presentation was made may have laughed at all the flaws in the study.

- The second reference is an attempt to acquire credibility for the product by linking it with a study from an esteemed scientific journal. This (mythical) study sounds as if it is related to Monsta Pump but actually isn't. The common element is nitric oxide—a chemical that Monsta Pump claims to stimulate (without any evidence that it does so). The real study may have investigated the outcomes in laboratory animals after the use of a drug that really does stimulate the production of nitric oxide. It is dishonest to use credible, rigorous science to lend status to a poor imposter.

CHECKLIST 14.1
How to evaluate dietary advice

- What recognised qualifications does the nutrition 'expert' have? Check with a sports dietitian if you are unsure.
- Does the advice promise results that are too good to be true? If so, they probably are!
- Is the advice based only on an idea or on case histories?
- Has the recommended practice or product been scientifically tested and reported in a reputable journal? Check with a sports dietitian if you're not sure.
  - Is the journal 'peer reviewed'—does it employ a process in which scientists scrutinise each other's work?
  - Do any studies quoted in support of the dietary advice relate closely to its essential features? Were such studies done with humans or animals? What other practices were the subjects following that might tend to bring about the reported results?

  - Did the study's design allow a successful treatment to make a detectable difference from no treatment at all? Did the study include a 'control' group ideally taking a fake treatment they believed to be the real thing (a placebo) so the power of positive thinking could be taken into account?
  - Do other studies support the findings of the one being quoted?
- Is the advice generally compatible with healthy nutrition guidelines? Is it supported by recognised nutrition authorities? Again, check with a sports dietitian.
- Is the support of any other organisation being used to promote the idea or product? Is this endorsement genuine? Is the organisation reputable?
- Is anyone involved in presenting the advice going to make money from people who follow it?

TABLE 14.1
Sample of one day's eating during the body-building training phase

Meal 1: Rolled oats and non-fat milk Omelette made with 10 egg whites Unsweetened apple juice Supplements	*Meal 4 (post-workout):* Protein shake 100 g rice cakes Supplements
Meal 2: 200 g tuna in spring water Protein shake Supplements	*Meal 5:* 400 g grilled chicken breast 1 cup brown rice 2 oranges Supplements
Meal 3: 400 g chicken breast 2 cups broccoli Protein bar Supplements	*Meal 6:* Protein bar Protein shake Supplements

Expert's Notes:

1. This meal plan is likely to provide > 500 g protein per day, well over 4 g/kg body. This is unnecessarily high

2. This meal plan is high in total energy intake, and is likely to promote weight gain in conjunction with training. However, it is expensive and boring to follow
3. Intakes of some micronutrients, from food sources at least, is compromised by the severely restricted food variety
4. The supplement plan is likely to be based on unproven products and also adds significant expense to the diet

TABLE 14.2
Sample of one day's eating during a post-contest binge by a female body-builder

1 brownie
2 cups 2 per cent milk
2 chocolate doughnuts
360 ml beer
1 cream popsicle
2 cups potato chips
30 g dip
1 Hardees biscuit (bacon, egg, cheese)
1 cup hash browns
1 cinnamon and raisin biscuit
2 cups Mountain Dew
2 cups Dr. Pepper
1 Big Mac hamburger
3 biscuits
1 brownie
1 piece pineapple cake
60 g barbecue ribs
9 scallops
1 cup steamed shrimp 4 crab legs
1.2 cup seafood casserole
½ cup corn
1 piece strawberry shortcake
1 piece cheesecake

(From a research paper by Janet Walberg-Rankin and colleagues, *International Journal of Sport Nutrition* 3:87–102, 1993)

TABLE 14.3
Joe Biceps' Body-building Pre-contest Diet

Hey, dudes, I start this eight weeks out from my contest to achieve a chiselled shredded look. It's the hardest thing about body-building.	
5.30 a.m.	Wake up, **Pre-workout supplements:** Silvers Fat Blaster, Silvers Mega Caffeine, Silvers Metabolean
6 a.m.	75 min weights followed by 12 capsules Silvers BCAAs 45 min cardio workout
8 a.m.	**Meal 1:** 1 cup oatmeal (measured dry) 40 g Silvers Whey Isolate and water **Supplements:** 1 g Silvers Vitamin C, 2 tablets Silvers Chromium Picolinate, 300 mg Silvers Alpha-Lipoic Acid, 8 tablets Silvers Liver, 2 tablets Silvers Minerals, 3 tablets Silvers Monsta Pump 10 g Silvers Glutamine, 5 g Silvers Creatine
10 a.m.	**Meal 2:** 180 g grilled chicken breast 1 tablespoon Silvers fish oil
12	**Meal 3:** 180 g chicken breast + 300 g steamed green beans Every third day: add 2 cups steamed brown rice to carb up **Supplements:** 1 g Silvers Vitamin C, 300 mg Silvers Alpha-Lipoic Acid, 8 tablets Silvers Liver, 2 tablets Silvers Multi Vitamin-Mineral
1.30 p.m.	**Pre-workout supplements**. See above
2 p.m.	Cardio workout—45 mins
3 p.m.	**Meal 4:** 180 g grilled chicken breast 1 tablespoon Silvers Flaxseed oil 10 g Silvers Glutamine, 5 g Silvers Creatine
5:30 p.m.	**Meal 5:** 180 g grilled chicken breast + 300 g steamed green beans **Supplements:** 1 g Silvers Vitamin C, 300 mg Silvers Alpha-Lipoic Acid, 8 tablets Silvers Liver, 2 tablets Silvers Milk Thistle
7 p.m.	**Meal 6:** 180 g lean grilled steak

8:30 p.m.	**Meal 7:** 180 g grilled chicken breast
10 p.m.	**Meal 8:** 180 g grilled chicken breast 1 tablespoon Silvers Fish Oil, 10 g Silvers Glutamine, 2 tablets Silvers ZMA, 3 tablets Silvers Monsta Pump

Expert's notes:

1. The diet is significantly reduced in energy compared to the usual training diet, but remains focused on protein so that it still highly exceeds requirements
2. Inadequate carbohydrate intake is likely to make the body-builder feel fatigued during training
3. There is a continued dependence on supplements whose efficacy is unproven. It is probable that this body-builder is sponsored by Silvers

Judo and boxing

Judo and boxing are combative sports in which athletes fight within weight divisions. The rules governing weight divisions and when they are assigned relative to competitions vary considerably across weight category; in the case of boxing, they vary considerably between amateur and professional codes.

There are seven weight divisions in judo, with different cut-offs for male and female contestants. The lightest female weight division is <48 kg and the heaviest 78 kg and above. Male weight divisions start at <60 kg, with the open division set at 100 kg and above. The duration of a judo bout is 5 min for adult males and females and 4 min for competitors under 20 years of age. A weight division is contested over a single session—generally 4–5 hours in length. Athletes can be required to contest 4–5 bouts during a competition before the eventual winner is decided. There is a minimum of 10 minutes is scheduled between bouts.

Boxing is done mostly by men and is run by a number of governing bodies. Amateur boxing has 11 weight divisions and professional boxing has 17. In general, weight divisions range from mini or light flyweight (48 kg) to heavy or super heavyweight (above 86 kg and 91 kg). An amateur boxing match is fought over four 2-min rounds. Professional bouts are contested over up to 12 rounds of 3–4 min depending on the federation and the terms of the contest as agreed between the two boxers. Amateur boxers are expected to fight daily or every second day during major competitions such as world championships and Olympic Games. They generally contest numerous events year-round, both domestically and internationally. Professional boxers, on the other hand, generally fight only 3–4 times a year and have extended lay-offs between contests.

Both sports feature relatively short bursts of high-intensity anaerobic effort against a background of continuous low-intensity aerobic activity. Although aerobic fitness is important to both judoists and boxers in helping recovery between bursts, the primary requirement for success in competition is the ability to generate muscular force quickly. Obviously, technique and tactical decisions are also important.

Training

The training of judoists and boxers depends on their mode of competition, whether in weekly bouts, multi-day tournaments, or single, isolated bouts. A professional boxer may have long periods during which time-specific training and even general fitness work may be suspended or reduced.

In the lead-up to a competition, judoists and boxers train daily, supplementing skill and technique sessions with various forms of aerobic training such as running and skipping. Weight training may be undertaken to increase muscular strength and power, but it becomes less important just before or during the competition phase. In the final preparation for competition, the athlete's attention turns to making weight. He may increase his aerobic training load to help reduce body-fat levels and diet strictly to achieve rapid weight-loss during final preparation.

Competition

As we have seen, competition may be organised in various ways. Weigh-in is normally completed on the morning of a competition, at least two hours before the start. Professional boxers may weigh in 24 hours before the scheduled fight, leaving plenty of time to rehydrate and refuel in preparation for the contest.

Recovery from bouts—and from repeated efforts to 'make weight'—is especially important in multi-day tournaments and weekly competitions. Athletes who compete at their natural weight have an advantage over those who must repeatedly cut weight just before competition, as they avoid the physical and mental consequences of drastically restricting fluid and food intake. In reality, however, many athletes cut weight in the final 24–36 hours before competition in order to compete in a lower weight division then their usual training weight. The ramifications of cutting weight are not fully understood and are likely to vary depending on the extent of weight loss and the time available for refuelling and rehydrating before the start of competition.

Physical characteristics

A wide range of body sizes is seen in these combative sports: the weight divisions are an attempt to level out the physical inequalities among competitors. Top judoists and boxers tend to have low body-fat levels, since they want maximal power and strength for their weight limit. In general, competitors benefit from having higher lean mass and arm 'reach' for any given body weight. In the heavyweight divisions of boxing, higher body-fat levels are sometimes seen.

Common nutritional issues

Training nutrition

Many judoists and boxers do not set themselves a routine training diet. Rather they move between the extremes of eating almost everything and eating almost nothing, depending on the phase of their competition. This may happen over a weekly cycle for those in a competition phase, or on a more extended cycle for those who compete sporadically in major contests. Clearly, such a roller-coaster is not ideal for either nutrition or weight management.

Read Chapters 1 and 2 for an overview of the elements of a healthy training diet. A well-chosen diet and moderate approach to eating and weight control will avoid the physical and mental stress of jumping between extremes.

Choosing a fighting weight

Combative athletes choose their fighting weight for many reasons, few of which are based on health or optimum performance level. In the case of professional athletes it may be to chase an opponent or a title, and such athletes often fight at a number of weight divisions depending on the rewards on offer. Judoists may select their weight division because it affords the only available spot on the club, regional or state judo team. Adolescents may be chosen or certified at one weight division at the beginning of a season, then fail to take into account growth and weight gain in the subsequent months.

Two views integral to combative sports continue to support such choices. The first is the belief that one gains advantages of strength, speed and leverage by fighting against a smaller opponent. By coming down a weight division, athletes (most notably boxers) may feel that they have gained an edge. Of course, this edge is wiped out if their opponent has done exactly the same thing, and if the methods used to cut weight actually impair performance. The second view is the acceptance of rapid weight-loss techniques. These have not only become a means to an end, they have also become ingrained in the language and culture of these sports. The restricted eating, the excessive training and the saunas have acquired an almost romantic aura, serving to bond athletes together through the shared experience of hardship. Read the account below to see just how institutionalised these practices have become and how high a price they exact from athletes.

The first step in addressing the situation is to set realistic competition weights based on weight and body-fat levels that are healthy and achievable for the athlete. For growing adolescents these may need to be continually reassessed. If you have body fat to spare, there may be leeway for weight loss; see Chapter 3 for a more detailed discussion. However, if you already have low body-fat levels, you should think carefully about the weight division you choose.

Making weight

'Making weight', 'cutting weight' or 'cutting up' all refer to the process of losing weight rapidly in the days or week leading up to a competition. It occurs in every sport in which there are weight divisions, the variables being how regularly competitions occur, how much time elapses between weigh-in and the event, and, in the case of sports with multi-bout or multi-day formats, whether athletes need to weigh in for their events. The sport that has been best studied in relation to weight making is wrestling—a popular sport in US high schools and colleges. There are many studies spanning decades that speak of wrestlers fasting, restricting fluids, sweating in saunas and sweat suits, and even resorting to self-induced vomiting or illegal use of diuretics to make sure that they tip the scales at their appointed weight. In some cases this goes on week after week during the competitive season, or against a backdrop of prolonged energy deficit and fat loss. Fewer studies have been done of boxing, judo and other combat sports, but they report similar practices.

The effects of these practices can range from neutral to serious. Chapter 3.8 identifies some of the situations of most concern, and some of the outcomes are illustrated in the Judo case study below. From the outside, it seems obvious that better selection of weight divisions and healthier weight-loss or weight-control programs would benefit combative sports by presenting athletes at their peak for competition and by reducing the negative effects of participation. Of course, it can be hard when you are close to a sport to see it completely objectively, or to believe that major changes in attitude are even possible. Nevertheless, it is up to all those involved—coaches, athletes and administrators—to push steadily for change.

Changing the culture of weight-making in a sport is difficult, but some headway seems to have been achieved in wrestling in the US, with strategies that combine 'reward' and 'punishment'. Educating athletes and coaches to understand and comply with healthier practices is a good start. However, checks also need to be instituted to back this up—for example, changing the weight categories, certifying wrestlers to a minimum weight cross-referenced to hydration and body-fat levels, banning forced dehydration and purging programs, and closing down the chance to recover after weigh-in to deter those tempted by severe weight loss. Recent studies suggest that progress is being made in reducing the amount of weight that wrestlers are prepared to drop before competition and the unhealthy practices used to achieve it. Unfortunately, it took the deaths of three college wrestlers in 1997 to generate enough official will to produce the successful programs. And there is still much to be done.

Read Chapter 3 for a clearer account of healthy weight-loss methods, including both long-term weight control and last-minute fine-tuning before a competition. If you can maintain a general training weight within a kilogram of so of your competition target, you will be able to shed the last grams without fuss or risk. This can be done both for a weekly competition and, as in the case of Daniel below, for a special tournament. While these healthier techniques might strip combative sports of some practices seen as traditions, who really needs these? The boxer's world can sound brave and wonderful in books and films, but the reality of diuretics, induced vomiting and sweat boxes is hardly glamorous.

Profile: Judo life

On the mat and in the journals

Judo (meaning 'gentle way') is a modern Japanese martial art whose competitive form was introduced into the Olympic Games for men in 1964, and for women in 1992. It was added to the Paralympics as a sport for the visually impaired in 1988. The leading nations in Olympic judo history are Japan, followed by France and South Korea. However, the sport now has contestants and medallists from all over the world. Australia's most successful judoist, or *judoka*, is Maria Pekli, who competed at five Olympic Games, and won the bronze medal in Sydney in 2000.

Two judo contestants face each other on a square mat (*tatami*), measuring 8 m × 8 m, over a contest lasting up to 5 min (4 min for under-20s and 3 min in youth competitions). The objectives of this contest are either to throw your opponent to the ground, immobilise him with a grappling manoeuvre, or force him to submit by joint-locking the elbow or applying a choke. These moves end a match immediately. Otherwise, judges award scores or penalties for other manoeuvres to decide the winner. A competition is held over a single day, with the draw dividing the contestant pool into two groups and a series of bouts based on an elimination system matching up the two final competitors. There are seven weight divisions for each sex, so the Olympic judo program lasts seven days as it moves through the divisions from the lightest to the heaviest.

Competition, both domestic and international, is scheduled throughout the year. As in other weight-division sports, judoists typically target a weight division that is below their off-season weight so as to gain a theoretical advantage over smaller opponents. Losses of ~5 per cent of body weight are typical. Think about that for a moment: it is usually equivalent to 3–4 kg! The rapid loss of body weight immediately before competition is often achieved through one or more of: very restricted diet, artificial means of dehydration, and excessive exercise. Weigh-ins are conducted over a one-hour period, starting two hours before competition. This provides the athlete with a small window to rehydrate and refuel before his bout starts. After a tournament, judoists are well-known for bingeing as they rebound from the rigours associated with making weight. This cycle of weight loss and regain is routinely repeated between tournaments throughout the competition season.

A number of studies have been published of the actual or likely outcomes of weight-making practices in judo. Most were carried out on Japanese or French competitors. Some of the results are summarised below:

- Ten French male judoists were asked to lose 5 per cent of body mass—an average of nearly 4 kg—over a seven-day period using their usual methods. They chose to restrict energy (by 4000 kJ or ~1000 Cal a day), carbohydrate and fluid. A battery of tests was undertaken at the start, after the 'weight-making' period, and just after the judoists completed a simulated competition of five 5-min bouts. After weight-making, the judoists scored higher for fatigue and tension and lower for vigour in psychological tests. This wouldn't exactly be regarded as a winning frame of mind! They also had lower hand-grip strength and performed worse on a 30-sec rowing task than a separate group of judoists who also prepared for the simulated competition, but without having to lose weight. Oddly enough, the weight-stable group were also found to be following a low-carbohydrate diet—old practices apparently die hard. The two groups had similar reductions in performance after the simulated competition.
- French judo athletes reduced their weight by 5 per cent over a two-month period with a self-selected diet; their food records

indicated a ~30 per cent reduction of energy, carbohydrate, and fluid intake during the seven days before competition. They were found to have lower left-hand grip strength and poorer performance on a 30-sec jumping task at the end of this period, but showed no difference in a 7-sec jump test or right-hand strength.

- Another study of 11 French judoists evaluated their diet and performance during a period of weight stability and after a seven-day period of rapid weight loss. Again, the athletes reported a low intake of carbohydrate whatever the period—and also failed to meet recommended intakes of vitamins and minerals. Food restriction reduced their left-arm strength and their performance in a 30-sec jumping test, but a 7-sec jumping test was not affected. Weight loss caused a disturbance to their psychological profiles.
- Elite Spanish judoists underwent a combination of gradual and rapid weight loss over a four-week period before a competition. One group reduced their body weight in these ways by an average of 4 per cent, while another group maintained a stable weight. Tests were done four weeks out from competition and the day before it. The weight-loss group were able to perform fewer reps of judo moves in 30 sec, and showed greater confusion and tension and less vigour. Performances of a squat jump, counter-move jump, and judo movement repetitions over 5 sec were not affected.
- Nearly 400 *judokas* (including both male and female athletes) were followed up after three consecutive competitions. A *judoka* was considered to be injured if he or she requested medical treatment or could not continue at a competition. Around 14 per cent of athletes sustained an injury, with the injury rate being similar between males and females and between athletes of different weight groups. However, there was a great risk of injury in athletes who lost 5 per cent or more of their body weight.
- Bone parameters were measured in 48 male and female *judokas* at the start of the judo season and after the round of weight-making, when they lost an average of 4 per cent of body

weight. Bone formation was disrupted during the weight-loss period and restored during the period of weight regain after the bout. Overall, however, the *judokas'* bone health was not different from that of a group of moderately active students. It seems that although weight-making is detrimental to bone metabolism, the strongly weight-bearing activities involved in judo help to protect bone.

- A series of studies of both French and Japanese judoists have found a deterioration in markers of immune health as a result of weight-making that can persist for a week after a competition.

These and other studies show that weight-making is associated with nutritional and health issues, though it does not have a consistent effect on performance. Dehydration does not appear to affect maximal muscular strength and power. Being lighter through dehydration may even increase power or ability to move against gravity (e.g. in jumping). By contrast, muscular endurance and prolonged anaerobic or aerobic performance are more likely to be impaired by weight loss, especially when dehydration also occurs. Some individuals seem to tolerate the effects of dehydration better than others. Just because these weight-loss techniques are an accepted part of judo, however, does not mean they are acceptable practices. It is hoped that with time and education, a fairer approach will be taken in such sports—fairer to the basic idea of matching equal opponents in competition, and fairer to the athletes in allowing them to reach optimum health and performance.

Profile: Daniel

Fighting fit and light

Daniel went to see a sports dietitian ten weeks before the state boxing championships. Things looked bleak. He was 8 kg overweight and needed to make his weight division of 65 kg. Life had been a little up and down in the past year. He'd broken his hand while sparring in the lead-up to a tournament several months back and had struggled ever since to get his weight under control. He hadn't been able to train fully for almost three months after his injury, and said he'd lost focus and gone a little 'crazy' with his eating.

During the forced lay-off, Daniel had drifted into bingeing on his forbidden foods and going out most weekends to party. He found himself re-establishing friendships with his old schoolmates—and loving it! He discovered that he liked having a social life and not always having to battle the bathroom scales. He wasn't too worried about the extra weight at first, figuring that it would come off easily once he got back into full training. But when he did return, he found that losing weight was harder than he remembered. He started feeling resentful about missing out on his favourite foods and an occasional beer with his mates. Could a dietitian get him down to 65 kg in ten weeks without it costing him his social life or his sanity?

The dietitian first assessed Daniel's body-fat levels to see exactly how much he had to shed. His skinfold score was 76 mm, so clearly he could afford to lose body fat. Paring off 40 mm, which would see him in 'trim' 35-mm fighting form, could well equate to the 8 kg he needed to lose. This meant that Daniel didn't need to jeopardise muscle mass to get down near his fighting weight. The dietitian listened to his training program and advised him that a slow but steady loss would be needed to ensure not only that he shed fat preferentially but that he'd consume enough carbs and nutrients to support his daily training requirements. It would be hard work, but he could do it without the usual problems of fatigue, irritability, and mental stress. His girlfriend and coach were also pleased with this news.

The dietitian devised a baseline menu plan of 8000 kJ (2000 Cal) that was easily adjusted to accommodate his daily training load. Daily energy (kilojoule) and carbohydrate intake was manipulated to reflect variations in training—allowing more on a hard-training day and less on a rest or light day. His daily menu was based around nutrient-rich foods and included a sprinkling of 'treat' foods that helped to put a sparkle in his day. One night a week, Daniel could have a meal out and a light beer to socialise with friends. After the beer he could enjoy a diet soft drink, so he wouldn't seem empty-handed among his mates. An outline of a plan for a rest day is presented in the table below.

Daniel was astounded—this was the first time he'd set out to lose weight without facing endless days of a limited menu with no variety. He felt more energetic in training than ever before, and enjoyed his occasional treat without feeling guilty. After five weeks he had lost 4 kg (skinfolds down by 18 mm), and at 8 weeks was within 2 kg of his weigh-in limit (skinfolds down by a total of 35 mm). At the beginning of the final week, he was within 1.5 kg of his target (weight 66.4 kg, skinfolds 39 mm), and under the dietitian's instructions he began to move into competition mode to shake off the last few grams.

For the final two days until the Saturday weigh-in, Daniel restricted his salt intake, making sure he wouldn't accumulate excess body fluid. All salt was cut from his meals (pepper helped to flavour the cooking), and he was careful to avoid salty foods such as cheese, nuts, chips, processed meats and salted crackers (not that these foods had been part of his diet for a while). On the Thursday, he ate his normal breakfast, then switched to a low-fibre meal plan for the remaining 36 hours. This involved replacing his evening meals with a liquid meal supplement (PowerBar Proteinplus) and using low-fibre options for breakfast and lunch. He was conscious of the overall weight of the food and fluids he consumed on the Friday and followed his pre-competition meal plan religiously. He woke up on Saturday morning feeling nervous but light and trim—and his flat stomach showed off the ripples from all his recent training.

Weigh-in was conducted before Daniel had eaten or drunk anything, and the scales rewarded him with a reading of 64.8 kg. For the remainder of the day, he rested and ate light snacks of carbohydrate-rich foods, topping up his fluid levels at frequent intervals. He was conscious not to overeat, as he realised that if he won today's fight he would be required to make weight again in the morning in preparation for his second-round bout.

He felt confident and strong both physically and mentally as he entered the ring and had the psychological boost of hearing that his opponent had spent two hours in the sauna before the weigh-in in order to make weight. He remembered all the times he'd had to resort to that himself, and how dreadful he had felt the time he took a diuretic (before this was declared illegal, of course). He won the match—and the next—feeling progressively stronger against his opponents.

While basking in the glory of his recovered state title, Daniel made himself a few promises. First, he decided to continue with some training even when no fights were in the offing. After all, he felt and looked good, and it would be a shame to throw that all away. And he'd have no trouble keeping his new dietary principles as a year-round plan. There was room and the excuse for a few celebratory meals over the next couple of days, and he could afford to increase his total kilojoule intake now that he was down to his target weight. But gone forever was the on-again, off-again feasting-and-fasting approach that had been part of his earlier career. He felt on top of the world, and he had the title to prove it!

TABLE 15.1
Typical day's eating for Daniel: weight-loss diet

Rest day:	
Breakfast (after training)	1–1½ cups mixed wholegrain cereal Low-fat milk 1 slice wholegrain toast + jam Unsweetened fruit juice or piece of fruit Tea with skim milk
Lunch	Thick sandwich or large roll—wholemeal bread, light spread of avocado, small amount of chicken, cottage cheese, salmon or lean roast meat Plenty of salad Piece of fruit Low-joule drink
Afternoon tea (before training)	Low-joule drink Piece of fruit Carton of low-fat fruit yoghurt or light Frûche
Tea	Lean meat, chicken or fish—150–200 g serve ¾ cup wholemeal rice or 1 cup pasta or large potato and slice of bread Plenty of other vegetables or salad Medium serve of fruit salad or low-fat fruit yoghurt
Energy: ~8000 kJ (2000 Cal) Carbohydrate: ~290 g (55–60 per cent of energy) Protein: ~100 g (~20 per cent of energy) Fat: ~40 g (15–20 per cent of energy) Vitamins and minerals: all above RDI level Training days: additional snacks were added to support exercise performance and promote recovery. Snacks were chosen to supply extra protein and carbohydrate, especially after the workout.	

Gymnastics and diving

Artistic gymnastics and diving are highly skilled sports in which performance is evaluated subjectively by a panel of judges. There are six events in an Olympic men's gymnastics program—floor, pommel horse, rings, vault, parallel bars and the high bar. The women's program features four events—floor, vault, uneven bars and the beam. The scoring system is reviewed after each Olympic Games, with points allocated according to technical difficulty, execution of skills and artistry of the routine. Gymnasts are required to demonstrate essential skills and are awarded additional points for linking two or more skills. There are separate titles for team competition and for individual performers, with the individual prizes being awarded for each event as well as the overall score.

All events in artistic gymnastics are anaerobic in nature, the longest being the floor (about a minute) and the shortest the vault (a few seconds, including the approach run). Skill, muscular strength and power relative to body weight are important components of success.

Diving is separated into springboard (1 m and 3 m) and platform (10 m) events for men and women. Recently, synchronised diving was adopted as an Olympic sport. It requires two divers to perform dives simultaneously. Divers are required to perform a set number of dives that involve various skills, including somersaults and twists in various directions and from different starting positions. They are judged on how well they complete all aspects of the dive and the amount of splash created by their entry to the water (the less the better). The degree of difficulty of a dive is determined by the starting position, flight movements, number of twists and the position in which the dive is performed. As in gymnastics, depletion of fuel stores is not a contributing factor to diving performance; it is skill and power that are the key determinants of success.

Male athletes peak much later than females in these sports. While most top male divers and gymnasts are aged 18–28, elite female competitors are much younger. In fact, rules are now in place to restrict females under certain ages (e.g. 14 or 16) from competing in international-level gymnastics or platform diving.

Training

The development of gymnastic skills takes years of intense practice and requires gymnasts to totally commit their lifestyle to the sport. Training begins at an early age, and even by the age of nine or ten gymnasts in elite development programs may train more than 20 hours a week. These programs now begin to prepare athletes four to eight years in advance of specific competitions, gradually building up to a full training load of 30–40 hours a week. Typically, eleven or twelve training sessions are done each week, with daily training sessions before and after school or work lasting two or more hours each.

The training load of an elite diver can be equally demanding, with three hours a day spent on water work, and another one to two hours on dry-land training. Training generally starts at an early age, reflecting the years of skill and strength development that are required. Occasionally, elite divers emerge from a gymnastics background, changing to diving at a later age after injury or lack of success have ended their gymnastics career.

In the non-competition season, or in the early development of the gymnast or diver, much of the training time is spent on acquiring skills through technique work and body conditioning. Supplementary weight training and conditioning is often undertaken, particularly by male athletes, and may make up to 25 per cent of total training time. As the athlete matures or as the competition season draws closer, progressively more time is spent on developing and refining the technical aspects of specific gymnastic routines or dives.

Competition

In Olympic and world championships, the competition is divided into three distinct sessions: team qualifying; team finals; and individual all-round finals and apparatus finals.

Gymnasts in the team qualifying round compete with their national squad on each piece of apparatus. The scores from this session are used to determine which teams qualify for the finals and which individual gymnasts advance to the all-round and apparatus finals. The program is typically spread over four days, with competition lasting about three hours a day for each competitor as they all rotate between types of apparatus. A warm-up of a similar length is usually completed before the start of competition, and between performances (from 5 min to 30 min apart) competitors may perform stretching exercises.

In diving contests, preliminary, semi-final and final rounds are held at world championship and Olympic competitions, with the top twelve competitors proceeding to the final. In semi-finals and finals, divers compete in reverse order according to their ranking from the previous round. All rounds are separate events, with scores starting at zero. Men perform six dives and women five, in springboard and platform events. Rules regulating the degree of difficulty and requirements of each dive performed vary slightly across 1 m springboard, 3 m springboard and platform competitions. A diving meet can last four to six days, with competitions on each of the boards being held on separate days.

Physical characteristics

Gymnasts are a physically homogeneous group, since the characteristics that make for success are very marked. The skill and agility of gymnastics call for athletes who are small and well muscled, with low levels of body fat. The physical profile of the female gymnast has changed since the 1970s, with champions such as Olga Korbut and Nadia Comaneci turning the spotlight away from mature physiques to a youthful, almost pre-pubescent look. In addition to the physical advantages of increased mechanical efficiency and power-to-weight ratio, being small and light conveys a more pleasing image to gymnastics judges. Divers have similar physical characteristics to gymnasts, with a compact frame and low body-fat level being important for both physical and aesthetic reasons.

Common nutritional issues

Body fat and size—are goals realistic?

Athletes in aesthetically judged skill sports—gymnastics, diving, figure skating, ballet dancing, etc.—are set strict guidelines on weight and body-fat (skinfold) levels. Females, especially, face an uphill battle to achieve or maintain the sparrow-like physique that is expected of them. They may have to fight against the fat deposition that accompanies puberty as they strive for body-fat levels that are more applicable to endurance athletes. Although these athletes spend many hours in training each week (and day), their practice is focused on skill and technique rather than kilojoule-burning aerobic exercise.

The secrets of body-fat loss are set out in Chapter 3; in essence, it requires increasing aerobic exercise and/or decreasing energy intake. When athletes are already training many hours each day, they may not have time for extra aerobic exercise, or their coach may be reluctant to allow the extra effort and the accompanying risk of injury. This leaves the athlete with only one recourse—a low-kilojoule diet. Even with a well-chosen meal plan, this may present difficulties, from inadequate intake of some nutrients to a lowering of the metabolic rate and increased energy efficiency. In some cases the athlete may enter a state of chronic low-grade starvation. Some athletes get caught up in the cycle of fad diets, disordered eating and eating disorders as they struggle to meet their body-fat targets. They face the consequences of undernutrition as well as the side-effects of the weight-loss methods used.

For males the problem is not so critical, since they are more likely to arrive naturally at the low body-fat levels associated with these sports. However, some will face similar challenges to their female counterparts.

Regardless of the athlete's sex, it is important that weight and body-fat targets be realistic. While low body-fat levels confer a physical advantage in skill sports, aesthetic values and peer pressure are also involved. Why should extremely thin or pre-pubescent athletes be judged better performers simply because of their appearance? Above all, the health and happiness of the athlete should be taken into account when setting body-fat goals. See Chapter 3 for more details.

Weight worries

Because of the need to get and stay trim, many gymnasts and divers weigh themselves many times a day. Sometimes weighing-in is a routine part of the training session. Coaches have valid reasons for fearing abrupt increases in body weight. It is dangerous for an athlete to attempt an intricate dive or gymnastics routine with the sudden addition of an extra 2 kg, which obviously upsets their balance and centre of gravity and other aspects of their finely honed skills. Coaches want to know if their athletes are at such a risk at any single training session, and to be forewarned of any creeping weight gain that might need to be checked.

However, scale-watching can lead to excessive concern, even obsession, about weight. Add a few misconceptions about weight and its fluctuations and you can end up with anxious athletes who take unhealthy measures in quest of impossible goals. For example, some athletes (and their coaches) do not realise that it is normal and healthy (and necessary) for weight to fluctuate each day—by as much as a kilogram in small-bodied athletes. Weight may be lost through sweating, gained temporarily because of food and fluids consumed (the gain equalling the weight of the food/drink) and lost again after going to the toilet. And this is without counting the weight of clothes and shoes that the athlete may or may not be wearing when she hops on the scales.

If you are a gymnast or diver, set yourself realistic body-fat goals and establish an eating plan that keeps you trim, performing well, and happy. A good plan will mean sizeable weight increases or decreases (2 kg or more) don't occur, and you won't need to resort to extremes (starving and not drinking, then overindulging later). Read the case history of Stacey below. Coaches too play an important role. They would do better to promote happy and healthy eating strategies for their charges rather than using the scales as a punishment tool. Even in an elite program, periodic weight checks (one or two a week) may provide all the information both athletes and coaches need and will reduce the misery of being a slave to the scales.

The nutritional needs of adolescence

Gymnastics and diving begin at an early age, often late childhood or adolescence. Growth and puberty make special nutritional demands, increasing the needs for energy and protein for growth, and calcium and iron for bones and blood. Where energy intake is chronically low, the athlete risks nutritional deficiencies and delayed growth and maturity.

A recent study of the physical characteristics of junior elite female gymnasts reported that those in the 7–10-year-old age group were of average height and weight for their age (around the 50th percentile), but that the 11–14-year-olds had slipped back to the 20th percentile in these measures. Muscle mass was high, but body-fat levels were below average in both groups. The drop in height and weight could indicate nutritional deficits, causing a delay in puberty and growth failure.

Alternatively, sports-specific factors may be selecting the gymnasts—that is, the smaller and lighter ones are progressing while heavier and bigger gymnasts drop out of the program. Or it may be that both factors are operating.

The same group of gymnasts would have to be followed through their careers to determine which factor was most important. However, this study suggests that young gymnasts are nutritionally vulnerable, and that their health and growth may be compromised if they adopt overly restrictive diets. It is hoped that gymnastics programs are not so dogmatic that they consciously 'bonsai' their young athletes—that is, deliberately restrict their growth by keeping them undernourished. Poor growth patterns are associated with more frequent sickness and general ill-health, including impaired bone development.

Amenorrhoea, calcium and bone impairment

Female athletes with low body-fat levels, particularly artificially contrived ones, may be at an increased risk of amenorrhoea. Amenorrhoea may take the form of a failure to start periods altogether, or the cessation of an already established menstrual cycle. The former condition appears to be a common pattern with elite gymnasts. A complication of amenorrhoea is reduced bone density, with perhaps an increased risk of stress fractures now, and osteoporosis later.

It is important that delayed onset of periods be reported to your sports medicine doctor so that issues such as bone health can be monitored. In many cases a healthy-eating gymnast will have good bone density, since exercise stimulates bone formation and may help counter the effect of hormone deprivation. A healthy, high-calcium diet (1000–1500 mg a day) should be part of the program for all gymnasts. There is some evidence that high calcium intakes, usually achieved by use of a calcium supplement on top of a good diet, can increase bone density in children before puberty.

Training nutrition: an overview

It has already been established that many gymnasts and divers are at risk of nutritional deprivation because of their restricted energy intake. Indeed, surveys of female gymnasts' dietary regimens have reported inadequate intakes of many vitamins and minerals. Read Chapters 1 and 2 for an overview of the nutritional goals of an athlete in heavy training.

Another factor that greatly influences the eating habits of these athletes is the great time commitment their sport demands. With the day divided between training, school and homework or a job, there is often little time for cooking and preparing meals—for the athletes or their families. The only people busier than young gymnasts are their parents—driving them to and from their training, and struggling to meet the needs of all the family members. Meals are often eaten in the car on the way to school, or on the way home from training. Gymnastics mums and dads must be creative to organise food that is nutritious, appealing, transportable and easily eaten.

Competition nutrition

Divers and gymnasts need a meal plan that will fit in with a competition schedule that's often spread over a number of days. Competition is not likely to threaten fluid or fuel stores, since routines are quite brief and low in intensity. However, each athlete needs to find a plan that sits comfortably both in his stomach and with his confidence. Challenges include the risk of weight gain if energy intake is not kept proportionate to the reduced energy expenditure of a lowered training load. When young gymnasts and divers travel away from their parents and personal coaches, lack of supervision at meals can also increase the risk of unhealthy eating patterns and weight gain. There is no need to carbo-load or change the diet radically in preparation for an event. Read Chapter 4.2 for an overview of nutrition before a competition and Chapter 4.4 for ideas about pre-event meals. The timing of meals will need to suit the daily schedule of training and competition sessions. This may vary from day to day.

Eating disorders

With so much pressure to be light and low in body fat, it is not surprising that much of the life, conversation and recreation of female gymnasts and divers revolve around food and weight loss. There is a relentless focus on what the athlete looks like, how much she weighs or how large her skinfold sum is, all of it reinforced by other athletes and often, unfortunately, by coaches and parents.

In this environment, it is not surprising that eating disorders and disordered eating become apparent, even common, among female athletes. How else can unrealistic goals be met? And how do you resist when everyone else is doing it? Read the account below to see how the problem ranges all the way from shared weight-loss efforts to desperate measures and pathological disturbances in eating behaviour. The hazards and the treatment will vary accordingly, but the needs for great patience, steadfast support and probably the input of various professionals are near certainties. The problem also occurs with male athletes but there is a much lower incidence.

Profile: Stacey

Starving for success?

When Stacey took up her new position as head gymnastics coach at the college, she immediately consulted a sports dietitian. She explained that her last job had caused her some unhappiness because of suspected eating disorders among some of the female gymnasts. In a new setting and with new students she wanted to tackle the issue with a fresh approach. What could be done to prevent the problem? Was there anything she had done to cause or worsen it? How could she detect which girls were having problems, and what should she do if difficulties were found?

The dietitian summarised the symptoms of the two major eating disorders, anorexia nervosa and bulimia. While anorexics deny themselves food and generally lose large amounts of body weight, the major feature of bulimia is uncontrolled eating followed by purging through vomiting or laxative use, resulting in big swings in body weight. While the syndromes can exist separately, many sufferers show symptoms of both, either simultaneously or in tandem. In all cases, psychological problems are obviously present, including disorders in body image and in feelings about food.

However, the dietitian went on, eating disorders are not always clear-cut. Not every athlete who skips a meal is anorexic, and not everyone who forces herself to vomit once or twice really has bulimia. Instead, there is a spectrum of eating-behaviour problems among athletes. At one end of the spectrum are people who have anorexia or bulimia as a primary disorder—that is, a classical psychological disturbance with nutritional consequences. What causes these disorders is unknown, but the symptoms are well recognised and the health implications can be serious. Death is the most extreme outcome—from starvation in anorexics, from severe electrolyte disturbances in those with bulimia, and from suicide in either group if depression is also present. These disorders also occur in the community, and their victims include some athletes. Extensive treatment is required for both these eating disorders, involving specialised attention from psychiatrists and counselling from both psychologists and dietitians, as well as a look at the sufferer's interpersonal relationships.

At the other end of the spectrum are athletes with 'occupational' eating disorders—those who have problems with their eating behaviour because they are under pressure to meet unrealistic nutritional, sporting or social expectations. Achieving or maintaining a low body weight or body-fat level is the most common issue, and disordered eating is more likely among athletes in sports that emphasise low body-fat levels. This is particularly true if athletes are not well informed about the consequences of meeting unrealistically low body-fat targets through bizarre diets, vomiting, laxative use or other damaging practices. The other factor that supports the behaviour is peer acceptance. In some sports, body-fat phobia is almost institutionalised, with athletes swapping ideas about weight-loss techniques and making destructive eating behaviours seem normal because 'everybody does it'.

It's important to know the difference between disordered eating and an eating disorder. For the true anorexic, starvation is the end, while for an athlete with an eating-behaviour problem, it is a means to the end. In many cases, when the athlete is removed from the pressure or the environment that condones the behaviour, she will revert to better eating habits and the problem will disappear. Others, however, may get caught up in a self-sustaining cycle and become enmeshed in a true eating disorder. When she loses the ability to stop the behaviour, even when there is no longer a need for it and it is causing her harm and injury, then a more serious problem is diagnosed. Athletes seem to be at greater risk of developing eating disorders than sedentary people, partly because of the way their sporting community regards issues of physique and fatness, but also because of their personalities. An obsessive, perfectionistic person who likes to tackle tasks with focus and determination has the psychological characteristics that help athletes make it to the top. At the same time, however, such a personality is considered to put people at high risk for developing an eating disorder.

After listening to this explanation, Stacey thought back to her gymnastics career and recalled how she too had been obsessed with her weight. In her case, the environment had certainly supported disordered eating practices. Having been set unreasonable body-fat and weight targets—by herself, her coach or the sport—she had become consumed by the desire to be light and lean. 'We all thought about food all the time,' she said. 'We weighed ourselves a dozen times a day, and looked at our tummies every time we passed a mirror or shiny surface. The only time I stopped thinking about my next meal, how many calories, and how much exercise I'd have to do to burn it off, was when I started thinking about my friend and whether she was thinner than I was.

'We were pretty miserable, although at the time I didn't know things could be any other way. We were always trying the latest diet, and everyone was very conscious of what the others ate. This was particularly true when we travelled to competitions and we all ate together. I distinctly remember being more competitive about eating the least at dinner than about the actual gymnastics. A couple of my friends could make themselves sick, but I was too frightened to try in case my mother found out.

'Funnily, I never considered I had a problem, and in fact when I stopped competing in gymnastics I stopped worrying so much. I still like to keep myself trim, but it's not the consuming passion that it used to be.'

The dietitian agreed that Stacey's experience fell within the range of eating-behaviour problems, and that at any level these carried disadvantages for physical and emotional health and for athletic performance. Even if such problems don't become life-threatening, many athletes worry too much about their food and their body-fat scores. While definite causes of disordered eating and eating disorders can often be neither pinpointed nor eradicated, it is important to recognise the roles played by both a perfectionistic attitude on the part of the athlete, and the pressurised environment created by coaches, parents and other athletes.

Profile: Monique

The scales—friend or foe?

Monique joined a new elite gymnastics program when her family moved interstate. As a young gymnast she had shown a lot of promise, but since her sixteenth birthday her performances had become less and less consistent, both in training and in competition. Worse, she no longer seemed to enjoy her sport. The long hours of training restricted her social life and her school activities. Of course, that was nothing new. It was just that everything seemed to have become a source of pressure rather than pleasure—especially the business of eating. She remembered the days when she could eat anything and never gave a thought to her weight. Then, almost overnight, everything had changed and the scales had taken over her life. The last year had been misery, trying hard in the gym and at the table but getting nowhere. Perhaps, she thought, a new club in a new city would give her a fresh start.

Monique found the routine of the new club quite different from what she was used to. For a start, there were scales at the gym, but only the older gymnasts were required to 'weigh in'—and that was usually once a week on Monday morning, not once or twice a day as they'd all done at her old gym. Of course, you were free to weigh yourself more frequently if you wanted to, but no one seemed to be in a panic about it. Body fat (skinfolds), weight and height were monitored and reviewed every month by the club's sports dietitian, who also measured arm girth—relaxed and flexed—along with mid-thigh girth, as these helped to better interpret weight and skinfold changes.

Monique was surprised to hear that she would negotiate her personal 'ideal skinfold measure' with the dietitian after six months of monitoring, and that this would include a small margin of variability that was still considered OK. At Monique's old club, everybody had to keep their skinfold sum below 40 mm, and the number loomed large in the minds of all the gymnasts. In Monique's case, it had seemed that the more she worried about her skinfolds, the more there was to worry about. Her skinfold sum had hovered around 32–34 mm for seven sites back in the good old days, but it had gradually inched up to 55 mm.

At her old club, it was always about weighing light. She based her whole diet on this goal and often copied what the other gymnasts were doing. It was a tough life, made bearable only by sharing the struggle with the others. The day started with breakfast, which varied in content according to whether Monique had been to the toilet on rising and thus felt 'light'. If so, she enjoyed a decent-sized bowl of cereal with low-fat milk and a small glass of orange juice. However, if the trip to the toilet had been unproductive and left her weighing 'heavy', Monique would eat a small bowl of cereal, dry, and skip the drink. The total weight of this breakfast: about 30 g.

This was worth a few brownie points at the weigh-in before training. By comparison, her full breakfast with milk and juice weighed about 450 g—which could put her above 44 kg on a 'heavy' morning. During the day she had to work hard to minimise the weight of all food and drink consumed. If successful, she could weigh in at afternoon training at around the same weight as at the morning session. Although her mother sent her off to school with a packed lunch, Monique usually threw this out. After all, a sandwich weighed 200 g or even more if full of salad, an apple almost the same, and a tub of yoghurt was a luxury at 200 g! Who could afford to consume a 600 g lunch and face the scales and the coach with most of that still on board at afternoon training? A chocolate bar (60 g) or a packet of chips (50 g) provided a smaller and lighter alternative.

It was hard to keep yourself to only a mouthful of drink, though. She would get pretty thirsty over the day. She might be able to steal away for a drink during the training session, but the coaches usually watched to make sure she only had a few sips. Once, one gymnast had drunk so much that she gained nearly a kilo on the spot. Water sure was fattening!

With afternoon training over, there was a brief chance to relax—although Mum was pretty careful about the evening meal. Monique could count on a small serve of meat or chicken and vegetables, followed by some fruit or fruit salad, and ice-cream twice a week. Of course, she still felt hungry afterwards, and often raided the pantry for biscuits, chocolates and lollies. As Monique had two younger brothers and an older sister, it was easy to disguise how much of these foods she ate. If her parents asked about it, she routinely denied eating any and blamed her younger brothers for the missing goodies. Her evening indulgence provided some joy in a day of self-discipline—and her splurges didn't weigh much, so what was the harm?

Saturday afternoon was the best time of the week. Once Monique left the gym, there were a whole 36 hours of freedom ahead. Saturday night was a night at the movies (a family pack of sweets and an ice-cream instead of dinner), or a sleep-over at a friend's house (where they'd cook slices or cakes). Sunday morning meant a special breakfast at home—pancakes. By Sunday afternoon the fear of facing the scales next morning usually brought on an attack of the guilts, followed by a run (all rugged up to help her sweat more). One of Monique's friends had a sauna at home, and sometimes they all met there to spend a couple of hours sweating off their weekend's excesses. Of course, sometimes there was no way to avoid facing a weight jump—a kilogram or even two. And then the week's strict regimen started again.

On their first trip away for competition, Monique was surprised to see the new club's sports dietitian coming too. At her old club, the team was only ever accompanied by the physiotherapist, to make sure they all remained injury free for the competition. The club dietitian did all the shopping and cooked the meals for the athletes and coaches. He was actually an excellent cook, and Monique fell in love with his Mexican chicken wraps. Meals with this club were strange, as everyone seemed to be relaxed and really enjoying themselves—not at all what meals had been like on trips with her old club.

After the camp, the coach had a chat with Monique and arranged for her to see the dietitian for an individual consultation. Unbeknown to Monique, he had spotted some unusual eating habits when they were on camp and thought it would be worthwhile to see if she had any issues or concerns about food. At their initial meeting, the dietitian listened carefully to Monique as she recounted what foods, and in what quantities, she had eaten in the past 24 hours. Monique, however, told the dietitian what she thought he'd want to hear, not what she actually ate—there was no way she was going to confess to eating chocolate biscuits and lollies to a dietitian.

The dietitian noted the differences between what Monique reported eating and what he'd observed while the team was away at camp. Given this disparity, he asked Monique to come back for a fortnightly review so he could help her achieve the skinfold and weight targets they'd discussed. On her first review session, the dietitian explained to Monique why there was such concern about body weight in her sport. He explained that gymnastics requires precise skills and balance—factors that could be thrown out by a sudden gain in weight or a slow gain in body-fat stores. Gradual changes in height and lean body mass through growth could be accommodated, he said, although in the end there was a mechanical bias towards gymnasts who remained small and lean even after puberty, when they were fully grown.

Monique was pleased to hear that the new talent identification programs in gymnastics concentrated on selection of children with the right genetic make-up. Monthly checks on weight, height and skinfolds helped to monitor progress. If problems were noted, such as a steady increase in skinfolds and weight, then steps could be taken to address the situation early. In Monique's new club, great pains were taken to make skinfold goals realistic and healthy for each gymnast—and to help rather than harass each gymnast if her skinfolds deviated much from her ideal range.

'But if I'm only weighing myself once a month, won't I get fat?' Monique asked, unconvinced. The dietitian assured her that the scales were available whenever she wanted feedback, but that weighing herself wouldn't prevent her from gaining body fat or help her lose it. Those results would come from understanding the importance of weight management for gymnastics, healthy eating strategies, and sound exercise practices. In fact, in the dietitian's experience, the more people weighed themselves the more they worried about the results rather than the action needed to achieve the results. The situation often developed into a vicious cycle of weighing, worrying, thinking about food, eating, then weighing and worrying again.

The twice-daily weighing had actually distracted Monique from the real issues. What's more, it had confused her into following the very patterns that made it easy to gain body fat by making her think that weight changes over the course of the day reflected her body-fat levels. Nothing could be further from the truth.

During a follow-up session, the dietitian reminded Monique of what she had learned in biology at school—that gaining body fat is a long-term project. Each kilogram of fat is equal to about 30 000 kJ of surplus energy. To lose or gain that amount of fat takes 1–2 weeks of consistent energy deficit or gain. Daily weight changes result mostly from the normal fluctuations in the amounts of food and fluid entering and leaving our bodies. Most people eat 1.5–4 kg of food each day, and the recommended 'eight glasses of water each day' alone weigh about 2 kg. (Of course, many athletes need to drink two or three times this amount to replace daily sweat losses.) If we are eating exactly our energy requirements, this food will be processed during the day and the waste products eliminated. Fluid is also in dynamic balance in the body, being lost through trips to the toilet, sweat, and even breathing. In the case of athletes who train in hot weather for long periods, 'weight' can drop 2–4 kg by the end of the session if no fluid is drunk. So at the end of the day net weight gain may be nil even though there have been continual 'deposits' and 'withdrawals'. In a small gymnast who is eating and drinking healthy foods and spreading this intake throughout the day, body weight may fluctuate by up to a kilogram each day. This will cause no problem for training performance.

But when gymnasts weigh themselves too often and react (especially with panic) to every small fluctuation, they can mix up the short-term view with the big picture. In Monique's case, she had been confusing the weight of her meals and drinks with their kilojoule value and their overall contribution to her nutritional requirements. Unfortunately, size doesn't correlate to kilojoules. For example, some foods that are 'small' and 'light' are also full of fat and kilojoules, with minimal vitamins and minerals (e.g. chocolate, lollies, biscuits). Fat content is a particularly tricky issue because fat is such a compact kilojoule source and because fat itself may be more 'fattening' than other nutrients per kilojoule. On the other hand, some 'heavy' foods, like fruit and vegetables, are low in fat and kilojoules and full of nutrients. Water is 'heavy' but has no energy value. What's more, plenty of fibre and fluid are essential for regular bowel habits.

When it was put this way, Monique could see how her 'small foods diet' had some flaws—but she still found it hard to comprehend that you could eat a lot of food and actually be taking in fewer kilojoules. As Monique started to trust the dietitian, she confessed to her true food and fluid intake. The dietitian did a computer analysis of a typical day of her old diet compared with a typical day of a new eating plan he had devised. The new plan included cereal and reduced-fat milk at breakfast, a yoghurt and piece of fruit for morning recess, a small roll or sandwich chock-a-block with various fillings and another piece of fruit for lunch, a couple of crackers and a slice of cheese before afternoon training, and Mum's dinner with some extra veggies after training. On one occasion, the dietitian asked Monique's mother to come in so they could discuss cooking techniques. He gave her a great cookbook that included her new-found favourite Mexican chicken wraps. After dinner on heavy training days, Monique was surprised to hear the dietitian suggest a treat. Her favourite on his list was a small carton of yoghurt (frozen so it would take ages to eat). There were even some treats for the weekend, and some new dessert ideas, including fruit kebabs with low-fat custard. Water was to be drunk at every meal and during training, so she would be constantly topping up rather than drying out and then drinking like a camel. To Monique it sounded almost too good to be true—she would not get hungry or empty the way she used to, her trips to the toilet would be more regular, and she would have more energy for training and school. The new plan was also just a little lower in kilojoules than her present needs so a small and continuous decline in skinfold measurements would result.

Despite the bright outlook, Monique at first found it hard to change her ways. The new diet involved a total inversion of her previous beliefs, but she stuck to it because she knew it would help her succeed in gymnastics. Her coach and the dietitian were encouraging and patient—

weaning her down to a weekly weigh-in, then fortnightly, then monthly. Once she couldn't help herself and hopped on the scales at the local pharmacy. The results were a bit scary—and prompted her to skip dinner that night. But her fortnightly appointment with the dietitian gave her an opportunity to talk through her fears and regain her confidence. After six months on the new program, Monique received some great rewards: a skinfold measurement back below 40 mm and an award for the most improved new gymnast at the club. At her end-of-year review she happily discussed a long-term skinfold goal with her coach and dietitian—and felt confident that 35–40 mm was a good target.

Monique is looking forward to her next year at the club, and has set herself a number of personal goals. There are some important competitions to do well in, and perhaps an overseas trip to aim for. But part of her plan is to keep working on her attitude to food—to reduce her fears so she can enjoy each meal more. Eventually she hopes to stop fretting about food and be confident that her healthy eating program means she doesn't need to worry.

Rowing

Rowing is a sport with a venerable tradition. Its international governing body, FISA (Fédération Internationale des Sociétés d'Aviron), is the oldest international federation in the Olympic movement. Many famous rowing events, such as the annual race between Cambridge and Oxford universities over a 6-km course on the Thames River, are more than 180 years old. In the United States, the annual Yale–Harvard race dates back more than 150 years.

The standard international rowing event is conducted over a 2000-m course, with teams divided into classes according to sex, the number of rowers in the boat (1, 2, 4, or 8), the presence or absence of a coxswain ('cox') to steer the boat and direct the rhythm of the strokes, and the way the oars are used. In sweep competition, each rower has a single large oar; in sculls, rowers use two shorter oars simultaneously on each side of the boat. At the international level there is a separate weight-based division for lightweight rowers.

In Australia, rowers generally start in the sport at school, where races are confined to the summer months. However, for top athletes, rowing is a year-round sport, with the major international competitions being the Olympic Games and the annual world championships. There are also many other international- and national-level regattas and World Cup events. Although rowing has been included on the Olympic program since the beginning of the modern era in 1896, women's rowing was introduced only in 1976, and lightweight rowing only in 1996. There are 14 boat classes on the Olympic program and 24 on the world championship program. Separate national and international competitions exist for different age groups, including the senior B competition (under 23 years), youth and juniors (under 18 years), and masters rowing (>27 years and following retirement from open rowing).

At elite levels, the time taken to complete the 2000-metre race ranges from over 7 min for the singles to around 5.5 min for the eights. Since rowers use both arms and legs, representing a large proportion of total body muscle mass, their bodies are subject to considerable cardiovascular and metabolic stresses. Rowing makes great demands on both the aerobic and anaerobic energy systems, and mean oxygen consumption in a top race can be close to the maximum achievable.

Training

Rowing training is long and intense. For eight to ten months of the year, rowers complete about twelve sessions a week: nine on the water and three in the gym. At times some crews make an even greater commitment, with two water sessions and a gym session in the same day. In a typical rowing session, the athletes cover about 20 km at a heart rate high enough to stress both aerobic and anaerobic (lactic) metabolism. Weight training sessions are often undertaken to improve muscular endurance. It may seem odd that such long hours of training should be required for a 5–7 min event, but rowing requires a unique mixture of technique, power and endurance of both aerobic and anaerobic energy systems, and this time is needed to bring each component of the skill to a peak.

Competition

Depending on the stature of the regatta, competition may last from three days to a week. Scullers and crews are first drawn in heats, with successful competitors progressing to semi-finals or finals and the remainder to a repêchage. Competitors successful in the repêchage may progress to a semi-final. In large competitions, rowers may be required to race only once a day, but they may have to race as hard on the first day as in the finals to keep progressing through the competition. Light training is undertaken on rest days. In lightweight competition, weigh-ins are conducted on the mornings of the events.

Physical characteristics

The biomechanical requirements of rowing favour athletes with long 'levers'—limbs—and a large muscle mass that is capable of producing high power outputs over a sustained period. Therefore, heavyweight rowers are tall and heavy, with strong muscles and long limbs. While muscle mass should account for most of these athletes' increased weight, body-fat levels are typically higher in heavyweight rowers, particularly females, than in other endurance-trained athletes (e.g. runners or cyclists). However, as in many sports, there has been a recent trend to greater leanness at the top level of competition.

In lightweight rowing, male rowers or scullers are not permitted to exceed 72.5 kg, with a crew average of 70 kg; the limits for women are 59 kg (maximum) and 57 kg (crew average). Lightweight crews are obviously smaller and lighter than their heavyweight counterparts, with lower body-fat levels showing the importance of a high power-to-weight ratio. As in most sports with weight divisions, many athletes 'sit on the fence' of the limits, being too small and light to compete successfully against bigger and stronger athletes, but struggling to fit into the lower weight class.

Common nutritional issues

Training nutrition: high energy and carbohydrate requirements

Energy and fuel requirements are increased by a large body size, a heavy training program and periods of physical growth. This trifecta commonly exists in rowing. Rowers can need enormous amounts of energy and carbohydrate to support heavy training loads and body-weight or strength goals. Male rowers often fight to maintain or increase their lean body mass during periods of heavy training, while all rowers must work hard to recover from one day to the next. The lifestyle of the rower can also interfere with meeting these huge demands. Time spent at training is time that isn't spent eating, and as in the case of Trent below, many rowers find it difficult simply to chomp through the amounts of food they need in a day.

Read Chapters 1 and 2 for details of the optimum training diet. A high-energy, well-fuelled, nutrient-rich eating plan is needed for both heavy training and specific needs to gain muscle size and strength. A pattern of frequent meals and snacks, including carbohydrate–protein combinations immediately after training, is the best plan of attack, providing both sufficient fuel (Chapter 3) and optimal recovery (Chapter 5). Of course, as Trent finds, this means being organised.

Matters of physique: gaining muscle mass

Gaining muscle size and strength is a key goal for rowers in the conditioning months before the competition season. To this end, male and female rowers usually undertake a heavy gym program. As Chapter 3 explains, the way to gain muscle mass is through a well-designed resistance program combined with adequate and properly timed nutrition support. It is even more important to fuel well before and during on-water sessions. Not only do rowers need the kilojoules to train well in the boat, but sufficient fuel helps to limit the breakdown of muscle in rowing sessions. It is obviously counterproductive to stimulate muscle-protein synthesis in the gym, then break it down on the water. See Chapter 3.7–3.8 for more background and some strategies for high-energy eating.

Matters of physique: losing body fat

Higher body-fat levels may not seem as great a disadvantage to a rower as they are to a distance runner. After all, it is an advantage to be heavy and strong, and body weight is supported in the boat. However, there is a limit to the excess baggage that can be carried. It is better to be 80 kg with a skinfold score of 50 mm, than 80 kg with skinfolds totalling 100 mm. Lightweight crews have a particular need to optimise their power-to-weight ratio. At some stage rowers may need to undertake special programs to lose body fat. See Chapter 3 for advice.

Fluid needs in training

Long training sessions on the water in hot weather cause heavy sweating. Good hydration practices involve drinking before training sessions, taking a water bottle to training, and rehydrating fully afterwards. Weighing yourself before and after training sessions will give you a clear picture of your body's fluid swings (see Figure 2.3). A sports drink will fuel as well as hydrate during long training sessions—your brain and muscles may both benefit, which will help you not only sustain high power outputs but maintain good technique. Carbohydrate support during workouts may also help conserve the gains made in the gym.

A study of fluid balance during elite rowing training by the Australian Institute of Sport reported average sweat-loss rates of 2 L an hour for male and 1.4 L an hour for female rowers in hot conditions (30°C); in cool conditions (10°C), average sweat rates were about 1.6 L/hr and 780 ml/hr respectively. Even though the rowers came prepared with their own water bottles, they were unable to drink enough fluid to keep pace with their sweat losses, especially in the hot conditions. Even when it was cold, they did not drink enough—perhaps because they underestimated their sweat losses. Problems included the need to carry large amounts of water on the boat (despite being surrounded by water, rowers can drink only from their own provisions), and the need to stop training to drink (two hands are needed on the oar to row!). Achieving good hydration in hot conditions might require athletes and coach to work out a plan. The coach could bring extra fluid out in the coach boat so empty water bottles could be topped up or replaced, or more drink breaks could be allowed during the session—a few seconds every 15 minutes or so would not disrupt the session too much, and might produce better performances.

Competition nutrition

Rowers should go into each race with fluid and fuel stores topped up and feeling comfortable after the last meal. With each regatta lasting a number of days, the challenge is not just to perform well but to recover between each day's sessions and between days of racing. Read Chapter 4 for advice about competition nutrition, and Chapter 5 for strategies to promote rapid recovery. Special care may be needed with pre-event eating—it can be very uncomfortable to race with a full stomach. Liquid meals such as Powerbar Proteinplus or Sustagen Sport may come in handy as a low-bulk pre-race meal or snack. With much of the day tied up in preparation and the race itself, there is usually neither time nor opportunity for rowers to consume their energy intake. Consequently, some rowers find that they quickly lose weight over the course of the regatta.

Whether it's for an energy boost or a well-timed post-race recovery snack, it makes good sense for rowers always to have nutritious food supplies on hand. This might mean organising suitable supplies both at the rowing site and at the competition accommodation. Don't rely on event organisers to consider your needs! Sandwiches, yoghurt, fruit, bars and special sports products (e.g. sports gels, liquid meal supplements) are low in bulk, nutritious and portable. Use your creativity to think up practical snacks, and your organisational skills to make sure you can put your hands on them when you need to.

Finally, don't neglect fluid needs. You may be dehydrated from your rowing efforts, your weight-making practices (see below), or just from sitting in the sun watching the rest of the competition. Carbohydrate-containing fluids such as sports drinks, juices and flavoured milk can be useful for both fluid and carb top-ups.

Lightweight rowing

As in other weight-matched sports, lightweight rowing competition often includes rowers who are clearly 'heavyweight'—that is, their usual training weight is well above the weight-division limits. This is a tricky situation, since it is clearly a successful strategy—most of the medals in the lightweight races in international competition are won by rowers who would normally compete in the open division. However, the reality is that for many lightweight rowers the experience ranges from challenging to damaging, with extreme dieting and obsession with food leading to disordered eating and eating disorders. This may be worsened by severe dehydration and food restriction in the days before weigh-in—practices that may be repeated for the duration of the regatta. Females seem to be most at risk, although these problems are also seen in male crews.

While some rowers seem able to survive and thrive as they cross back and forward between their normal weight and competition weight, others are affected—physically and mentally, with consequences for both health and performance. From the performance perspective, a rowing competition is an extremely severe exercise challenge that should not be attempted with less than optimal preparation. The long-term consequences of persistent weight-making may include disturbed metabolic efficiency, poor bone health and an unhealthy attitude to food. It is not unusual to find rowers complaining that losing weight gets harder as time goes on, until even with heavy training and a sparrow's diet, they seem to be in perpetual energy balance. There are many additional ill effects on health and nutritional status.

Read Chapter 3 and Amy's story below for alternative ways to deal with the issue. Commonsense is often overlooked because crazy weight-control practices become entrenched in a sport. Unfortunately, such behaviour can even be glorified. From the commentary box during the 1990 World Rowing Championships in Australia came the following encouragement: 'And let's give a big hand to the crew from X. These girls have not eaten anything for four days to make it into this final. What a heroic effort.'

The life of the cox

The coxswain's life is not easy. He may be under pressure to lose weight (the crew obviously wants the cox to be as light as possible), and he also bears the responsibility of keeping the crew together in stroke and spirit. It takes a distinctive personality to rule over a boat. Weight control is made all the more difficult for coxes by the fact that their job does not consume energy: they are more or less along for the ride.

Since a cox may be involved in many hours of other people's training each day, he often has little time or incentive to do extra aerobic exercise. As a result, many are tempted simply to cut down on food, and get caught up in a vicious cycle of weight gain/loss or a general food and weight obsession. As in other sports, this is harmful to health. As with lightweight rowers, the body may develop an undesired energy balance, making the weight even harder to lose.

The keys to weight loss are detailed in Chapter 3. They include sensible targets; healthy nutrition and exercise plans; and avoidance of severe dehydration and food restriction before competitions. If you won't do it for yourself, do it for the team. The last thing a top crew needs at an important competition is an irritable and fatigued cox!

Profile: Trent

Fitting enough food into the day—and the stomach

Trent was living in a university college and rowing with the university coxed fours. The training schedule leading into the competition season was intense—ten water sessions and three weight-training sessions each week. The energy requirements were obviously enormous, and Trent was fighting a losing battle to keep his weight up. Not only was he becoming tired, he was now about 5 kg below the average crew weight. He was careful to eat a high-carbohydrate diet. He had learned all about that in the nutrition classes that were part of his sports science degree course. But he could not seem to find the time or the stomach room to increase his energy intake enough. He was already suffering from heartburn, especially when he bent over the oars, and a couple of times he had even vomited. Naturally, he was reluctant to enlarge his meals any further.

After the third consecutive drop in his skinfold measures, he went to see a sports dietitian. She took a detailed account of his typical daily training and eating habits. She told Trent he obviously understood which foods were good for fuel and had made these the focus of all his meals. As to why he wasn't eating enough, she came up with two reasons. First, he was limited to eating three times a day, because that's all the university dining hall catered for, and because his time between meals was tied up. Training and class or study together took up eight to ten hours a day. As a result, Trent was often caught between eating too little and the fear of aggravating his heartburn with huge meals.

The dietitian suggested some practical ways to increase eating opportunities and reduce the bulkiness of Trent's meals. With six or seven meals and snacks a day, and with the clever use of nutritious drinks (low in bulk and high in energy) he could consume all the kilojoules he needed without distressing his gut.

First, Trent needed greater access to food. The dietitian and Trent met with the chef at the university dining hall and together they negotiated a plan to meet Trent's special needs. The chef was keen for the college to be lauded for having a winning athlete, and said he'd be happy to give Trent food to take to his room—all rooms in the college had a small fridge and tea-making facilities. Trent could take up supplies of breakfast cereal, milk, fresh and canned fruit, and cereal bars. And he was encouraged to order two bagged lunches each day—one to be eaten during the morning classes and study blocks, and the other to cover lunchtime and the afternoon. Sandwiches, buns and fruit were easily eaten in the back of class, so he could nibble his way through this food over several hours, thus avoiding the discomfort of a gigantic lunch. To keep things interesting, the chef agreed to swap around sandwich fillings, bread types and muffins/fruit buns/pikelets. Trent was also encouraged to look at the cafeteria menu a couple of times a week so he could add a hot item to the mix—not pies or sausage rolls, but a noodle stir fry or laksa, or a sizzling salad. As for the evening meal, the chef made plans to keep one waiting on the nights when Trent would get back to college late.

The dietitian also said Trent needed to be aggressive with recovery eating—consuming nutrients before, during and after each workout to promote performance in the session and adaptation afterwards. This included having a snack before on-water sessions, fuelling during these sessions, and having carbohydrate–protein snacks after both water and gym- or land-based training. These could include everyday foods but might also make the most of the convenience of sports foods. While they were more expensive than regular foods, sports foods were usually portable, relatively non-perishable, ready to go and easy to consume.

The final item on the agenda was for Trent to learn how to make nutritious high-energy drinks. He was encouraged to buy a hand-held blender so he could mix up delicious concoctions of milk, fruit, and low-fat yoghurt or ice-cream, with a boost from skim-milk powder or a powdered liquid meal. He could do this in his room for an evening snack, and the chefs could also make something similar for the breakfast menu. Nutrient-rich kilojoules that didn't require chewing would allow Trent to cut down the size of his meals and feel more comfortable. Table 17.1 summarises a day of his 'after plan'.

After following this plan consistently for a while, Trent began to regain the kilos and find new vigour at training. The heartburn and bloating after meals were also greatly reduced, making him feel better in the boat. It was sometimes a nuisance having to be so organised, and unless he kept varying his drink concoctions he got bored with the same thing three times a day. But as long as he stayed one jump ahead of himself, he was streets ahead in performance.

Profile: Amy

Rowing lightweight

Amy tried out for selection in the state rowing squad as a lightweight single sculler. She did well in the physiological testing and was assessed as having a good stroke technique. Inevitably, however, the scales poked their way into the assessment, and the news was discouraging. At 63.5 kg, she was nearly 5 kg over the competition weight limit of 59 kg. Some of the other girls were even worse off—two weighed nearly 69 kg. One of these girls had collapsed in her last race, clearly exhausted and dehydrated, and had to go to the medical tent for intravenous rehydration.

Amy was steadily losing her own battle with the scales. When she'd started rowing four years ago she had hovered around 60–61 kg, and needed only a small extra effort in competition week to make the weight limit. At first the business of making weight had seemed exciting and even a bit mystical. She had watched the pairs and fours going through their weight-loss rituals together, and thought it must really bond them as a team. Later, though, as it got harder and harder to get the weight off, she realised that weeks of starving, and days of sitting in saunas or running in thick tracksuits, made teams irritable and argumentative rather than close and cohesive. The crews were allowed to average their weights, so there was always niggling within the team about who should lose more weight and who was letting the others down.

These days, Amy's fretting about weight was no longer confined to the week leading up to competition. It had become a full-time obsession. She was constantly trying to shed the kilos, but the harder she tried the harder it got. If worry was supposed to make you lose weight, she shouldn't have any problem. Thoughts of food and the scales filled her every waking hour, but all to no avail. The frustration drained away all her enjoyment of her sport.

She didn't tell this to the selection coach, but then she didn't need to. The trials and tribulations of lightweight rowing were no news to him. He was well aware of the constant dieting, and of the dangerous sweating and fasting that went on during competition. He explained to Amy that he was not prepared to tolerate this. He was only interested in recruiting girls who could safely and healthily row in the lightweight division. While it might seem cruel to turn people away, he did not want to be part of the misery or the damage.

The coach looked at Amy's skinfold measurements—81 mm over seven sites. This was higher than it needed to be, which meant Amy had a real chance to make it into the lightweight-class without harming her health. He also took into consideration that she had not yet had a mishap during competition. Amy had always rowed well, and could truthfully say that she had never resorted to diuretics, laxatives and vomiting like some of her fellow rowers. The final decision was to award Amy a temporary scholarship, to be revised in ten weeks. The conditions were that she see a sports dietitian and reduce her training weight to 60–61 kg, with a decline in her skinfold measurements.

Amy agreed to this trial, but wondered what good seeing a dietitian could do. What could a dietitian tell her about weight loss that she didn't already know? Nevertheless, she kept to her side of the bargain and went along.

Listening to Amy's story, the dietitian said her years of restricted kilojoule intake and yo-yoing weight had probably reduced her energy requirements. Amy's diet was low in kilojoules and did not provide enough protein, iron, calcium or other minerals. It was a wonder she was able to keep up her training load on such a small intake of carbohydrate and energy. The dietitian suggested that Amy was probably not always aware of the extent of her splurges—and would be surprised to know how wildly her total energy intake fluctuated.

Feeling she had nothing to lose, Amy agreed to try the dietitian's meal plan. It included more protein, carbohydrate and minerals to support training and health requirements; a small treat each week; a low-dose multivitamin/mineral tablet each day to ensure that all nutrient RDIs were met; portable foods, such as a breakfast that could be eaten on the way to work (see summary below); and the minimum kilojoule intake that could be regarded as healthy and unlikely to cause metabolic adaptations.

As suggested in Chapter 3.4, Amy was to try an energy intake of about 4320 kJ plus the energy cost of training. The sums worked out like this:

Training = 8 sessions a week × 60 min

Energy cost of training (assume rowing is equivalent to moderate running @ 50 kJ per minute) = 24 000 kJ/week or 3430 kJ/day.

Therefore, suggested energy intake = 7748 kJ/day (1850 Cal/day).

The dietitian told Amy her greatest need was to begin to let go of her fears and worries, and to think more positively about her food and weight. With confidence and a happier outlook, she would be less likely to get out of control and splurge. This would need a lot of self-talk and support—after all, she would need to reverse years of misery and frustration. The dietitian scheduled a weekly appointment for Amy to discuss her progress and promised that no scales would appear during that time. The emphasis would be on how Amy was feeling and coping.

Progress was slow but sure. Amy needed a lot of encouragement to change her old way of thinking. She was happy with the meal plan, but said she needed to remind herself that a small treat was OK now and then, and that she didn't need to watch the scales or have all the weight off within a week.

The first weight and skinfold check-in was scheduled a month into the new program. The results were encouraging—Amy's weight was down to 62 kg and her skinfolds down to 65 mm. At the end of the second month, she'd lost another kilogram and 10 mm off her skinfold total. A fortnight later she weighed in at 60.5 kg. With a little fine-tuning before competition, and the nerves that went with big races, she would easily be inside the event limits. The rewards for her effort were not only a full rowing scholarship but a totally changed outlook on life and her sport.

TABLE 17.1
A high-energy day in the life of Trent

Before	
6.30–8.00 a.m.	Rowing at river. Drinks water Often has heartburn from too much food the previous evening.
8.30 a.m.	Back to university college for as much breakfast as can be scoffed in 25 minutes: Cereal + tinned fruit + milk Fruit juice Toast + baked beans/spaghetti/eggs

9.15–12.30	Study or uni classes Often suffers indigestion and heartburn
12.45 p.m.	Lunch at university cafeteria (packed lunch provided by university college): Sandwiches/rolls with meat and salad fillings Fruit bun Fruit juice Sometimes has to cut back the amount if heartburn is bad—can't risk too much discomfort for evening session
1.30–4.00 p.m.	Study or uni classes
5.00–7.30 p.m.	Training at river Weights sessions 3 times a week before rowing—often training goes past 8 p.m.
8.30 p.m.	Early nights—arrives at the university dining hall just in time for late meal sitting: Meat/fish/chicken—large serves (often 2 meals) Rice or potatoes—sometimes pasta Veggies or salad Bread Jelly/fruit salad/rice pudding/icecream Late nights—misses the official meal time. Makes jam sandwiches in tea room—sometimes almost a loaf of bread. Probably eats too much, but what else can he do?
9.00–10.00 p.m.	Study, if he can keep his eyes open
After	
6.00 a.m.	PowerBar and some water on the drive to training
6.30–8.00 a.m.	Training. Sports drink during session. To also trial gels for an extra fuel boost 2 Tetra Paks of Sustagen Sport and banana on drive home from training

8.30 a.m.	University breakfast—can afford to eat more slowly and reduce the size of meals Cereal + tinned fruit + milk Smoothie—juice, yoghurt, fresh fruit and skim-milk powder Toast + eggs/baked beans/spaghetti
9.15–12.30	Lunch bag 1 during university study/classes Sandwiches/wraps/rolls, flavoured milk, muffins
12.45 p.m.	Starting lunch bag 2, often adding item from university cafeteria to promote more variety (e.g. take away noodle dish or sizzling salad) Large flavoured milk
1.30–4.00 p.m.	Study/uni Finishing lunch bag 2. PowerBar on the way to training
5.00–7.30 p.m.	Sports drink during session. Between on-water training and gym session—2 Tetra Paks of Sustagen sport Trip home: flavoured yoghurt and fruit
8.30 p.m.	University meal—smaller portion than previously
9.30 p.m.	Sip on supersmoothie while getting ready for next day's activities Try not to study after training—get sleep to make next day more productive

CHECKLIST 17.1
Slowing down the rate of eating

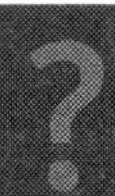

Use the following tips to increase your experience of eating, reduce the likelihood of overeating or getting into binge mode, and help to calm you down if you start feeling anxious about food

1 **Make it chunky and chewy**

- Create meals and snacks with lots of veggies and salad or watery fruits (strawberries and melons). This increases the volume of the meal and makes it slower to consume. It also reduces the number of calories per mouthful and adds a bonus of vitamins and antioxidants.

Ideas:

- Add plenty of salad to a sandwich
- Eat a large salad or veggies with your meal
  - —Add them as a side serve (especially in restaurants, where you may want to have an entrée or just a small amount of a main course but still feel full)
  - —Mix them into the meal by having a main meal salad or a stir-fry or pasta/lasagne sauce with extra veggies added the recipe
- Add lots of veggies to your soups, and leave them in chunks
- Make a veggie platter with protein dips as a light meal or snack
- Make a fruit platter with yoghurt dip as a dessert or snack

2 Make it hot (temperature)

- If your foods and drinks are served boiling or sizzling hot, you will have to eat more slowly or burn your mouth

Ideas:

- Serve your soup boiling hot
- Serve hot main meals hot rather than lukewarm
- Have a skinny hot chocolate as a snack or dessert

3 Make it hot (spicy)

- You will find it hard to overload on spicy foods—and drinking water with the meal will also slow you down and fill you up

Ideas:

- Add just enough spice to your main meals—chilli, curry powder, wasabi. Add it at the plate if others you are eating with don't share your sense of adventure!
- Add spice to your dips or soups

4 Eat it frozen

- Many foods freeze well and can make a longer-lasting dessert or snack
- It's a refreshing idea for summer eating

Ideas:

- Freeze a carton of yoghurt as part of a snack or dessert
- Freeze fruit chunks or pieces as a dessert or snack—suitable fruits include grapes, mango segments, berries, orange and mandarin segments
- Make a home-made frappé with a cup of skim milk, ice cubes and cocoa powder or chocolate protein powder (or buy a skinny frappuccino without cream at a coffee outlet)
- Freeze diet soft drinks in a large cup and drink it as it begins to thaw
- Make icy poles with low-cal cordial or soft drink

Australian Rules football

Australian Rules football is played predominantly by males, and the major league, the Australian Football League, organises a national competition. It is played from primary school upwards, at a variety of levels both amateur and professional. A game is made up of four 20-min quarters, with time (usually 5–10 min) added for the time that the ball is out of play. The first and third quarters are separated by a short break, and there is a longer break at half-time. Each team consists of eighteen players on the ground and four interchange players, who may be swapped at any time with players on the field. Rules are often adjusted in the pre-season competition to promote the evolution of the game.

The traditional line-up sees five lines of three players spread from one end of the ground (backs) towards the other (forwards), with the final three players set to follow the play. However, as the style of play has become more mobile and fluid, these traditional lines have lost much of their former meaning. In addition to running, players must leap to mark or punch the ball. Heavy physical contact and tackling also increase the demands on players.

Training

The football year can be divided into three sections: pre-season, season, and off-season. The length of each section will vary with the level of competition. A typical schedule might be:

- Off-season: October onwards for 6 weeks (professionals) to 3 months (lower-level players).
- Pre-season: 2–4 months. Training starts in November for professional clubs and culminates with pre-season competition over the final month. At the highest levels, players train 5–6 days a week, often with several training sessions, or training and a meeting, on the same day. Individual players are often selected for specific programs according to the requirements of their position or their individual weaknesses. In general, training revolves around a running program to build up an aerobic base and then develop anaerobic speed and endurance. Weight training is important, especially for players who need to build bulk and strength. Other sports such as boxing or swimming may also be included. The emphasis on skills and match play in training increases as the pre-season progresses, with practice matches and the pre-season competition leading into the season.
- Competitive season: There are roughly six days between matches. Most professional clubs schedule a recovery session the day after the match and two conditioning and weight sessions during the week, with lighter skill-oriented sessions near the end of the week.

Competition

The AFL season consists of 22 games played both at home and away, with one game played each weekend from March to August. A final series involving the top-finishing teams is played in September, and culminates in the Grand Final between the top two teams. At the elite level, games are played on Friday nights or on weekend afternoons and evenings. At lower and junior levels, there may be a set time for the weekly match, but at the professional level there is a variable schedule involving interstate travel and six to eight days between matches.

An Australian Rules football match lasts about two hours, and its physiological demands vary considerably depending on players' field positions and the playing style of the team. On-ball players may run 12–20 km in a match, although new rules allowing unlimited use of the interchange bench have increased the speed and number of repeated sprints players undertake before being rotated off the field. These players have high fuel requirements. Full-forwards and full-backs perform brief, fast sprints, which use mostly anaerobic energy and impose lower total fuel demands. Repeated physical contact between players and the resulting damage to muscle fibres must also be taken into consideration in the recovery between matches.

Physical characteristics

An Australian Rules team is a mixed bag of field positions and playing skills, and players' physiques are similarly varied, from 200-cm rucks to 175-cm on-ballers. Lower body-fat levels are expected among running players. Indeed, over the past 20 years there has been a dramatic reduction in the body-fat levels of professional players and an increase in muscle mass. Greater height and muscle mass are expected in key positions where players directly contest the ball.

Common nutritional issues

The weekly routine of nutrition needs

In the old days, footballers worried only about what they ate the night before the game or for the pre-match meal—if they worried at all. Many thought they should eat protein at the beginning of the week and carbohydrate at the end. The modern view of football nutrition is to tailor eating patterns to the individual needs of each player and the demands of the training or match schedule. Chapters 1 and 2 discuss nutrition for training, while Chapter 5 covers recovery between training sessions. Modern Australian Rules footballers now recognise the benefits of proactively addressing the significant fuel, fluid, muscle-repair and adaptation requirements of their game.

Each player needs to have a customised plan that will take him from each day's training all the way to long-term goals. Covering all the issues can take fairly complex planning, and most top teams have a sports dietitian in their training services crew (see Profile below). Other players who need help in honing their plan may need to find their own way to a sports dietitian. For a developing player who wants to get the best from his talents, this may be a sound investment.

General nutritional knowledge and cooking skills

The top football leagues begin to recruit new players as young as 16 or 17. Sometimes, recruitment means relocating to a new city. Lodging is often arranged with local families, but many new players and even some older ones share houses in which no one has any real nutritional knowledge or cooking skills.

At the lower levels of play, footballers may have full-time work or study commitments. Professional players generally have a crowded week of training, meetings and other club activities, and many also work part time or study with a post-football career in mind. One way or another, the life of a football player can be busy, leaving little time for food shopping and preparation. A pattern of skipped meals and reliance on take-aways is common.

Australian Rules football players should be screened to identify those whose diets are below par. Basic nutritional education and cooking lessons could do a great deal to improve diet and, as a result, well-being and performance (see Rugby chapter).

Weight and body-fat control

Over the past decade, interest has grown in optimising body-fat levels to suit Australian Rules' increasingly mobile style of play. Most high-level clubs routinely monitor players' skinfold measurements, though not all use accredited professionals for the task (see Chapter 3). In some teams, inaccurately taken measurements have been compounded by misinterpreted results. Some teams set skinfold targets that all players must achieve. Some players compete to have the lowest skinfold totals in the team. An individual approach is needed that allows for the specific needs of a position, the player's genetic background, and the change in body-fat levels that can be expected from his growth and training load. Body-fat levels should be monitored at strategic times of the football year and individual profiles and targets set for each player (see Chapter 3.2, 3.3). It can take several seasons for a player to identify his best features and develop them fully.

There are times, of course, when players need to reduce body-fat levels, such as pre-season or on return from illness or injury. Young players, or players living in a disorganised household, may have high body-fat levels because they lack a long-term and sensible to eating and training. Footballers are notorious for using crash and fad diets to lose weight. Chapter 3.4 and Checklist 3.2 present a better approach to steady and permanent fat loss, and Robbie's story below shows how this can work in real life.

Gaining muscle mass

At the other end of the spectrum is the young, slightly built recruit who wants to gain weight to withstand the physical rigours of the game. As Chapters 3.7–3.8 and Checklist 3.4 make clear, bulking up requires an appropriate weights program, a high-energy diet and realistic expectations. In addition, specialist coaching may help slender players adopt body-positioning and playing skills that help protect them from bumps and collisions.

Alcohol intake

The alcohol intake of many footballers is a good example of the victory of peer pressure over good nutrition—and even good sense. The past and present drinking patterns of Australian Rules players are examined below. Although some players rationalise such habits as normal, alcohol misuse and abuse impairs performance in a number of ways. A better approach to alcohol in sport is presented in Chapter 1.6 and in Checklist 18.1.

Take-aways and restaurants

Take-away foods are typical fare on weekends after the game and may become a staple for footballers who can't cook for themselves. Better cooking skills should enable such players to make quick and easy meals at home. However, players should also be educated about good choices with take-aways, and how to dine well in restaurants. It is inevitable that players will occasionally eat from such sources, but with careful selection they should be able to do so without thwarting their nutritional goals. See the section on take-aways in the Basketball chapter, and on eating out in the Golf chapter.

Pre-match preparation

The demands of the match will challenge many players' muscle carbohydrate stores. These players should top up their glycogen levels before each match, focusing on carbohydrate-rich foods from the end of the last team training session of the week to the start of the match. Other players may need less attention to glycogen stores yet still need to be adequately fuelled for the match. Chapters 4.2–4.3 provide some guidelines for match preparation.

The pre-match meal is the last opportunity to fine-tune fuel and fluid levels. Each player will need to develop a plan of carbohydrate-rich meals or snacks that suits the timing of the match and their individual preferences (see Chapter 4.4). Most players like to have a larger meal 3–4 hours before the match, with perhaps a top-up just before the warm-up. Teams that travel to another town for match day often organise their own, catered pre-event meal.

Fluid intake during training and matches

Many people think of Aussie Rules as a winter sport. However, the late-summer start of the pre-season competition and the popularity of the game in the northern states of Australia mean many football matches (and training sessions) take place in warm to hot weather. Even in winter, players should be on guard against dehydration. Our experience in monitoring fluid losses over the course of matches and longer skills-training sessions shows that a substantial number of players will develop a fluid deficit of more than 2 per cent body weight. In a sport involving fast decision-making and skilful execution, such dehydration can be expected to cause fatigue; this in turn can affect the outcome of a game.

Although the demands of playing Aussie Rules can create large sweat losses, the breaks at the end of each quarter provide an opportunity to rehydrate, trainers are allowed onto the ground to bring drinks to those not actively involved in the play, and time spent on the interchange bench can also be a time for drinking. It is useful for players to weigh themselves before and after each match to keep track of fluid losses. Improving hydration requires some effort on the part of the club (to provide the trainers, the drink bottles and player education). But it also requires the players to take advantage of drinking opportunities. Chapter 4.6 sets out the basis of good fluid-intake practices.

Many studies of soccer and other stop-start sports have shown the benefits of refuelling during play. It can help players run longer or faster in the second half or last quarter, or help minimise fewer tactical mistakes and fumbles in this crucial part of the game. This should be especially important for the on-ball players. Chapter 4.7 and Checklist 4.4 discuss the range of drinks and sports products that can be used to keep muscles and brain fuelled right until the final siren.

Profile: AFL

Champion of sports nutrition in Australia

In 2008, the 150th anniversary of Australian Rules football provided the occasion to reflect on the game's contribution to sports nutrition and to the career path of one of the authors of this book (LB):

The first appointment of a sports dietitian to the medical team of an AFL club occurred in 1980. Melbourne-based Karen Inge was invited to provide regular nutritional advice for Collingwood, a highly successful team. Inge needed a project to undertake as part of her postgraduate studies, and Collingwood was smarting from its loss in the previous year's Grand Final. The players had used special fructose tablets before that important game, and some had overindulged and suffered from gastrointestinal distress. As a result, the medical team at Collingwood thought it would be good to get some nutritional advice from a reputable source. Collingwood made it into the 1980 Grand Final but lost.

Coincidentally, the club at the bottom of the premiership ladder, St. Kilda, also invested in sports nutrition in 1980. The Saints had won only one premiership in the history of the competition and sorely tried the patience of their fans. One fan, in the last year of a degree in dietetics, wrote to the team's star to convince him of the importance of sound eating to optimal performance. The player, Trevor Barker, not only read the letter but passed it on to the club doctor, who contacted the student.

That piece of serendipity started my career.

So what was it like working for a professional football club in the 1980s? The pre-event meal was the main focus of performance nutrition at the time. Many players felt that eating the right foods in the right quantity at the right time before the game (with their lucky knife and fork) would overcome a week of poor eating and turn them into champions. Recovery was not yet a concept and post-game activities mostly revolved around alcohol and partying. At the end of each season, players would disappear for several months and return many kilograms overweight. Their major reason for seeing the club dietitian was to get advice on weight loss. Counselling might take place in one part of the club rooms while in another section players were enjoying a sausage sizzle and a few beers. It would be fair to say that the Saints and I weren't ready for each other.

The culture and physiology of the game have changed over the past 30 years. In the 1980s, most good players were skilled rather than athletic. Even though AFL was a professional code, most players held full-time jobs as physical education teachers, bank workers or salesmen. Training sessions were held late in the afternoon to accommodate work commitments, and all games in the 12-team competition were played at the same time (on Saturday afternoons). There were no travel issues to worry about—all teams in the country's major competition were located within 100 km of Melbourne. Each team played with 20 players—18 who took the field at the start of the match in set positions and two reserves who were brought on to replace injured or fatigued players. Trainers carried half-filled cups of water onto the ground during the breaks between quarters, and doctors administered glucose tablets for energy.

The game of 2008 is much faster and highly athletic. The differences between positions are blurred, and players are generally seen as forwards, defenders, and midfielders. The midfield players who wear GPS devices during the match typically log 12–16 km of running during a game of four ~30-min quarters, with exceptional players clocking over 20 km. Because the 18 players on the field can now be constantly rotated on and off via four interchange players, however, the emphasis is more on sustained high speeds than on total running distance. Most of the teams are still based in Melbourne, but with six of the 16 teams coming from interstate and matches held in all states and territories, the challenges of travel and play in a variety of climates are now part of the game. Thirteen of the teams now have sports dietitians on their fitness or medical-support teams. Typically, each dietitian spends one or two days at the club each week and plays a variety of roles on match day. Some dietitians travel to all interstate games and sit on the team bench during play, monitoring hydration status and the like. The dietitian's job might include:

- Making anthropometric assessments of body composition
- Counselling players individually
- Conducting group lectures and meetings
- Supermarket shopping and label reading
- Holding cooking classes
- Conducting specialised educational and induction programs for young players
- Organising catering during interstate trips
- Managing of supplement programs and policies
- Contributing to 'innovation' committees
- Attending medical-services meetings
- Setting up individualised plans for match-day nutrition
- Organising match-day nutrition needs and post-match recovery eating
- Monitoring hydration status during matches and training sessions and from day to day
- Attending next-day recovery sessions for match feedback
- Running a nutrition education/message notice board
- Organising catering on some training days

This list highlights a number of apparent changes in views about how nutrition can affect the performance of AFL players. Sound eating practices are now part of players' preparation across the board. The club dietitian plays an important role in facilitating or implementing the nutrition program and is recognised as part of the fitness or medical-support staff. Players and coaches also now expect a case-management approach to individualised players' nutritional needs and goals, rather than having a 'one size fits all' plan for all players.

I have had the opportunity to witness this change firsthand, having returned to the Saints from season 2006–2008 to coordinate a nutrition program. (Well, they still hadn't won that elusive premiership, so I felt the need to roll up my sleeves again.)

There's a funny sense of déjà vu at the club because the rooms and facilities haven't changed but the attitudes to nutrition and diet have. I have a lovely reminder of my past whenever I am at the club. My childhood hero, Trevor Barker, succumbed to cancer many years ago at the age of 39, but his father, Jack, still attends all training sessions and matches. During the winter months I organise hot soup and bread rolls for the players after the main training session of the week, and 81-year-old Jack comes in to serve them. He often tells me that Trevor listened to my advice about eating vegetables or not eating too many desserts! And I often tell him that without Trevor, who knows what I would be doing today?

Profile: Booze

Drinking to your sports success

In 1983, a study was done of alcohol intake among players in one of the top clubs in the Australian Football League. Fifty-four players took part in the study, which required them to record their food intake, including all alcohol consumed, over a typical week during the season. The players were then interviewed about their usual drinking patterns. Finally, since people often under-report or exaggerate their alcohol intake on questionnaires, blood samples were taken from 41 players at a Sunday morning training session and their alcohol content was used to gauge how much the players had consumed the previous evening, after the match.

Most players followed the club policy of drinking alcohol only on weekends. They reported that they drank on Saturday nights after the game and on Sundays. They admitted that they made up for the week's abstinence on those occasions, but claimed heavy alcohol intake was part of team bonding and helped them unwind after the game. During the off-season, when the club policy was not in effect, the frequency of alcohol binges would increase. Only five of the footballers interviewed in the study described themselves as non-drinkers.

The players' food records showed an average daily alcohol intake of 20 g—equivalent to two standard drinks (see Figure 1.1). This sounds moderate on paper, but of course the 'average' figure covered up the fact that the entire week's intake was fitted into a weekend. Players who consumed alcohol on the Saturday night drank an average of 120 g or 12 standard drinks. However, individual intakes ranged from 37 g to 368 g—almost 40 standard drinks. In an extreme case, alcohol provided 43 per cent of the kilojoules consumed that day, but on average it supplied almost one-fifth of each player's total energy intake on the Saturday.

The results of the blood-alcohol readings supported the story of the Saturday-night binge. Fourteen players still had alcohol in their blood at 10 a.m. the next morning, with readings from 0.001 g/100 ml to 0.113 g/100 ml. Four players had blood alcohol readings over 0.05 g/100 ml—the legal limit for driving a car in the state of Victoria. Clearly, some players had drunk a lot of alcohol the previous evening.

You might ask how professional athletes, paid to perform at their best, could have such an unprofessional attitude to alcohol misuse. Back in the 1980s, football tradition and peer-group influence heavily supported drinking to excess. It was the norm rather than the exception. It was also encouraged by some clubs and pubs, which lured players to their venues with free drink cards, supported by the media and tolerated by the public. They all covered up or excused the problems created by excessive drinking (drink driving charges, violence, accidents). They rationalised that 'boys will be boys' and even romanticised the drinking binges. One Victorian hotel we know has a plaque commemorating the time a high-profile football player consumed '37 × 375 ml cans of [beer] in two hours. Witnessed by hotel patrons, teammates and a very nervous doctor'. Within the team, people would say 'everybody does it'—a poor excuse at best. Other rationalisations included: 'I only do it once a week', 'It's part of cultivating team spirit', 'Beer is good for carbs', and 'I can sweat it out the next day'.

Fast-forward 25 years. Binge drinking among football players is now a major issue. Newspapers carry frequent reports of binge drinking after games, on 'Mad Monday' (the first day after a team has finished its season), and on club trips in the off-season. The highly publicised activities that have taken place on these occasions include deaths and serious injuries to high-level players caused by drink driving, violence leading to injuries and criminal records, and arrests for other criminal activities. The public no longer supports binge drinking, but it appears that this disapproval is not having much impact within sport. Administrators of football competitions and individual clubs now realise that such antics are directly hurting their 'brand' and their bottom line, if not causing social, financial and physical harm to players. Read Chapter 1.6 for the facts about alcohol and sports performance. It is a difficult problem to address, since the culture of alcohol use among clubs and many players is longstanding and resistant to change. However, the AFL is one of the signatories to a new program aimed at reducing the misuse and abuse of alcohol and drugs in sport. It involves:

- Identifying the practices that encourage dangerous drinking and binge drinking in the club environment and team culture
- Changing any club policies, practices or culture that suggest drinking alcohol is an 'all or none' activity
- Educating players about the personal risks they run in binge drinking, including loss of earnings through the damage to their reputation when bad behaviour is publicised, and accidents and violence, which can lead to criminal charges, injury and death
- Having players develop their own code of conduct, one that incorporates safe drinking practices and the principle of looking after team-mates on outings involving drinking (see Checklist 18.1)
- Implementing punishments for breaches of the player-developed code of conduct
- Ensuring that all club functions and activities provide low-alcohol and non-alcoholic drinks and forbid under-age drinking
- Encouraging players to drink either in their own homes or at private club activities
- Creating good role models in players with a moderate and healthy approach to drinking.

Watch this space to see whether this new initiative does help footballers develop safe and sensible drinking practices that are consistent with the performance goals in which clubs invest so heavily.

Profile: Robbie

Losing kilos to befit a 'smaller' jumper

At 22 years of age, Robbie was moving up fast at his top AFL club. After a couple of years as a rookie, he had made his way into the first senior team and played all but one match in the previous year. In fact, he'd finished third in the club best and fairest competition—vindicating the judgement of the recruitment manager, who had first spotted him playing in a country schools competition. When he'd come to the club as an 18-year-old, Robbie had been lean and spindly. His first three seasons were spent in the gym and in the offices of the fitness staff, scrounging bottles of protein powder and sports bars to help him gain weight.

After the end-of-season club trip to Bali, Robbie went back home for the off-season, hanging out with his old mates and catching up on the fun he'd missed. His football commitments had kept him away from several mates' 21st-birthday parties over the previous year, but he soon made up for lost time. Between parties and the celebrations for his developing footy career (everywhere he went, one of his Dad's buddies would insist on toasting his newfound success), he always seemed to have a beer in his hand. It was nice to hang out with the old crowd and get back to country living. No rocket salads and fancy but microscopic meals on giant plates around here, he laughed, as he told his mates about his dining-out experiences in the city. For two months, he soaked up roasts and barbecues and his Gran's famous trifle. It was nice to have some real time away from the focus and discipline of the football club.

It wasn't so nice when he arrived back at the club to find that the staff had a new member—a sports dietitian—and that he'd gained 4 kg. He had succeeded in filling out his frame to an adult size, and then some! It was a novel experience to find himself worrying about having the pre-season 'skinnies' (body fat) assessment done. In previous years he had joined the laughter and teasing as names were added to the Fatty Club list on the team noticeboard—to join, your skinfold scores had to add up to over 50 mm. The punishment included fines, extra running, ridicule and crash dieting. The new dietitian did the skinfold measurements in a way he hadn't seen before, involving tape measures and marker-pen lines on various parts of his body. He expected there might be some change from his previous low-40s skinfold totals, but the measurement of 68 mm floored him. He vowed to get out of the Fatty Club as soon as he could. Luckily, the dietitian had so many new people to meet that Robbie was able to avoid face-to-face contact with her. He thought he would sort out the weight thing for himself in a fortnight and then start his relationship with the dietitian on a positive note.

Unfortunately, shifting the weight was harder than he thought. It bounced all over the place—down 2 kg in a single morning after training, then up again after the weekend. After a week, it was hard to say how much progress he'd really made. He was hardly eating anything, avoiding bread and carbs like the plague, and was hungry all the time. This made him grumpy, and he only got grumpier when he found himself falling behind everyone else at training. The team had done the first of their 3-km test runs in the second week, and he was a whole 50 sec down on his time from the previous season. What made things even more embarrassing was that several of the older players in the club had retired at the end of last season, leaving some of the 'higher' numbers vacant. He had been presented with No. 3 to replace his rookie 42. With this sign of the club's high expectations and his own greater public visibility, Robbie felt very frustrated. He redoubled his efforts to cut kilojoules, eating only one meal a day, at night. Then he had a dizzy spell in a gym session and was literally dragged into the dietitian's office to discuss what was going on.

What Robbie expected to be an uncomfortable encounter turned out to be an encouraging one. The dietitian listened carefully to his story and commiserated that he had fallen for the oldest trick in the book—overeating and overindulging in alcohol while underexercising in the off-season. If he could learn from the lesson, it would be a mistake worth making once. But now he had some work to do, and a new way to think about himself. He was still living with a foster family, so he was in a good food environment. During the season, there would be time to move out and look after himself, as well as to review how well he was addressing 'performance nutrition' issues for match day. Right now, he needed to settle in to training and careful eating to lose the weight sensibly once and for all.

The dietitian explained to Robbie that football clubs were often a haven for macho attitudes to weight control. She had the support of the coach and the head of training services to bring in a new culture. There would be no more false expectations or crazy dieting practices. Rather than starving himself, Robbie needed to understand the fuel demands of his training—without meeting them, he wouldn't be able to train well. This rang a bell! She also explained that the scales measured total weight, including body water and gut contents, which went up and down each day separately from changes in body fat. She suggested Robbie weigh himself several times a week at home, first thing in the morning. This information would provide a clue about real changes in weight. Even so, urine samples would be taken as part of the hydration monitoring at the club to see how well he was replacing sweat losses over the day. Monitoring weight changes before and after each training session were also part of the club program. But instead of seeing a big 'loss' as a sign of weight loss, Robbie needed to see it as representing dehydration—a sign he needed to replace lost fluid. Skinfolds would be measured every fortnight, and even then he needed to build a possible error of 2–3 mm into the final figure. His progress would also be gauged by how well he was following a meal plan.

Robbie and the dietitian worked out a meal plan that involved his favourite foods (meat, meat and meat), the items he liked on his foster family's dinner menu (mostly good choices) and carbohydrate sources to fuel his training. He was happy to swap his usual bacon and egg breakfast for one of cereal and milk, or, on the morning before weights, a couple of poached eggs on toast. Apart from the fuel factor, the new choices were quicker and sat more easily in his stomach when eaten before a running/skills session. Sandwiches were still on the agenda for lunch, but the fillings were leaner—slices of chicken breast, roast beef or ham—than his previous favourite, chicken schnitzel.

Dinner involved not so much a change in menu as a change in portion sizes. Robbie's meat serve was halved (the dietitian assured him there was still plenty of protein in his day), and the vegetable component was increased so he still had a full plate. Rice, pasta or bread completed the meal, with the amount increasing or decreasing according to the training load. His 'farm boy' background and former need to bulk up had got Robbie used to drinking milk with every meal—up to 3 L a day, not including his protein recovery shakes at the club. Now he cut back to a small shake after his key workouts for the week and, for the moment, switched to water as his main fluid source. There was still plenty of dairy in his diet—yoghurt or custard with fruit for dessert. But now he went for the low-fat brands.

Alcohol was the final part of the plan. Or, to be more accurate, it was not part of the plan. Robbie had been on the wagon since his return to training, and actually preferred this to having a couple of beers each week. However, Christmas was coming up and he would be returning home to his mates and no doubt some parties. The dietitian suggested they make a plan for this period once Robbie had made some progress and felt motivated for a new challenge.

Robbie settled into the diet plan at once. He felt secure knowing what to do, and the plan actually wasn't that difficult to follow. He felt satisfied after meals and snacks, and he had plenty of energy for training. He noticed that his weight continued to jump around a little from day to day—and he had to talk to the dietitian again about his hydration practices during training—but overall his weight was on a downward trend. After four weeks, he'd lost nearly 3 kg and his skinfold total was down to the low 50s. At six weeks, as he prepared to go home for the break, he recorded a PB in the 3 x 1 km time trial. He had lost no more weight, but his skinfolds now totalled 46 mm. This suggested that he might have gained a little muscle mass (he was certainly stronger in the gym) as he regained his former leanness.

With newfound confidence, Robbie worked out a plan with the dietitian for the Christmas break. It had a little more flexibility and a few treats to suit the festive season. They spent most time talking about the behaviours and tactics needed to make it work—with particular emphasis on sensible serving sizes, avoiding the Christmas nibblies, and taking a sane approach to alcohol. A realistic goal would be to avoid weight gain over this time and return in January for a month of fine-tuning physique and fitness before practice matches started.

Robbie returned to the club with his goals met. It had turned out to be easier to cut out alcohol than he had anticipated. He'd made himself the designated driver and won lots of votes. Christmas Day was the only real blot on his copybook, and once it was over, he got straight back to his program. The most unexpected challenge had turned out to be his mum. She loved to fuss over him and kept telling him he was looking too thin. She had filled the pantry with his favourite foods, but Robbie had the confidence to let her know she was the best mother in the world without having to eat mountains of shortbread. In fact, he had escaped back to the city without a single Tupperware container of anything!

Having got on top of his weight issue, Robbie asked the dietitian about using better nutrition to boost his performance. He had a feeling that the new No. 3 would be getting plenty of notice in the season ahead.

CHECKLIST 18.1
Surviving a big night out

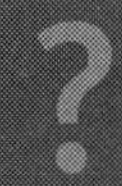

- Plan in advance:
  - Know what you are up for and how you will handle it
- Eat and rehydrate before going out. This will:
  - Look after your nutritional needs for the day's training/competition effort
  - Reduce the rate of absorption of alcohol because you have food in your gut
- If you are injured, consider it a non-drinking night
- Pace yourself:
  - Have one drink at a time so you can keep track of what you've consumed
  - Space alcoholic drinks with non-alcoholic ones
  - Keep yourself busy
- Select low-alcohol drinks:
  - Order low-alcohol beer
  - Have spirits in large glasses of juice or soft drinks
- Be the designated driver to ensure you stick to your no-alcohol or low-alcohol rule
- Avoid rounds or shouts!
- Don't take any drugs or unfamiliar substances and don't leave your drinks unattended
- Look out for your team-mates:
  - Develop a buddy system
  - Recognise when a team-mate has drunk to excess—don't leave him alone, and get him help if need be
- Rehydrate before bedtime!

Rugby League and Union

Rugby Union and Rugby League are contact sports, dominated by short bursts of running, heavy tackling and tactical kicking. Competition starts at the school level, where the rules are modified to prevent injuries during scrums, and advances to professional leagues and international competition. Both codes share a reliance on strength, skill and speed. Rugby League involves a team of 13 on the field (six forming the forward pack and the rest making up the back-line). In contrast, Rugby Union involves 15 players (seven backs and eight forwards). Each game is played over two 40-min halves. Differences in rules and playing style mean the physical requirements of each code differ, as do those of the various on-field positions. Other popular variants include Rugby Sevens, with seven players per side and shortened game time, and Touch Rugby, where 'tackles' are made by simply touching the ball carrier with two hands.

Rugby League (League) is the most popular football code in the Australian Capital Territory, New South Wales and Queensland. The National Rugby League, which evolved from the Sydney competition to become the top club competition in the Southern Hemisphere, involves 15 Australian sides and one New Zealand team. Other competitions under the eye of the Australian Rugby League include the State of Origin (an annual best-of-three games series) and the international program undertaken by Australia's national team, the Kangaroos.

The Super 14 is the largest club competition for Rugby Union (known as rugby) in the southern hemisphere, consisting of four state teams from Australia, five New Zealand franchises and five teams from

South Africa. Major international competitions in which Australia's Wallabies are involved include the World Cup every four years, the Tri Nations Cup, and the Bledisloe Cup against the New Zealand All Blacks.

Training

As in Australian Rules football, the rugby year is broken into three phases: pre-season, competition and off-season. Again, the length of these phases depends on the competition level. The top professional teams in Rugby League follow this typical pattern:

- Off-season: May be as short as a month. There is usually a break from all team training during this time, although some players may do their own conditioning work. At lower levels, a prolonged off-season can be a time of loss of fitness and gain of body fat.
- Pre-season: Can start in late November–early December. Training includes running and weights work, often specifically set for each player or each playing position. Four to six practice matches may be played in January and February.
- Competition season: March to September. Typically, four to five training sessions are scheduled for the six days between games. Some sessions are devoted to strength training, while others will involve running, drills and other skill work.

For elite players, sessions are scheduled at different times throughout the day and supplemented with other club activities. At lower levels of play, sessions may be scheduled in the late afternoon to accommodate work and study schedules.

Competition

The rugby codes are regularly played in both seasonal fixture and tournament format. The National Rugby League season runs from March to August, with the final series being held in September. Each team plays one game each weekend, with games spread from Friday nights to Monday nights. With the supplementary pre-season competition and the State of Origin series that is played in the middle of the season, some players compete in almost 30 matches each year. Travel is involved, since the teams are spread around Australia and in New Zealand. Periodically, an international tour may be organised, sending an Australian representative side to play games against English and French teams. This poses a great challenge to the elite players involved, requiring them to extend their competition peak right through two domestic seasons.

The Super 14 fixture for Rugby Union consists of a 14-week draw from February to May, followed by a short final series between the top teams. With teams from South Africa, New Zealand and Australia, this competition is played across an extraordinary number of time zones. Games are played on weekends, with weekdays accommodating training and the considerable travel schedule. Although the seasonal fixture is shorter than in other codes, there are greater opportunities in Rugby Union for international tournaments and matches. Competitions such as the Bledisloe Cup matches between Australia and New Zealand were once an irregular occurrence, but now happen annually in a two or three-match fixture, often included within the Tri Nations competition with South Africa. The Rugby World Cup tournament, held every four years over six or seven weeks, is considered the fourth largest sporting event in the world. Pre-tournament matches in the years preceding each World Cup are used to qualify teams. A pool system slots teams to play against each other, with the top eight teams moving forward to a knockout draw to decide the overall winner. Games are played every 6–7 days, and because the Cup is allocated to a country or region, players must usually travel between these matches.

Rugby League and Union are games involving short bursts of play. In Union, the ball is typically in play for only about 30 min of the 80-min game, with the remaining time being taken up by injury stoppages, periods when the ball is out of play, the setting up of scrums and line-outs, and kicking for penalty goals and try conversions. In fact, 95 per cent of all the activities that make up a match last less than 30 sec, with a generous recovery interval between bursts of play.

The ball winners are the large and powerful forwards, who engage in brief, high-intensity activities in contact with or in close proximity to the opposition team to gain possession of the ball. Meanwhile, the backs (known as the ball carriers) stand and walk until required to sprint—either to move the ball forward, provide decoy running lines, or run back to cover defence. The typical distance covered during a game is 5.8 km, with 2.2 km at walking pace, 1.6 km jogging, and 2.0 km sprinting. The typical sprint distance is ~20 m, with the backs covering greater distances, both in total and at sprinting speeds. Most high-intensity activities of the forwards involve body contact rather than running.

As a result, a rugby match is not demanding in terms of energy. Fuel stores would not normally be depleted during a game, provided that muscle glycogen levels have been successfully restored since the previous game and maintained over the week of training. However, the game is physically challenging because of injuries, soft-tissue damage and bruising caused by heavy body contact and tackling.

Physical characteristics

Rugby forwards need to be able to run the ball offensively and to tackle. The typical forward is heavy, with large muscle mass and a higher body-fat level than his back-line counterpart. Backs are typically 10–20 kg lighter and, in keeping with the running requirements of their game, have lower body-fat levels.

Common nutritional issues

The rugby codes share many nutrition concerns with Australian Rules football. The Australian Rules chapter outlines common nutritional concerns in high-contact team sports. Special attention should be paid to the discussions concerning alcohol intake, and to general nutritional knowledge and cooking skills.

In general, single players who don't live in a family situation are at high risk of poor nutrition. Lack of knowledge and cooking skills can be compounded by lack of time and post-training fatigue, making irregular meals and fast foods an easy pattern to fall into. As in the case of Tim below, dietary counselling can help players to find their way around the supermarket and kitchen. An astute football club will screen its team to identify players in need of nutritional education and support. Why waste talent simply because of poor eating habits?

Although the fuel requirements of a Rugby League or Union game are lower than those of Australian Rules, a typical Australian diet may not provide the right amounts of carbohydrate for training and match play—or at the right times. As in Australian Rules Football, players need to promote recovery from each key training session or match by consuming carbohydrate and protein immediately afterwards. When muscle damage has occurred—something to be expected in a sport involving such heavy body contact—even greater carbohydrate intake is required to help refill muscle fuel stores.

Fluid and fuel intake

The extended rugby seasons, the inclusion of teams from northern states, and the siting of matches in tropical climates (a recent Bledisloe Cup match was held in Hong Kong) means that training sessions and matches may be held in hot weather. With large muscle mass, and perhaps relatively high body-fat levels, Union and League players might be expected to have poorer heat tolerance than other athletes. Heavy jumpers and/or padding can also trap heat and add to the resulting stress.

Like AFL, rugby codes allow players to have access to fluids on the field during matches and at the half-time break. Many clubs now organise hydration testing sessions during training sessions and practice matches, and monitor weight changes over regular games to keep an eye on hydration issues. Such activities help to pinpoint individual players or game situations in which fluid deficits climb above 2 per cent of body weight. While some players still need to drink more during games, training often poses the greater risk of dehydration and heat stress. In summer, particularly, teams may conduct prolonged and intense training sessions in the hot afternoon sun, with little concern about sweat losses. Even in winter, fluid losses should be taken into account: the old tradition of toughening players by not letting them drink during training is both unscientific and unsafe. Improving fluid intake habits may require a change of attitude on the part of players and coaching staff, as well as practical arrangements to make drinks available during and after training as well as games. Individual drink bottles help prevent the spread of viruses and bacteria among players and make it easier to keep track of how much fluid is being consumed.

The fuel requirements of a rugby match may be met by well-stocked body stores. However, for some players, and in situations where good preparation is not possible, a little extra fuel during the game or training may delay fatigue and boost performance. Sports drinks may be a good choice in this regard, though water will suffice when fluid needs are the only concern.

Bulking up

Muscle mass and strength play a larger role in rugby codes than in AFL and soccer, and bulking up may be a key goal of both training and diet. Some teams assign a playing weight for their players and considerable effort may be needed during pre-season to reach it. See Chapters 3.7–3.8 and Checklist 3.4 for hints on bulking up. The necessary high energy intake from nutritious foods may sound great, but it is often hard to fit frequent meals and snacks into busy days of work and training. The travel schedules required for a domestic and international seasonal fixture often throw a spanner in the works. In addition, the international matches and tournaments scheduled between seasons can bite into the pre-season time that is traditionally used for bulking up.

Nutrition during injury

At some stage in their sports career, most athletes have an injury that restricts or stops their training or competition for some time. Injuries are double-sided in body-contact sports such as Rugby League and Union—they arise not just from what you do to yourself in training or a game but from what other players do to you.

Nutritional considerations during injury and rehabilitation can vary between situations and individuals. First, changes in energy expenditure need to be taken into account, particularly if the lay-off from exercise is prolonged. An injured player may not automatically reduce his food intake to match the sudden cessation of exercise. This can result in a significant increase in body-fat levels, making returning to form more difficult.

Muscle mass will be lost when strength-training athletes take time off their weights work or when surgery requires body parts to be immobilised. In the latter situation, muscles can atrophy badly. A focus on the principles of training and eating to build muscle mass may be needed during rehabilitation (see Chapters 3.7 and 3.8). In any case, it is important to eat nutritiously while recovering from injury. Severe injury or extensive surgery will significantly increase the requirements for energy, protein and other nutrients—and failing to meet these will delay recovery.

Even with the best of intentions, many players find it difficult to look after their nutritional needs during rehabilitation. Limited mobility can interfere with normal shopping and cooking. Injuries to the head and neck can also directly interfere with eating, particularly if chewing and swallowing are restricted. A fractured jaw poses a special challenge—staying well nourished while eating through a straw for six to eight weeks. Liquid meal supplements and nutritious milk drinks play a crucial role in such circumstances, and whenever eating or preparing solid food is difficult. See a sports dietitian for specialised help.

Profile: Tim

Learning to cook in four easy steps

Tim was in his second year with a second-tier Rugby League team. Being recruited from a country zone meant relocating to the city, a move that had been made easier in his first year by boarding with a family. Now, however, Tim was sharing a house with a friend from work, and an ideal domestic situation it was not. Tim had been too well looked after by his mum and then his house mother. His only experience of housework to date had been making his bed.

After six weeks of pre-season training, it was clear that something was amiss. Tim had lost 4 kg, was well under his normal playing weight, and his training performances were sluggish. The club doctor sent him to a sports dietitian to see where the problem lay. It was only after she'd done her assessment that the full picture of Tim's eating pattern—or perhaps more correctly the lack of one—became apparent. The first problem the dietitian identified was a lack of food in the house. Tim and his housemate had not organised regular shopping expeditions. Instead, they made sporadic trips to the supermarket when motivated and midnight trips to the 7-Eleven when desperate. With no schedule of food buying, Tim would often get to the breakfast table to find no milk, no bread, and Weet-Bix dust in the bottom of the packet. He'd have to buy something from the vending machine at his part-time work, or from the biscuit barrel in the tea room. So as to leave work early for training, Tim took only a half-hour break for lunch. This was well spent in the nearby sandwich bar, but there was a limit to how much he could chew in 30 minutes.

The next opportunity to eat was after training, and Tim admitted he was often too tired to eat, let alone cook. Only twice a week or so did he find the food and the energy to cook a real meal. His cooking repertoire was, in his own words, 'nothing flash'—sausages, steak or chops, with mashed potatoes and peas. On other nights he made toasted sandwiches or opened a can of soup. To save money he tried to limit take-aways to weekends and kept the Dial-a-Pizza number beside the telephone. 'Pretty disorganised,' he said when he read through his dietary interview. 'How can I learn to cook?'

The dietitian agreed that Tim's eating habits were hit and miss, and that he was not meeting his nutritional needs in terms of total kilojoules and carbohydrate, and possibly other nutrients as well. She suggested this plan to improve Tim's cooking skills and domestic organisation as well as his diet.

CHECKLIST 19.1
Four steps to quick and healthy cooking (adapted from *Survival from the Fittest*[1])

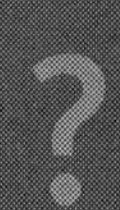

Step 1 Use teamwork

- If you share a house, call a team meeting to organise tasks that are shared. When time or money is scarce, it helps to pool resources.
- Don't worry if conflicting timetables mean you meet up only a few times a week. Use your time together to plan and roster shopping and cooking. Use lists to communicate what is needed.
- Use your rest day to do shopping and cooking tasks that help other housemates. You will be pleased to enjoy the same assistance on your busy days.

Step 2 Acquire new skills

- Gradually master new cooking skills. Use recipes in athlete-friendly cookbooks (Table 19.1) to learn a style of cooking (eg. risotto or a stir-fry), then branch out on your own by changing a few ingredients. Practice makes perfect!
- Look out for tips from other athletes or good cooks. Take information from a variety of sources and adapt it to your own needs.

Step 3 Plan ahead and manage your time well

- Start with a well-organised and clean kitchen. This makes cooking quick and easy.
- Make a list of useful items for the freezer, fridge and pantry and keep these in on hand (Checklist 19.2). Note when stocks are running low and take advantage of supermarket specials to grab multiples of these items.
- Plan your meals for the week ahead and note the required ingredients. Make a shopping list from this and add your general food-stock needs.
- Avoid supermarkets in peak hours. Shop late or early to save time.
- Avoid shopping when you are hungry or tired—the shopping list is likely to go out the window.
- Buy goods only if you can use them before their use-by date. Choose good-quality products that have been appropriately stored.
- Plan your meals to take advantage of leftovers or batch cooking. For example, if you are having rice as an accompaniment one night, cook extra and make it into fried rice the following evening. Pasta sauces can be served the next night as a filling for potatoes.
- Use your rest day to cook ahead for the week. Cook up one or two dishes that can be refrigerated or frozen. It's great when you come home late and tired from training to find that the hard work has been done.
- Even if you are cooking a meal for just one or two people, cook

the whole recipe to ensure there are leftovers. (Cook double quantities if you are feeding a few.) This may save you from cooking again the next night, but you can also freeze leftovers in single portions. These will thaw or reheat quickly so you can have a meal in a few minutes. Invest in a good set of clear plastic containers that you can label and stack in the freezer.

- Prepare as much of the meal as you can before training (e.g. make the pasta sauce or chop the ingredients for a stir-fry) as this will speed up the cooking process when you get home.
- Plan snacks that can be eaten on the run or taken with you on your busy day—for example, single-serve cereals, cartons of yoghurt, cereal bars, fruit and even some leftovers will travel.
- Make up a loaf of sandwiches when you have roast meat or deli meats on hand. Meat or cheese sandwiches freeze well and can have salad added when thawed.

Step 4 Use creative shortcuts

- Invest in a few good cooking tools or household items that save time and produce quality outcomes. A good wok, large non-stick frying pan, microwave, sharp knives, lasagne dish and pizza trays (and cutter) are all good purchases. A rice cooker may also be useful.
- Make use of nutritious time-saver products available in supermarkets. There are many that can make a good meal or form a base for quickly cooking a meal (see Checklist 19.2).
- It sometimes helps to buy meat already trimmed or diced for a stir-fry, or frozen and fresh vegetable stir-fry mixes. They can cost a little extra, but often the time you save in meal preparation is worth this expense.
- Soften vegetables such as potato, pumpkin and carrots that need to be chopped for a recipe by placing them for 1–2 min in the microwave to make them easier to cut.
- Leftover rice and pasta can be frozen. To reheat, microwave or pour boiling water over it and drain.

- Fresh pasta cooks more quickly than dried varieties. Gnocchi cooks in a minute, while fresh lasagne sheets cut the baking time in half. Hokkien noodles and couscous are other alternatives—just add boiling water and they 'cook' in minutes.
- If you are not adventurous with flavourings, make use of prepared pasta and stir-fry sauces and even fresh soups. These can be used as the flavouring base of a dish to which you add your own choice of meat and vegetables.
- Jars of minced herbs provide authentic flavour and save you having to chop or grate items such as garlic or ginger and waste the unused portions. Some fresh herbs, for example parsley or coriander, are worth buying, and you can also freeze them in small portions for later use.
- Be versatile. Know which ingredients are vital for a recipe and which can easily be replaced. Replace recipe ingredients with similar ones that you have in your fridge or pantry or that are in season or 'on special' in the supermarket.
- Choose recipes that are complete meals for single-portion freezing. If the dish is self-contained, with meat, vegetables and a carbohydrate choice, you will need no meal preparation other than reheating—and you may even be able to eat it straight from the container, saving on the dishes!

CHECKLIST 19.2
Lists for a well-stocked pantry and fridge

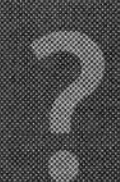

Nutritious time-saving products

- Fresh pasta and noodles, Hokkien noodles
- Tomato-based pasta sauces
- Some stir-fry and casserole sauces (check the label for the fat content)
- Fresh or frozen pizza bases

- Pizza and tomato paste
- Frozen vegetables, vegetable medleys and stir-fry mixes
- Most fresh and some canned soups (check fat content)
- Canned beans, chickpeas and other legumes
- Canned tuna, salmon
- BBQ chicken—skin removed
- Diced or stir-fry-prepared meats
- Lean deli meats
- Canned tomatoes, corn
- Long-life milk
- Evaporated low-fat milk
- Custards and rice puddings in cartons
- Pancake, muffin and bread mixes
- Spray-on oil

Other things for the freezer

- Skinless chicken, lean mince, lean beef, lamb or pork fillets, fish fillets
- Breads, muffins, crumpets
- Filo pastry
- Grated reduced-fat cheese

Other things for the fridge

- Fresh fruit and vegetables
- Juices
- Reduced-fat cheese
- Low-fat yoghurt/custard/Frûche/creamed rice
- Milk
- Eggs
- Margarine
- Sauces (chilli, plum, chutney tomato paste), minced herbs (garlic,

ginger, curry paste) and condiments (mustard, low oil dressings and mayonnaise)

List for the pantry

- Pasta, rice, couscous
- Oats, breakfast cereal
- Tortilla/burrito breads
- Canned spaghetti
- Creamed rice
- Sauces, herbs, spices
- Cereal bars, muesli bars
- Baking goods (sugar, flour, cornflour, custard powder, essences, cocoa)

TABLE 19.1
Athlete-friendly recipe books

- *Survival for the Fittest* (AIS cookbook 1), Murdoch Magazines, 2000
- *Survival from the Fittest* (AIS cookbook 2), Murdoch Magazines, 2001
- *Survival Around the World* (AIS cookbook 3), FPC Custom Media, 2004
- *Survival for Families* (AIS cookbook 4), Allen & Unwin, 2010.

Soccer (football) and field hockey

Football and field hockey are team games played on rectangular fields—the soccer field is slightly larger—and usually on grass or artificial turf. Both have eleven players to a team (ten mobile players and a goal-keeper), both are physical but technically non-contact sports, and both involve intermittent high-intensity exercise underpinned by skill and tactics. Games are played in two halves of 45 min (soccer) and 35 min (hockey), with a short break between halves. Men and women participate in both games at all levels, including the Olympic Games and world championship/Cup. Hockey also features in the Commonwealth Games program.

Soccer is enjoying a surge in popularity in Australia, so much so that its national governing body has officially changed the description of the game it manages to 'football'. This is in line with global usage: soccer is not only the world's largest and most lucrative code of football but apparently the most widely played sport. Although it might be confusing to the traditionalists in Australia, we will refer to the game as football.

In Australia, children's participation rates in football continue to grow even faster than those in AFL and the rugby codes. The Socceroos have become one of the country's most recognised and supported national teams, thanks to their return to the performance levels needed to qualify for the World Cup and, in 2006, even make the quarter-finals. Outside their national team duties, many of Australia's top players are contracted to the elite football clubs overseas such as those of the English Premier League, and are among the highest-earning Australian sportsmen. A professional domestic competition exists for men (A League) and women (W League) and there is also a National Youth League. The Australian football scene now sees year-round play, with the national leagues being conducted over the summer months and state/club competitions continuing as winter sports.

While hockey has lower participation rates and a lower profile, it is also played across all ages (from the modified-rules Rookey at school right through to masters level) and performance levels (recreational to international). The national men's (Kookaburras) and women's (Hockeyroos) teams rank among Australia's best-performing teams. The women have won three Olympic gold medals in recent years (1988, 1996 and 2000), while the men's team was triumphant in Athens in 2004. While one can talk about hockey in Australia without major misunderstandings, in North America the name 'field hockey' is used to differentiate it from the (ice) hockey that is a dominant winter sport there. Hockey is traditionally a winter sport. At lower levels it exists as a seasonal fixture, though the Australian Hockey League plays several shorter formats. In some years the state teams play each other in a four week home-and-away season culminating in a finals week. In other years, they play a two-week tournament that simulates the Olympic competition schedule.

Training

With games played in seasons, training varies between the off-season, the pre-season and competition itself. The time and duration of the three parts of the season vary depending on the level of play. The typical features of each are described in detail in the AFL chapter.

As in the other field-based team games covered in this book, pre-season training in both hockey and football involves general conditioning work, weight training and skill practice. Concentration on skills and match practice will increase as the season approaches. During the season, two to four training sessions are generally scheduled between matches. Mid-week sessions involve lengthy match practice, and the training load gradually eases towards the end of the week to prepare for the next match.

Players at the elite level who play in a number of competition formats, or move between a number of competitions (domestic leagues, national team representation and even a professional contract with an overseas team), may find it difficult to juggle their conditioning work between competition schedules. They may go for prolonged periods without a full 'pre-season preparation'. National team representation usually involves specialised training camps, often before a major tournament, in which daily training sessions are the norm.

Competition

Depending whether football or hockey is played as a seasonal or tournament fixture, the interval between games may vary from a day to a week. National competitions can involve team travel and some double-header fixtures. At the international level, extensive travel may also be involved.

Each match of hockey or football is a fast game with bursts of intensive play interspersed by light activity. While rules restrict tackling and body contact, players in both games can have significant amounts of physical contact, with the potential for contact injuries. Time-and-motion studies of football have determined that the average distance covered in a match by national and international players varies with position and playing style. However, midfielders typically cover 9 to 11 km per match, compared with 8 to 9 km for the outfielders. Only about 10 per cent, or around 2 km, of this distance is covered at a sprint pace, a quarter is covered at walking speeds, and around half at jogging or cruising pace. Goalkeepers typically cover about 4 km.

Even when such studies are available, it must be borne in mind that information about player distances and speeds underestimates some of the true challenges of these sports. After all, the energy costs of running are increased when a player is required to accelerate, decelerate, change direction, run at an angle, or handle the ball. In fact, each player in a football match is involved in over 1000 discrete activities, with a change in activity occurring every 5–6 sec. The typical movement pattern requires the player to be able to run every 30 sec, with a 15-m sprint every 90 sec and a rest period lasting about 3 sec every couple of minutes. Clearly, this is fatiguing, since both the total distance covered and the time spent in high-intensity activities decrease in the second half of matches.

Generally, football and hockey players rely on anaerobic fuel sources, with contributions from aerobic energy during the recovery between bursts. As well as drawing heavily on muscle-fuel stores, games played under hot conditions may leave players dehydrated.

Physical characteristics

Hockey and football players, as well as being skilful, must be agile and fast. Players vary widely in body size, and differences in physical characteristics may not so much limit performance as determine position on the field or style of play. While most players tend to be well muscled regardless of height or weight, a low body-fat level is also an advantage for speed and agility. Over the past decade, there has been a strong trend towards lower body-fat levels in elite players of both sexes. David Beckham may be a fashion icon off the field, but his lean torso on the field attracts just as much attention.

Common nutritional issues

Body-fat levels

There are several reasons and situations in which a player might want to lose fat. At the elite level, most hockey and football players are lean and athletic. Women, who are required to compete in figure-hugging bodysuits, have extra reasons for wanting to live up to this ideal. Even at a lower level of play, being lighter and leaner can pay off in speed and stamina. Some players may not reach their ideal physique easily. Others may return from the off-season looking like twice the player they used to be. Or, as in the case of Jimmy below, an injury may have kept them inactive and gaining weight.

For healthy and permanent fat-loss methods, read Chapter 3. Controlling weight all year round requires an awareness of changes in your energy requirements. At the end of the season, you may need to eat less to match the decrease in training—or you may choose to keep up some activity to give you a head start on next season.

The training diet: week-long recovery

Recovery is difficult when there are only one or two days between matches in a tournament, or where a lot of training must be done between weekly matches. One study of elite football players found that their muscle glycogen levels recovered very slowly in the days after a match owing to a combination of inadequate carbohydrate intake and continued training. Muscle damage arising from the match may also slow the rate of glycogen storage.

Read Chapters 1 and 2 for an overview of all aspects of the training diet, but pay special attention to the idea of periodising carbohydrate and nutrient intakes according to your actual needs. When you are in heavy training, it makes sense to start recovery-nutrition tactics immediately after each session to maximise the outcomes. Read Chapter 5 for guidelines.

Match preparation

With good post-practice recovery measures, muscle fuel stores should gradually increase over the week. Light training at the end of the week, and strategically timed high-carbohydrate meals, will top up muscle and liver glycogen stores. Read Chapter 4.2 for general ideas, and make sure that your fuelling-up menu is as high in carbohydrate as you need it to be. Chapters 1.3 and 2.2 provide practical ideas about carbohydrate foods.

The pre-match meal is eaten to top up carbohydrate (and fluid) stores on the day of the event. Experiment with the type, timing and amount of food to find out exactly what suits your game schedule and individual preferences. Don't let match nerves and travel requirements prevent you from eating what you need, and if a certain meal suits you—regardless of how 'scientific' or not it seems—then stick to what you like. Most players have adopted high-carbohydrate, low-fat meals, but for others the tradition of the high-protein (and high-fat) meal is hard to shake. The most important thing about the pre-event meal is that you should feel comfortable and confident with your choice. See Chapter 4.4 for more details, and see how CJ successfully solved his match-day food problems below.

Fluid for training and matches

Although football and hockey are technically winter sports, there are many scenarios—altered seasons, pre-season training and competitions in hot countries—in which training and match play occur in a hot environment. Recent studies of hydration practices during training in elite football and hockey teams made some interesting findings. First, many players appeared to have trouble drinking enough fluid in hot weather, producing urine samples that were consistent with dehydration. Second, sweat rates and fluid deficits vary fairly widely even across a training session. Although most high-level clubs have the infrastructure to support good hydration practices during a training session (individual drink bottles, trainers taking drinks to players, breaks in the session), not all players seem able to keep the net loss under 2 per cent of body mass. Even where losses during the session are mild, they may be worsened by pre-existing dehydration. Third, although players sweat less during cold-weather sessions than in the heat, they often drink less in these conditions and thus still incur a fluid deficit.

Few studies have been done on hydration during match play in elite hockey and football—understandably, since top teams don't want to be disturbed by research projects. However, the scanty research that is available on match play suggests that the issues mirror those of the training situation.

The rules and customs of these sports make fluid maintenance something of a challenge. Until 1994, the code of the Fédération Internationale de Football Association (FIFA) allowed for drinks only at the half-time break—after 45 min of play. Since substituted players can't return to the field, this severely limited opportunities for fluid intake during standard football games. FIFA rules have since been amended to improve those opportunities—up to a point. 'Players are entitled to take liquid refreshments during a stoppage in the match, but only on the touch line. It is not permitted to throw plastic water bags or any other water containers onto the field.' Smart teams, however, can work around this. Bottles can be left at strategic points around the perimeter of the field so that players can take advantage of a small break in play following a goal, injury or rule infraction to run over and grab a drink. In addition, in matches played in extreme conditions, referees may sometimes permit a short drink break in the middle of a half.

The rules of hockey are a more supportive of hydration practices. The length of the half is shorter, and players are rotated on and off the bench. In hot-weather play, these rotations are managed so players can come off the field for a brief break. The reduction in workload not only reduces body-heat production but also provides an opportunity for cooling strategies (iced towels, fans) and fluid intake.

Studies of the effects of dehydration on performance suggest that keeping fluid deficits low in hockey and football has a variety of benefits. In hot environments, fluid losses of 2 per cent of body mass or more are associated with a detectable reduction in work outputs during simulations of team sport. This takes the form of slower running speeds and shorter distances run during stop-start sprinting protocols. In addition, there is some evidence that dehydration leads to impaired concentration and skill. These ill-effects are less apparent in cold conditions.

Of course, most studies are limited by the difficulty in detecting small yet significant changes in performance. In the real world, matches (and tournaments) are won and lost by tiny margins—sometimes by a penalty shoot-out at the end of nearly two hours of play, preceded by 2–4 weeks of hard-fought games. The outcome may rest on a slight loss of accuracy that lets a ball through or misses a target, or a tiny loss in speed that gets the player to the ball a split second too late. Dehydration can bring on such losses gradually, rather than in a black-or-white process. Best practice should be to keep players' fluid deficits to a level that can be comfortably managed. Chapter 4.6 sets out sensible drinking practices, and Figure 2.3 shows a way to track sweat losses during training and matches.

Fuel needs in matches

Studies of footballers have shown that the game makes heavy demands on the fuel stores of the midfield and running players, particularly when there is a carry-over effect from matches played in close proximity (e.g. a tournament or mid-week fixture). This is less well studied in hockey. However, there are some characteristics of hockey play that may reduce the fuel challenge: the game time is shorter and players can be rotated in and out of play. In any case, low muscle glycogen levels are likely to interfere with both endurance and high-intensity exercise capacity—and indeed, in football studies, players with depleted muscle glycogen stores were found to have slower average speed and cover less ground than their teammates in the second half of the match. Studies on first-class football players suggest that depleted brain fuel stores may also affect performance, perhaps by reducing the speed and accuracy of mental processing—and thus skill level.

In support of these findings, several studies of actual or simulated football have reported an improvement in players' performance when they consume carbohydrate just before the game as well as during half-time. The effect has been attributed to both more energetic movement during the second half of the game (better muscle carbohydrate availability) and better skills/fewer mistakes during this period (prevention of central nervous system fatigue).

If you are a running player, you may find it helps to be proactive with fuel intake during a game. Sports drinks may be of value to hockey or football players, since they attend to fluid and carbohydrate needs simultaneously. Sports gels are another easily consumed and quickly digested fuel source. Fluid and carbohydrate losses may be compounded during tournament situations, requiring more aggressive strategies both during each match and in the between-match recovery period. Chapter 4.7 gives the lowdown on fuel intake during exercise.

Post-match recovery

Recovery should begin straight after the match—a time that tends to be swallowed up in celebrations, commiserations or general relaxation rather than attention to nutritional needs. But with the next match a maximum of six days away and a tough training session scheduled in 48 hours, players' carbohydrate and fluid losses need replenishing immediately. There may also be bruising and other tissue damage to repair. See Chapter 5 for an explanation of recovery processes and how best to time eating after exhausting exercise.

Having the whole team arrange for suitable drinks and snacks to be available after the match means everyone can enjoy the benefits. A spread of sandwiches, fruit, soup and carbohydrate drinks in the club, or a box of supplies in the bus on the way back from 'away' matches, can get recovery off to a good start. Players may be left to make their own decisions about how they spend the rest of the evening, but a team recovery snack will provide a lesson and a statement about the club's priorities, and hopefully kick-start effective recovery.

Alcohol intake

It's a tradition in some team sports for alcohol drinking—often excessive drinking—to follow a match. Chapter 1.6 discusses the sensible use of alcohol in sport, particularly during post-match recovery. There is no need to be a teetotaller, but excessive intake (even once a week with 'everyone' doing it) cannot be condoned as professional behaviour. If you have bruising or soft-tissue injuries from the match, a large dose of alcohol will significantly increase the damage and delay healing and rehabilitation. If a lot of drinking is going on, it's also unlikely that people will be paying attention to practices such as ice, elevation and compression.

Tournaments and travelling

Hockey and football tournaments may involve many games in quick succession, placing great importance on the recovery strategies already discussed. The plan, in a nutshell, is to recover as quickly after a match as possible—repairing tissue damage, refilling muscle glycogen stores, and rehydrating. Chapter 5 sets out how to attend to these needs.

Tournament play may also increase the importance of nutrition during the match—inadequate time for recovery, even when good practices are in place, may mean fluid and fuel deficits are carried from one game into the next.

Of course, when the competition means being away from home or travelling on a tour, the challenge of refuelling becomes greater, as does the importance of being organised. For help on the road, read Checklist 22.1 in the Tennis chapter (the travelling athlete), and the Golf chapter (eating in restaurants).

Profile: Jimmy

Injury, frustration and fat gain

Jimmy couldn't believe it. In three months, his hockey career had turned from bright to uncertain, and his body from trim and taut to—frankly—cuddly. The irony was that he had spent most of his teen years as a beanpole, able to put anything into his mouth and never gain a gram. It was only in recent years, with his heavy training and weight work, that his body had filled out. Then he'd been diagnosed with a stress fracture of the tibia. In the ten weeks he'd been off nursing it, his skinfolds had climbed from 47 mm to 78 mm, and his weight had rocketed by 7 kg. At his latest medical check, the doctor had recommended that he see the clinic's sports dietitian. The extra weight, the doc warned, was not only bad for his game but put an additional load on his weakened leg. This had probably already delayed his recovery. After the usual six-week rest, Jimmy had tried to resume light training, but his leg hurt so much he had to stop.

Jimmy explained his plight to the dietitian, complaining that he had never had to worry about his weight or food intake before. Why was there suddenly a problem? After a full assessment of the situation, the dietitian offered a simple explanation: 'energy in' was greater than 'energy out'. A number of factors were causing this:

- A change in Jimmy's metabolic rate as he got older. As an adolescent, he had burnt up many thousands of kilojoules each day to cope with the needs of growth and training. Now that both had slowed down, he needed to ease up on the 'bottomless pit' eating habits he had learned.
- A drastic change in activity level. Playing club-level hockey and training with the state team had kept Jimmy busy with training or matches every day of the week. The sudden stop meant his energy requirements had nose-dived. Jimmy admitted that he had taken things a little too easy in his rehabilitation. Although the physiotherapist had suggested swimming and cycling as alternative forms of exercise, Jimmy had not enjoyed either and had let the program slide.
- Poor general dietary habits. Jimmy had always thought that if your weight was OK, then you must be eating well. Never having had to worry about his skinfold measurements before, he had turned a deaf ear to advice about good nutrition. The dietitian told Jimmy that his diet was high in fat—and kilojoules.
- Boredom eating and drinking. Being injured left Jimmy a lot of time to sit around the house feeling sorry for himself. Not

used to being home straight after work—he usually went to training—Jimmy had begun having afternoon snacks and a beer after work. He'd also had quite a few commiseration sessions with friends at the pub. The alcohol and 'comfort foods' were sneaking in far more kilojoules than he had realised.

Jimmy committed himself to a full plan of rehabilitation—both for his leg and for his abdominal skinfolds. It was time to take stock of his new energy requirements, and to change his energy balance in favour of body-fat loss—at least until he could resume full training. A proper plan of swimming, upper-body weight work and cycling was organised. Not only did this burn up some kilojoules, but it kept Jimmy out of the house (and the fridge) and gave him a focus, with encouragement and help in goal-setting. A dietary plan was written, limiting food quantities in general, and fat and oil intake in particular. There was even a weekly quota of light beer so Jimmy could continue his social life without interfering with his sporting goals.

Within six weeks, Jimmy had lost the bulk of his excess fat and was back in half-training. Food quantities were adjusted as his energy requirements and body-fat goals changed. The dietitian promised Jimmy that not only was his new eating pattern good for weight control now and in the future, but with his new understanding of how to match fuel intake with fuel needs, he could expect action-packed training and matches. Jimmy can't wait to put this to the test in his first game back in a few weeks' time.

Profile: CJ

The pre-match meal

When CJ moved up into the senior team at his football club, his father gave him some advice: 'You'll need a lot of stamina at this level, son, especially with the game kicking off at 3 p.m. When I used to play I always had a big breakfast for energy—steak, eggs and toast. I'll get your mother onto it.'

The next Sunday, CJ sat down to his father's tried and true pre-match meal. At 1 p.m., when they left for the ground, his stomach was full of food and butterflies. In the first half he felt sick, at half-time he was sick, and in the second half he wandered around the field feeling empty and a bit tired.

The following week CJ went back to the breakfast he had eaten in his junior league days—a couple of pieces of toast and honey and some fruit juice. This was light and compact and had served him well in an 11 a.m. match. However, when eaten at 9 in the morning it didn't seem substantial enough to get him through an afternoon match. By midday he was feeling hungry again, and by match time he was finding it hard to concentrate on his game above the rumbling of his stomach.

Asking the coach for some advice, he learned that a sports dietitian was coming to the club to talk about this very topic. With a revamped and expanded league this season, the coach was worried about having to face some new match-day conditions. The inclusion of some new clubs would mean a four-hour bus trip to some of the away matches. The coach wondered whether he should organise a team breakfast along the road to break up the trip, or whether they should take some food supplies on the bus. Later in the year, the team might play in a country league tournament with matches at various times of the day over a week or so of competition. Should his players eat differently for morning matches and evening ones? Time for some expert advice!

The dietitian explained to the coach and players that the role of the pre-match meal was to tie up the loose ends of the weekly eating efforts—it wasn't a magic wand for super performance. She asked the players whether they were happy with their present pre-match meal routines, or whether they thought there was room for improvement. About a third of the team admitted they had experienced problems at some time. Some, like CJ, had trouble figuring out how much and at what time to eat. Others suffered so badly with pre-game nerves that they were unable to eat anything.

The dietitian listed all the types of foods the players chose for their pre-event meal, and presented it for discussion. Their rituals ranged from two small meals to a late-morning brunch, and from cooked breakfasts to a piece of toast. Clearly, each person had his own approach—and different plans suited different players.

The dietitian outlined the aims of the pre-event meal:

- to top up liver and perhaps muscle glycogen stores;
- to top up fluid levels;
- to leave players feeling comfortable (neither too full nor too hungry), and to avoid foods that disagreed with them; and
- to ensure the players felt confident and ready for action.

For footballers, the most obvious way to fulfil these goals was with a carbohydrate-rich meal, and the dietitian listed some suitable food combinations—from typical breakfast fare such as cereal, toast and fruit to more elaborate meals such as pasta and tomato-based sauces, pancakes and syrup, and rice pudding. She also discussed the carbohydrate-poor or high-fat foods that some athletes had put onto the pre-event menu—including steak, bacon and eggs, and oily lasagnes.

Were these foods bad? the dietitian was asked. She agreed they fitted traditional rather than the scientific ideas of an ideal pre-game meal, but suggested that for some players they didn't seem to cause ill effects. She recounted the tale of an American swimmer who had eaten an amazing spread of hamburgers and cookies before swimming to a gold medal, and concluded that the effects of the last meal were psychological as well as nutritional.

Most players were interested in experimenting with the low-fat, high-carbohydrate menu plans, although a couple of die-hards decided to stick to their 'lucky steaks'. The dietitian said the amount and timing of meals on match morning were also individual preferences, and suggested that each player use his everyday breakfast routine as the basis for a pre-match plan. For example, someone who usually ate a hearty breakfast of cereal and six rounds of toast might need a bigger meal than someone who was satisfied with a muffin and fruit juice.

Whatever time the match was played, the meal should end at least two hours before. For afternoon matches, the choice between a single (larger) meal and an early breakfast followed by a snack would rest on individual comfort as well as the match travel arrangements. For home games it might not be necessary to leave for the ground until the early afternoon, whereas many of the 'away' games required an early departure from home. The dietitian suggested that for long trips to matches, an organised meal-stop en route could be good for team morale as well as nutrition. She suggested that a regular venue be chosen and supplied with a menu, and that a buffet format would make it easier for players to cater for their individual likes and needs.

What about players who needed a small top-up to breakfast, either at the ground or at home? Light snacks could include sandwiches, fruit, or liquid meals such as PowerBar Proteinplus or Sustagen Sport. There were other ready-to-go flavoured milk drinks in Tetra Paks that provided an easy-to-digest alternative to solid meals. The final item on the checklist was fluid intake, which needed special attention on hot and humid days. With all players trained to drink during their stretching and the warm-up to the match, hydration needs seemed to be well looked-after.

The players at CJ's club now eat their own 'secret weapon' breakfasts—either at their own homes or, on occasion, on the road. They like the team eating, since it is a good chance to bond and to go over the team plan. Now they all know that once they take to the field they are ready for anything. The pre-event meal is the icing on the cake of a week's good training and nutrition.

Profile

FIFA promotes the role of nutrition in the 'beautiful game'

Football is the most popular sport in the world today, and every four years, it hosts the largest single sporting competition on the planet, the World Cup. With so much at stake, it is pleasing to see that football's international governing body (FIFA) and its Medical Commission (F-MARC) are actively promoting the role of nutrition in the game.

In preparation for the 2006 World Cup, FIFA and F-MARC hosted a Consensus Conference on Nutrition for Football. This meeting, held at FIFA headquarters in Zurich, Switzerland, in September 2005, aimed to produce a summary of important nutritional issues in football and to create some education resources to help football players achieve these nutrition goals. The meeting was based on the successful formula of similar meetings held by the International Olympic Committee (IOC), the IAAF (the governing body for track and field) and FINA (the governing body for aquatic sports).

Among many interesting papers and discussions, conference-goers learned that the rules of soccer limit players' access to fluid and carbohydrate replacement during the game, yet during a 90-min game of high-intensity football, hydration and refuelling are likely to be important to the performance of midfield players. This is particularly important in the case of the professional player who plays in a match every 3–7 days during the competition season. But the plight of the referee, who is also involved in a prolonged high-intensity activity involving skill and decision-making, can be even more challenging. While top-level football teams have doctors, dietitians and trainers to provide sports drinks, monitor hydration levels and educate players about their needs, the referees usually participate in a match without any organised support. Many recommendations were made of changes to conditions and practices that might enhance the health, well-being and performance of all involved in the game.

At the end of the meeting, a summary of the main nutritional issues for players was presented to FIFA-FMARC. It can now be found on the FIFA website as an overview of the new nutritional guidelines for soccer.

A booklet was later published on *Nutrition for Football*, to translate the messages from the conference into practical and targeted strategies for players and coaches.[1] It can also be downloaded from the FIFA website. (http://www.fifa.com/aboutfifa/developing/medical/newsid=513876.html)

More recently, FIFA has looked at a specific challenge in sports nutrition—the practice of fasting during Ramadan, the ninth month of the Islamic calendar. All Muslims are enjoined in this month to abstain from eating or drinking from sunrise to sunset, and to undertake a special program of prayers. Many top athletes are Muslims and choose to fast during Ramadan. Such a practice would be expected to affect hydration, sleep, training and performance. Since the Islamic calendar advances each year, Ramadan can fall during any month of the Gregorian calendar and may coincide with a period of heavy training or competition. For example, the 2012 Olympic Games in London will take place during Ramadan. FIFA recently funded a large study to observe the effects of fasting on football players. A series of papers describing the results was published in a supplement to the *Journal of Sports Science* in 2008.

These activities of FIFA and F-MARC help to provide football players—and other athletes—with up-to-date and practical ideas for improving sports nutrition practices. It is good to see a sporting organisation recognise the importance of nutrition to the health and performance of its athletes and take steps to strengthen that nutritional foundation.

CHECKLIST 20.1 Nutrition for Football: the FIFA/F-MARC Consensus Statement

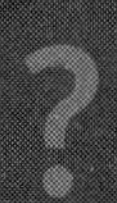

Football players can stay healthy, avoid injury and achieve their performance goals by adopting good dietary habits. Players should choose foods that support consistent, intensive training and optimise match performance. What a player eats and drinks in the days and hours before a game, as well as during the game itself, can influence the result by reducing the effects of fatigue and allowing players to make the most of their physical and tactical skills. Food and fluid taken soon after a game and training can optimise recovery. All players should have a nutrition plan that takes account of individual needs.

The energetic and metabolic demands of football training and match play vary across the season, with the level of competition and with individual characteristics. Typical energy costs of training or match play in elite players are about 6 MJ (1500 kcal) per day for men and about 4 MJ (1000 kcal) for women. The football player should eat a wide variety of foods that provide sufficient carbohydrate to fuel the training and competition program, meet all nutrient requirements, and allow manipulation of energy or nutrient balance to achieve changes in lean body mass, body fat or growth. Low energy availability causes disturbances to hormonal, metabolic and immune function and to bone health. An adequate carbohydrate intake is the primary strategy to maintain optimum function. Players may need 5–7 grams of carbohydrate per kg body mass during periods of moderate training and up to about 10 g/kg during intense training or match play.

Nutritional interventions that modify the acute responses to endurance, sprint and resistance training have the potential to influence chronic training adaptations. The everyday diet should promote strategic intake of carbohydrate and protein before and after key training sessions to optimise adaptation and enhance recovery. Solid or liquid carbohydrate consumption should begin during the first hour after training or match play to speed recovery of glycogen. Taking food or drinks that contain protein at this time may promote recovery processes.

Match-day nutrition needs are influenced by the time since the last training session or game. Players should try to ensure good hydration status prior to kick-off and use opportunities to consume carbohydrate and fluids before and during the game according to their nutrition plan. Fatigue impairs both physical and mental performance, but intake of carbohydrate and other nutrients can reduce the negative effects of fatigue.

Training for and playing football lead to sweat loss even in cool environments. Failure to replace water and electrolyte losses can lead to fatigue and impaired performance of skilled tasks. Breaks in play currently provide limited opportunities for carbohydrate and fluid intake, and may not be adequate in some conditions. Football is a team sport, but the variability in players' sweating responses dictates that monitoring to determine individual requirements should be an essential part of a player's hydration and nutrition strategy.

There is no evidence to support the current widespread use of dietary supplements in football, and so the indiscriminate use of dietary supplements is strongly discouraged. Therefore, supplements should be used only on the advice of a qualified sports nutrition professional.

Female players should ensure that they eat foods rich in calcium and iron within their energy budget. Young players have specific energy and nutrient requirements to promote growth and development, as well as fuelling the energy needs of their sport. Many female and youth players need to increase carbohydrate intake and develop dietary habits that will sustain the demands of training and competition.

Players may be at increased risk of illness during periods of heavy training and stress. For several hours after heavy exertion, components of both the innate and adaptive immune system exhibit suppressed function. Carbohydrate supplementation during heavy exercise has emerged as a partial countermeasure.

Heat, cold, high altitude and travel across time zones act as stressors that alter normal physiological function, homeostasis, metabolism, and whole-body nutrient balance. Rather than accepting performance decrements as inevitable, well-informed coaches and athletes should plan strategies for training and competition that offset environmental challenges.

Alcohol is not an essential part of the human diet. Recovery and all aspects of performance may be impaired for some time after alcohol use. Binge drinking should be avoided at all times.

The needs of the referee are often overlooked, but high standards of fitness and decision-making are expected of all referees. At every level of competition, training regimens and nutritional strategies, including fluid intake during the game, should be similar to those followed by players.

Talent and dedication to training are no longer enough to achieve success in football. Good nutrition has much to offer players and match officials, including improved performance, better health, and enjoyment of a wide range of foods.

Zurich, September 2, 2005

Basketball and netball

Basketball and netball are team ball games, played both on indoor and outdoor courts. While basketball is played at a high level by both males and females, netball is predominantly a female participation sport, played throughout the Commonwealth. Australia and New Zealand enjoy a fierce rivalry matching that of the Wallabies and the All Blacks in Rugby Union. Strong international competition exists in both sports—basketball is an Olympic sport, and both sports hold world championships.

Basketball is played by teams of up to ten players, with five appearing on the court at one time. Each player has a specific role on the court, but all are mobile, covering the whole court and being involved in both offensive and defensive plays. Players are continually substituted from the bench throughout the game. A basketball game can be played in 12-min quarters, or in 20-min halves, with a break of 10–15 min at half-time. Since the timing clock stops when the ball is out of play, the duration of each game is considerably longer.

A netball team is composed of seven players, each in a specific position with a defined role and a defined court space. Reserve players are allowed, but once a substitution is made a benched player cannot return to the court unless she is replacing an injured teammate. A netball game can be played as a game of 15-min quarters or 20-min halves, again with a short break at the halfway point.

At the elite level, netball and basketball are fast-paced games of skill and physicality, in spite of rules against direct contact between opponents. The stop-start nature of play places considerable demands on anaerobic energy systems, with aerobic fitness assisting recovery between short bursts of high-activity exercise.

Training

Basketball and netball are generally played in competition seasons, and national leagues exist in both sports. The competition season for the National Basketball League (NBL) runs from September to February, with the play-offs for the finals in March. The Women's National Basketball League (WNBL) has its season from October to February, with plays-offs in March. The Australian Netball League has undergone many changes over recent years, but its competitive season currently extends from July to September. International games and tours are scheduled year-round for high-level teams. Typically, each league provides a break of 2–3 months between one season and pre-season training for the next. Most players at the elite level will remain active for the whole year, keeping fit with personal training when the team is not conducting official practice. At lower levels, players may have longer breaks between seasons, with consequent risks of weight gain and loss of fitness.

Elite players train every day, in some cases—for example, on training camps for national teams—twice a day. In the pre-season, the emphasis is on building a fitness base, and training involves more running and strength work than at other times of the year. Younger male athletes are often required to 'bulk up' and may do up to 3–4 weight-training sessions each week during the pre-season to match the muscle mass and strength of their more seasoned opponents. Skills work and practice matches, where set plays are drilled, are undertaken year-round and are the dominant mode of training. The number of training sessions each week will vary with the number of games played. The team will normally meet for 3–4 sessions a week, and players may train individually or in small groups at other sessions, concentrating on weaknesses and specific tasks relevant to their roles on court.

At the non-elite level, training loads vary. Many basketball and netball players do their own programs to keep fit and to practise skills, and then play in a weekly competition supplemented with perhaps one or two team training sessions a week.

Competition

Like football codes, court sports can be played in both a seasonal fixture and a tournament format. As such, competition outcomes are decided by a series of games with recovery intervals from 1–7 days. The seasonal fixture usually involves a series of games to decide the top teams, who then go on to play in a final series.

NBL games are scheduled mid-week and weekends. Players typically play one to two games each week, while an interstate road trip may involve two or three games in quick succession (Wednesday night, Friday night and Sunday afternoon). This presents a great challenge, in terms both of recovery between games and of the interruption to sleep, diet and training caused by travelling.

WNBL and National Netball League games are routinely scheduled on Friday nights or other weekend slots. Typically, games are played a week apart, although the schedule may also require teams to play two games over a single weekend. At sub-elite and recreational level, most players take part in a weekly competition. However, others may play for a number of teams, or in a number of competitions, building up to a weekly commitment of two or three matches. This may pose a similar challenge of recovery to that faced by elite athletes, but against the background of a lifestyle that is less sympathetic to the needs of the sport.

Tournaments for major competitions and championship events such as the Olympic Games and world championships are conducted over 10–12 days, with recovery time between games of one or two days. Many young players and recreational players compete in shorter tournaments over a weekend or throughout a week which sometimes schedule more than one game in a day.

Physical characteristics

Height is the most noticeable physical characteristic in court-based team games, particularly basketball, with a gradual increase in height from the small but skilled guards who make the plays, to the forwards and centres who dominate the air space around the goal. In netball, there is greater allowance for shorter players in some positions, particularly where the ball is played close to the ground (e.g. centre position). However, netball players are generally of above average height.

Lower body-fat levels confer greater agility and speed and assist in jumping and reaching. The body-fat levels of elite players may be relatively low, reflecting both the training load and the considered advantages of being lean. However, they are not usually as low as those of endurance athletes. At lower levels many players, while skilled, may be less trim and fit.

Common nutritional issues

Daily energy and fuel needs—being organised over a busy day

Energy requirements in basketball and netball can be high, but this often reflects the size and growth needs of players rather than the energy cost of their exercise program. Training and matches, while they take up much of the day, are generally not as energy-intensive as they might appear, owing to the emphasis on skills practice and stop-start play. Therefore, the energy needs of some players, particularly females, may not be particularly high. On the other hand, it can be hard keeping up with the huge energy requirements of a teenage basketball player as he grows into a 200-cm giant. The principles of training nutrition are explained in Chapters 1 and 2, with emphasis on the individuality of energy and nutrient needs. Chapter 3 discusses situations of low and high energy needs, and suggests ways to tailor meal plans to suit each type of energy budget.

A single game of netball or basketball does not pose much threat to the fuel stores of a trained athlete. However, players often struggle to recover fuel stores from one day to the next, and gradually accumulate fatigue from the carry-over effects of a daily schedule of practice and matches. Players can find it hard to set an organised meal plan because of their hectic and unpredictable lifestyle, and this may result in a mismatch between daily fuel demands and daily food and fluid intake. Training sessions and matches are generally held at night—and often late into the night. For those with full-time jobs, or even those who are full-time athletes, this can mean a crowded day.

How do you spread your eating through the day to meet the nutritional and logistical demands of your sport—such as not eating too close to a game—but also fit in with the eating schedule followed by your family and just about everyone else? Juggled meals can often mean disorganised nutrition. An evening game may finish late at night, leaving the player unmotivated to cook, unable to find anywhere to eat out, or wary of eating a big meal just before bed. Since the player may have been reluctant or unable to eat a well-planned meal before the game, the whole day may become a series of grabbed snacks—often poor in nutritional quality. If this is the pattern for the week, overall nutritional status can be jeopardised, as can body-fat and weight goals. Busy players may find that their schedule of games, training and meetings leaves only one night of the week for a home-cooked meal.

It is a major task for many players to organise a meal routine that meets all their nutritional targets. It helps to plan the week ahead, noting commitments and 'down times', the 'black-out' times where it is impractical to eat, and the best nooks and crannies into which to tuck extra small meals and snacks. You may need to use nights at home to catch up on cooking for the week, preparing meals that can be frozen and quickly zapped onto the table on game nights. You may need to experiment with the pre-game meal plan, splitting your food into a pre-event snack and a post-event top-up. You might even like to switch the focus on those days, making lunch the main meal and having lighter meals for the rest of the day.

Losing body fat

The off-season can be a time of weight gain as players' reduced energy intake conspires with a catch-up in social eating. An energy mismatch can also occur when a player is injured or simply disorganised—unable to keep track of his total food intake. Some female players struggle endlessly to reach and maintain an ideal playing weight.

Although low to moderate body-fat levels are valuable for some players in mobile sports or positions, basketball and netball generally tolerate a range of body-fat levels among players. In recent years, however, the 'look' among female players has grown leaner, though more for aesthetic than performance reasons. The catalyst for this appears to be have been the introduction of revealing bodysuits as competition uniforms. These uniforms might make the game seem more contemporary and increase the appeal of the game to spectators and television viewers. However, some players feel uncomfortable with their 'lumps and bumps' on show. Hopefully, players will be able to find a weight and body-fat level that lets them eat well, play well, and feel comfortable with their body image. It is often valuable to see a sports dietitian for specific advice. Chapter 3 outlines safe and sensible ideas for fat loss. See, too, Paula's story below.

Iron

Low iron levels may be a problem for female players and some males, too. Contacts and impacts—such as hitting other players or landing hard on the floor—may increase iron losses through increased destruction of red blood cells. In any case, female athletes and athletes on weight-loss diets are at risk of iron deficiency. See Chapter 2.5 for a discussion of iron requirements and ways to ensure a high iron intake.

Match preparation: the pre-event meal

In theory, the pre-event meal or snack should be a light, carbohydrate-rich meal, eaten at least two hours before the match. There are many menus to fit this description and each player should experiment to find something that suits her needs. Since it is likely that you will play matches at various times of the day or night, you may need to be versatile with meal ideas to suit a range of occasions. See Chapter 4.4 for general ideas on the pre-event meal.

Fluid intake at matches and in training

If you are working hard and the stadium is warm to hot, you may sweat out a significant amount of fluid. Fluid losses for the rest of a day will depend on the weather, your other daily activities, and how hot you get. Read the general guidelines for daily fluid intake (Chapter 1.4, Checklist 1.5), and for drinking practices during games and practice (Checklist 4.4). Our work has helped us to prepare specific fact sheets on 'Fluid and Fuel for Basketball and Netball' (*www.ausport.gov.au/ais/nutrition*). These are summarised in the Fluid-science profile below.

Tournament nutrition

Tournament schedules are often challenging, requiring you to play a number of matches over a short period. Travelling may also be part of the deal. The effects of failing to prepare well before each game and recover fully after it, may not be apparent in the early part of the schedule. However, the carry-over effect may gradually edge you into the fatigue zone just as the performance challenge is peaking. Often, victory does not go to the best team but to the best recovering team.

All this requires planning and preparation. As soon as you know your likely schedule of matches, begin to plan a meal routine. You will need to take into account suitable pre-event meals (Chapter 4.4) and post-event recovery strategies (Chapter 5). If you are on the move, or playing in other countries, then the notes on the travelling athlete will be of help (see Tennis chapter). It may pay to be more aggressive with nutrition during the game—both to prevent fluid and fuel deficits from building up and to counteract the effects of deficits that are carried into a game.

On the road again

Being on the road is tough work. Not only does it disrupt your normal eating, sleeping and training schedule, but you may be required to play two or three games over three days. This will challenge your abilities of recovery and organisation. See the Tennis chapter for a three-pronged plan of attack, which includes knowing your nutrition goals, planning ahead, and being assertive to make things happen the way that you want them to.

Some teams arrange a dining schedule for the road trip, with most meals eaten as a team and menus organised by a team manager or the captain. In other clubs, players are responsible for most of their own eating and are given a *per diem* (daily allowance) for their food. For financial and practical reasons (where else can you eat late at night?), take-aways and fast foods can make up a big part of the weekend's eating. These foods have a bad reputation, nutritionally speaking, that is not always deserved. Read the account below to learn about fitting them into your lifestyle and your nutritional goals.

Profile: Paula

Lose body fat, once and for all!

In her first year of university, after moving into a college dorm, Paula gained 6 kg. For the first time in her life, she had full control over what she ate and drank. Meals were served up three times a day in the college dining room, with the buffet presentation allowing her to eat her fill. And there always seemed to be parties to attend—opportunities, as Paula saw it, to make new friends. As her university life flourished, Paula found herself losing sight of her aspiration of playing in the state netball league and maybe even joining the national team in the coveted role of centre.

It wasn't that she lacked talent—her high school netball coach had rated her as a potential state-level player. But the mobility required of a centre is sabotaged by extra body fat. And at nineteen years of age, Paula had stopped growing up and started to grow out.

Paula trained with her team three times a week and squeezed in a 30-min run on the other weekdays. Her weekends were busy, what with a Saturday job, study and socialising with friends and college mates. Her weight gain didn't seem fair, especially when she compared herself to her sedentary peers. One college friend in particular drove her mad with envy, since she ate whatever she wanted, was always the last home from a big night out, and didn't carry a gram of excess body fat.

When Paula decided it was time to take control of her dwindling netball prospects, she started dieting to lose weight. A couple of her friends were carb-phobic and suggested she try a high-protein diet. Cereal was dropped from the menu at breakfast, tuna salad was her staple for lunch, and carbs were forbidden at dinner—no more rice, pasta or potato on her plate. Paula found her new low-carb diet amazingly effective at reducing her weight, but she gained it back quickly if she took even a minor break. She could lose 2 kg in a week, but a weekend visit to her parents (and Mum's famous risotto and chocolate cake) saw her back to normal by Monday morning. Importantly, even with less weight to carry, she found it impossible to train consistently. Her longtime coach had watched her struggle to control her weight, but jumped when she noticed her lacklustre performance at practice. She insisted Paula adopt a healthier and more long-term approach to weight control and suggested she phone a sports dietitian who was herself a former elite netball player.

The dietitian found Paula's plight all too familiar, and reassured her that she wasn't the only player who needed to find a balance between her sporting aspirations and her social life. Although Paula's energy needs might be lower than others', there was no point comparing herself to other girls, the dietitian said. That would not solve the problem. Instead, she had to look at her own situation carefully and find ways to increase energy expenditure and decrease her energy intake from food.

Although Paula acknowledged that it would be ideal if she could do some formal training on weekends, the demands of university and part-time work made that difficult. This meant that most of the solution to her recent weight gain would have to come from changes in her diet. Paula described her usual meal patterns to the dietitian and detailed her recent attempts to lose weight.

First, the dietitian suggested some ways for Paula to manage her alcohol intake on social occasions. Paula was surprised to learn how much a night on the town contributed to her daily energy intake. It couldn't be true (could it?) that a 375-ml bottle of pre-mixed spirit and soft drink had the same kilojoule content as a standard chocolate bar. Paula only ever ate one chocolate bar at a time, but on a night out with friends she had no trouble drinking five or six Vodka Cruisers or other alcopop concoctions. Now she resolved to be more careful with her alcohol intake, spacing these alcoholic drinks with a diet cola or a soda drink to cut the kilojoule total in half. On some nights it made sense to appoint herself the designated driver and select low-energy, non-alcoholic drinks all night. Her wallet, her energy budget and her friends would all appreciate the effort.

Second, Paula learned about the importance of portion control. This notion had gone out the window with her college diet—first because of the buffet-style meal service, and later because of her belief that as long as it wasn't a carbohydrate food she could eat as much as she liked. Together Paula and the dietitian worked out a meal plan, complete with appropriate serving sizes of various foods. This was cemented with useful tools such as how to gauge amounts according to volume (e.g. cups, tablespoons) or visualisation (e.g. size of a deck of cards, or a tennis ball or the palm of her hand).

The sports dietitian reminded Paula that since carbohydrate foods provided the most important fuel for exercise, and she should not neglect them. She encouraged the idea of tracking Paula's daily intake of carbohydrate against her daily activity and training demands. Paula understood the message that carbohydrate intake on heavy training days was crucial to support performance and assist recovery. It wasn't about eating a 'high carbohydrate' diet (a bit scary in the context of Paula's recent ideas) but about matching fuel intake to fuel needs. Paula was shown how to scale up carbohydrate by adding some foods and drinks around training sessions—for example, a carton of flavoured yoghurt before an early-morning weights session or a small container of dried fruit and nut mix before afternoon training. This helped to support the specific needs of a session as well as adding extra fuel on the days when it was most needed.

The plan worked well. Paula noticed almost immediately that she had extra spark at training, with extra stamina for extended hard workouts. Within eight weeks she had lost most of the excess weight, and the dietitian recorded a 20-mm drop in her skinfold measurements. Paula was still able to have a social life—in fact, many of her friends became interested in her netball success and resolved to come and watch her play.

Profile

Fast food doesn't need to be junk food!

When you live life in the fast lane, it's inevitable that fast food will be part of it. Take-away foods can provide a quick mid-afternoon snack before training, a late-night meal after an evening game, or a staple of the travelling diet when cooking facilities are not available and restaurants are beyond your budget. Maybe, after a hard week of work and training, you just want a day when you don't have to bother with domestic duties. And after a period of careful eating, take-aways may be high on your personal reward list. Many athletes in weight-making sports go on a 'take-away bender' following a major tournament or competition.

Despite their convenience, fast foods and take-aways do not generally have a good reputation. 'Junk food' is a frequent description for them, although that doesn't stop people from eating (or liking) them. Most people feel a little guilty about making take-aways a big part of their diet, and some feel guilty about eating them at all. Is their reputation really warranted?

Many fast foods work against the principles of healthy nutrition and the optimal training diet. Nutritional assessments of popular take-away foods—for example, the menus at the big hamburger chains and fried chicken outlets—find that the most popular items are high in saturated fat, salt, sugar and kilojoules, and low in fibre and some vitamins, particularly vitamins A and C. In addition, many take-aways may lack sufficient carbohydrate to meet the fuel needs of athletes in heavy training. These facts make many nutrition experts fairly hostile to take-away food, with pet hates including:

- 'Do you want fries with that?'
- Meal deals, which give apparent 'discounts' if you add something deep-fried or sugary, plus a soft drink, to the fries and original item
- Encouragement to upsize your serve, also at a bargain price
- Special 'limited offer' items that are heavily promoted on TV. These items usually feature the challenge of eating 'double meat', 'double cheese' or other combinations that deliver more than a day's budget of energy and saturated fat in a single item

Recent attempts have been made by some fast-food outlets to redesign their menus along healthier lines. On the whole, these modifications have created better choices for athletes—with less fat and more carbohydrate. From the financial point of view, a take-away meal is more expensive than a home-prepared one, though you may not notice this on a once-off occasion. However, take-aways are less expensive than restaurants generally, and may suit the timetable or *per diem* budget of the athlete on the move.

The bottom line is that indiscriminate use of take-aways may keep you from achieving your nutritional goals. However, with some forethought and good nutritional knowledge, take-aways can play a useful role in your diet (see Checklist 21.1).

Profile

The science of fluid and fuel for court sports

At the Australian Institute of Sport, we've had the chance to study the hydration demands and drinking patterns of elite basketball and netball players, ranging from our junior elite players all the way up to national teams. We've monitored hydration status at the start of each day by looking at the characteristics of players' urine. We've also looked at practices and games to see typical sweat losses and rate players' success in staying hydrated over the session (see Figure 2.3).

We found that elite male basketball players at an intensive training camp lost an average of 900 ml of sweat per hour during practice on a cold day (temperatures inside the stadium were about 12°C). Even though all the players were doing the same workout, their sweat rates varied between 600–1200 ml per hour. Courtside drink bottles and opportunities for a fluid break between scrimmages allowed players to drink at a rate that typically replaced half of their losses. By the end of the two-hour session, the average fluid deficit was just over 1 per cent of body weight—which is within the guidelines for good hydration practices. However, the deficit exceeded 2 per cent in several players, and we judged that 15 of 17 players started the session dehydrated from the previous day's activities. This suggests that poor drinking practices by some players may allow a level of dehydration to develop that detracts from their performance at practice. Clearly, it is difficult to stay well-hydrated with two practices a day—even during winter.

Other work with AIS basketball players has shown us that, as might be predicted, sweat losses during games and practices are higher in summer than in winter, even though the conditions on court did not vary nearly as much as the weather outside. However, we also saw that players drank less in cooler conditions, so their overall fluid deficit was similar or even greater in winter sessions. Sweat rates were higher in games than in practices, and male players' sweat rates were higher than those of female players. Again, even though average figures might not give much cause for concerns, some players clearly not staying well hydrated. Similar results were found when we studied AIS netball players.

How important is it to refuel and rehydrate during basketball and netball activities? Several studies involving 'stop-start' exercise protocols or sports (e.g. in tennis, soccer and cricket) show that dehydration and inadequate fuel cause fatigue over the course of the exercise session. When players consume fluid and carbohydrate during the session, this fatigue is reduced. Benefits include more even power outputs (greater distances covered at higher speeds in the later parts of a game) and better maintenance of skill and concentration. Several studies have focused specifically on basketball players.

- Adolescent males played two simulated '2 on 2' full-court games over 40 min in which a series of skills and physical tests were repeated. In one game, the players drank water to replace their sweat losses. In the other game, no fluid was consumed, and a fluid deficit of ~2 per cent of body weight was accumulated by the end of play. Dehydration did not affect the height of players' jumps, but it did impair performance of a 30-sec jump test (19 per cent decline in score) and the accuracy of field goals (8 per cent decline). These differences could affect the outcome of a real game.[1]
- Skilled male players did drills simulating a basketball game over 4 × 12-min quarters in three sessions. In one, players started the game with a fluid deficit of 2 per cent of body weight, while in other games they drank water or a sports drink to remain in fluid balance. Shooting scores were 45 per cent in the dehydration trial, 53 per cent in the water trial and 60 per cent with sports drink. Dehydration also reduced on-court sprinting performance, but drinking sports drink with added carbohydrate improved performance. Changes in the performance of other skills and drills also showed the damaging effects of a fluid deficit and the additional benefits of consuming a sports drink compared with water.[2]
- College-aged male basketball players exercised in the heat on five separate occasions. They received varying amounts to drink so they achieved either fluid balance or a fluid deficit of 1 per cent, 2 per cent, 3 per cent or 4 per cent of body weight. Following a short recovery, they played a simulated game of basketball drills. The results showed that as fluid deficit increased, there was a progressive decline in the players' performance of on-court sprints and shooting in comparison to the session when they were fully hydrated.[3]

Of course, the duration and intensity of a single game of netball or basketball may not be enough to cause nutritional fatigue in all players. This may need to be judged for each individual. Tournament play is likely to involve the greatest risk of nutritional fatigue, since players may have difficulty fully rehydrating and refuelling between games. However, during intensive training periods, some players may not fully rehydrate or refuel between practice sessions, and this may lead to fatigue. It makes sense for players to be monitored periodically to assess their fluid needs and how well they meet them, and also for players to consider refuelling during a game by choosing a sports drink instead of water. Some players may not like the taste or may need to watch their energy intake, but those who are on court a lot in situations like tournaments or a busy game schedule will likely notice the benefit.

CHECKLIST 21.1
Putting fast foods in your nutrition playbook

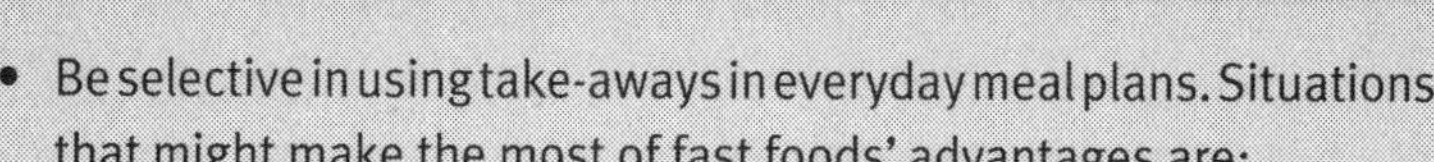

- Be selective in using take-aways in everyday meal plans. Situations that might make the most of fast foods' advantages are:
  - On the road when you're on a limited budget, have limited time or opportunity to eat at restaurants or cook for yourself, and may need to eat at unusual times
  - In a country where there may be some concerns about food and fluid hygiene or about the 'exotic' menu. Multinational fast-food chains can offer relatively clean, predictable meal choices.
  - In a social situation with friends when you really want to enjoy yourself.
- Think beyond the best-known chains. There are some 'healthy' take-away chains, and you can buy a sandwich, the quintessential healthy fast food, almost anywhere.
- Look for the better options on the menu. Many chains now offer 'light and healthy' selections, and provide information about the nutritional content of menu items.
- Avoid meal deals or options that look like a bargain. The 'cheap' extras are almost always high in fat and/or sugar, with little nutritional value.

- Don't even think about the Monster, Whopper Extravaganza special offer with double or triple layers. You'll just be compounding everything that take-aways are criticised for.
- When fuel intake is important, look for:
  - Roll- or bread-based choices—such as a burger, sandwich or souvlaki
  - Pizza—not pan fried
  - Baked potato—with salsa and a small serve of sour cream
  - Steamed rice as a base for an Asian dish
  - Pasta on the go—but only if the sauce is well chosen (i.e. tomato based)
  - Fruit juice
  - Low-fat yoghurt, flavoured milk and fruit smoothies
  - Fruit salad
- To reduce fat content:
  - Avoid battered choices
  - Avoid pastry
  - Choose grilled or steamed rather than fried or deep-fried
  - Take care with sauces and dressings. If a low-fat option isn't available, have accompaniments served on the side so you can limit the amount you eat
  - Avoid thin fries—if you must have chips, choose thick wedges
  - Limit cheese
- To reduce energy or increase nutritional value:
  - Choose salad fillings, a salad side serve, or a 'big salad'—based meal
  - Choose wholemeal options
  - Avoid soft drinks—if you need fuel, a juice or flavoured milk is better, while if your energy budget is small, go for water or low-calorie drinks so your energy choices can be chewed slowly rather than gulped

Tennis

Tennis is played by both men and women, in singles and in doubles competition (same-sex and mixed-sex pairs), and at levels varying from a social hit to the lucrative international circuit. It is played on various court surfaces, and both indoors and out. Tennis is a game of skill, speed, agility and concentration—and, often, endurance. Men's matches at international tournaments are often marathon efforts of four or five hours, with long rallies for each point and many sets going to tie-breakers. While the exercise itself is made up of brief bursts, such a game is likely to challenge the players' carbohydrate fuel stores and require great discipline to maintain concentration.

Training

For professional players, tennis is a full-time job. Between tournaments, 20–40 hours a week may be spent in training, most of it on court. Most players will supplement this with about an hour a day of off-court conditioning work, such as running, weight training and agility work. This training may vary according to the player's stage of preparation and the specific weaknesses in his game. Further down the competition ladder, tennis players may not have the luxury of spending hours training. Nevertheless, most of the time available is spent on court practice.

Competition

Most competitive tennis in Australia is played in the form of graded pennant competitions, with teams (four members) meeting each other in a weekly draw. A final series among the top finishing teams determines the pennant winner. The other form of competition is tournament tennis. This begins at the sub-elite level with weekend tournaments, and continues from satellite tournaments to the elite circuit of Grand Prix and Grand Slam events.

Typically, tournaments are played using a knockout system. Players are pooled, then seeded to play each other, with the winner of each match progressing to the next round until the last two players contest the trophy. The competition draw in the Grand Slam events (Wimbledon, Australian Open, French Open, and US Open) involves 128 players, with the top players battling through seven matches spread over a fortnight of competition. At this level, players typically undertake matches every second day to progress to the final. Other competitions are conducted with a smaller draw of players and in a shorter time frame (7–10 days) and generally require daily match play. Of course, many players may enter more than one competition within a tournament (singles, doubles, and, in the case of Grand Slams, mixed doubles), meaning that they often play more than once each day.

At the elite level, tennis is a fast and mobile game, characterised by bursts of intense exercise against a background of quiet movement. The length of rallies varies according to the surface and the players' style: longer ones are associated with slower surfaces and baseline playing. Typically, however, the average tennis point lasts 2–10 sec, with the longest points, even at world-class level, rarely lasting more than half a minute. There is a long ratio of recovery time to active time, with standard rest periods between games, when players change ends, as well as time between points when the ball is being retrieved and one player prepares to serve. Thus players rely mostly on anaerobic energy systems, although a developed aerobic capacity is an advantage in terms of recovery between points, stamina, and tolerance to heat.

A tennis match is decided on the best of three or five sets for men, and the best of three sets for women. The length of a match varies greatly, from 30 min to three hours for a three-set match, and from 80 min to more than five hours for a five-set competition. (The 2004 French Open final, between Arnaud Clément and Fabrice Santoro, went for 6 hr 33 min.) The fuel and fluid demands of a match vary accordingly. However, in tournament tennis, the nutritional focus is not so much on the effects of a single match as on the carry-over effects of playing so many matches in succession.

Tournament tennis sets an extremely tough schedule for players, with the time between matches varying from hours to more than a day. While muscle glycogen levels and hydration status may survive one match, the relentless schedule can make it a challenge for athletes to fully recover between matches. Compounding the difficulty of recovery is the uncertain match schedule for much of the tournament. Matches often start at the whim of the preceding match and the vagaries of the weather, and may end, at least in some tournaments, in the early hours of the morning.

For the world's top tennis players, life is a continual program of tournaments and exhibition matches, and most take only a short break after each venture onto the circuit to recover and prepare for the next. On average, an elite player participates in 20 tournaments a year.

Physical characteristics

Physical characteristics that are helpful in tennis include long arms and a relatively low centre of gravity (short legs in proportion to the trunk). These features should give a player extra reach for playing strokes and height for serving, and greater mobility on the court.

Other physical characteristics do not so much limit performance as help determine the style of game a player is best suited to. For example, tall, muscular players might best use their height and power in an aggressive serve-and-volley game, while shorter, agile players may do better with a mobile court-covering game.

In general, the body-fat levels of tennis players are relatively low, since excess fat can reduce both stamina and heat tolerance. In women's tennis, this hasn't always been the 'look'. In earlier times, many top females were skilled but relatively fat and lacking in aerobic fitness. Martina Navratilova set a trend in women's tennis by trimming down and developing her strength and fitness until she became almost invincible during the 1980s. The Williams sisters, Venus and Serena, have continued this tradition with their impressive muscularity.

Common nutritional issues

Training nutrition

During the 1980s, champions Ivan Lendl and Martina Navratilova publicised the importance of nutrition in their game preparation and paved the way for the professionalism of present-day players. The training and playing schedules of many elite players set up variable energy and carbohydrate requirements. They may be large in the case of males with multi-hour matches, but quite modest for some females who can finish a power game in less than 60 min. See Chapters 1 and 2 for a full account of the optimal training diet, and the guidelines for scaling up and down nutrient intakes according to need.

Body-fat levels

You can almost bet on it: stories emanating from the Australian Open in the quiet news month of January invariably include comments (usually by a male ex-player) to the effect that a female tennis player (or two) is out of shape. Many players, especially females, do not come naturally to the body-fat level that does them justice on the court. Several unique challenges exist in the world of tennis—being constantly on tour and away from home, having very little time in the year for conditioning, and practising aggressive nutritional preparation for matches that are ultimately very brief.

Nevertheless, carrying extra body fat carries more penalties than an unflattering photo in the papers. It reduces your speed and stamina, and increases your suffering during hot days on the court. If you need to lose body fat, read Chapter 3 for advice on setting suitable goals and adopting a healthy plan of eating and exercise.

Fluid intake during matches and training

Tennis is often played in sweltering heat. The Australian Open is well known for exposing players to ambient temperatures of 35°C to 40°C; court temperatures may exceed 50°C because of the enclosure of the space and the retention of heat in the playing surface. Most years there is at least one report of a player withdrawing because of heat distress or illness. When matches drag out to three hours or more, and rallies are long and intense, players can accumulate large sweat losses. The casualties of a large fluid deficit include a lowered work rate, increased perception of fatigue and reductions in skills and concentration.

To reduce the risk and effects of dehydration, players should follow a plan of fluid intake before, during and after matches that includes having cool and palatable drinks courtside. Even though players can drink during breaks between sets and at the change of ends every second game, it can be difficult to stay in touch with hydration needs when sweat rates exceed 1–1.5 L an hour. After the match, the remaining fluid deficit needs to be replaced—hopefully before the next match—to prevent the problems of chronic dehydration.

While water is adequate to replace fluid losses, there may be additional advantages in having some carbohydrate during long, intense matches, especially if you are gradually becoming glycogen-depleted over a long week of tournament matches. Carbohydrate intake during the match may help to boost flagging fuel stores and delay the fatigue of muscles and brain. A sports drink will provide carbohydrate and fluid needs simultaneously, but for a more concentrated fuel boost, some players will also turn to sports gels. Read more in Chapters 4.6 and 4.7.

Life on the circuit

Elite tennis players can look forward to a life of travelling—around Australia and around the world. While this can be exciting, it can also be stressful. It is often hard to meet nutritional needs in unfamiliar surroundings, especially when time and finances are limited. Read the accounts below for practical advice on travelling nutrition.

Tournament tennis

Tournament tennis is challenging from many nutritional viewpoints. Apart from the fact that it takes players away from home—even for a weekend tournament—the tournament schedule calls for forward thinking and clever nutritional strategies for games and for speedy recovery. Not only must players be committed to looking after their bodies' fluid and carbohydrate needs between matches, but they must do so without a definite timetable of their day's activities.

Since each day's match draw is determined by the results of the previous day's play, players receive short notice about their daily schedule. Forward planning is also made difficult by the loose nature of the daily timetable. While the first match of each session may have a set starting time, all other matches simply follow in succession. The impossibility of guessing the duration of matches means players must often simply wait—while being ready to play at any time. As in the case of Suzi below, tournament players must learn to be adaptable with their eating plans—having a clear idea of their nutritional goals for competition but being prepared to handle a great deal of unpredictability.

Profile: The travelling athlete

Accidental tourists

Take a modern athlete and you probably also have a seasoned traveller. At the elite level, frequent international competition is demanded by both the economics and performance standards of many sports. In addition to big events such as world championships and the Olympic and Commonwealth games, many top athletes undertake regular training/competition tours overseas, in search of better weather during Southern Hemisphere winters, specialised training such as altitude training, or general fame and fortune on the competition circuit. National competitions and championships, too, involve travel. In some sports these no longer mean a single annual national titles event, but, rather, a week-by-week requirement to go on the road. Even recreational athletes can be caught up in this mobility. Who hasn't travelled away to a basketball tournament, triathlon or tennis competition? Some athletes even choose to combine an overseas event with their recreational or business travel—

for example, for their annual holiday they might go to New York to run the marathon, or do a triathlon in Fiji.

While travel provides its own rewards and opportunities, for the athlete with special nutritional goals it can also pose some challenges. Some of the food-related problems you may face as a travelling athlete are:

- Being in a country with an unfamiliar food supply and different eating customs. As a result, it may be difficult to find the types of foods that you like and that you are sure will meet your dietary goals. It can be hard to find out the composition of restaurant dishes and packaged foods, especially if you don't speak the language. Many an athlete with a fussy palate has lost weight because she did not find the local fare to her liking, while others have struggled to find enough carbohydrate sources to load up for an endurance event.
- Food safety and hygiene. Many countries have lower standards of hygiene and food quality control than you enjoy at home. Finding safe foods and drinks, in particular, can use up a lot of your resources, patience and time. The consequences can be gastrointestinal upsets ranging in seriousness from a nuisance to a disaster.
- Being unable to prepare your own foods—needing to rely on restaurants and take-aways. Often when you are on a short trip you will be staying in a hotel or other accommodation that provides minimal facilities for food preparation or storage. Not only is it expensive to buy all your meals individually, but you are often compromised by the types of food outlets available and the times when you can be served.
- Communal eating. So, you are staying in a Games Village or on campus in an institution. You might be lucky enough to be provided with unlimited access to a menu designed for athletes. Foolproof? Unfortunately not. There are many pitfalls to eating in a communal setting, including being mesmerised by the quantities and varieties of food and being distracted by the eating habits of those around you.
- Distraction. Sometimes, just being away from home creates a holiday atmosphere. Indeed, for some athletes the trip may

actually be doubling as a vacation. As a result, many athletes find their trips away sabotaged by a 'let's just enjoy ourselves' attitude.

- Travelling itself. What you eat and what you need to eat can be at odds when you are on the move. Travelling can be stressful, involving long hours, changes in your body clock, and disruption to your training schedule.

It is easy to see how an athlete under these circumstances would end up failing to eat—and thus compete or train—at an optimal level.

Eating well as a travelling athlete requires a three-pronged attack. First, you should be clear about your nutritional goals and how these might change at various times in training and competition. Read through the appropriate sections in Part I of this book. Next, plan ahead and prepare for your trip. It is often possible to pre-organise foods and dining opportunities to suit your needs. Finally, while you are away, be assertive to make sure your nutritional goals are achieved. Guidelines for preparing and implementing your plan are summarised in Checklist 22.1. If you apply the same dietary commitment during your travels as you do while at home, then your trip should reward you with sporting success in addition to new stamps in your passport!

Profile: Suzi

Tournaments and travel

Suzi was sure she knew what she needed to eat and drink for competition, but turning theory into practice in tournament tennis was a difficult task. Still, she was determined to do it. She was convinced that good nutrition played a crucial role in sustaining her performance level over the week of competition. Too many times she had watched the final being fought out between players she should have beaten, after bowing out in the middle of the tournament. Often she'd felt that the effects of poor eating over the week had gradually taken their toll, leaving her tired and unable to play at anywhere near her best.

Of course, it wasn't only food that caused problems. Life on the circuit often meant lack of sleep, homesickness, and more stress and hassles than were good for her game. It was especially hard in her early days on the satellite circuit. Not only had the lifestyle been new and bewildering, but conditions were harder for unknowns like her. Being short of cash usually meant staying in cheap accommodation away from the tennis centre and having to spend precious time on public transport to get to and from matches. Access to food, at least the right sort of food, was limited by both time and money and often many days passed before she managed to eat a properly planned meal. In those circumstances it had been hard to keep coming up day after day, particularly if the three or four days of the tournament were preceded by qualifying rounds.

In the really early days of her career, Suzi had battled hard with her weight. Being away from Mum meant it was easy to stray from a good nutrition plan. At first she had simply taken advantage of the opportunity to eat whatever she liked without a stern eye watching. Later on, even when she wanted to eat well, she hadn't really known how to choose well. It had been so easy to leave it all to Mum. She'd also felt she needed to fuel up aggressively for every match lest she 'run out of juice' against the hard-running senior players on the circuit. As her frustrations about her fluctuating performances, homesickness and weight battles intensified, she had added to the problem by comfort eating. But then a miracle had occurred, in the guise of referral from a fellow player to a sympathetic sports dietitian.

Suzi had worked hard with the dietitian to understand her real needs and take a long-term approach to achieving a leaner shape. After a year, she was rewarded with a climb up the rankings, and now she'd made it to the Grand Prix circuit. She was entitled to stay in good hotels close to the competition venues, and caterers provided a spread of food in the player facilities at the courts. Now that good food was more accessible, the biggest challenges lay in the unpredictable nature of tennis.

Suzi talked the situation over again with a sports dietitian and they agreed that the main principles of tournament nutrition were:

- Understand your real needs based on actual match play—neither under-fuelling nor over-fuelling
- Maximise and speed up your recovery after each match—particularly if it's been a long, gruelling battle. Have a feel for your sweat losses and fuel needs. As soon as practical replace fluid, carbohydrate and protein with well-chosen snacks or meals.

- When there is a long gap between matches—overnight or a rest day—continue to eat nutritiously, with the emphasis on meeting real needs for energy and carbohydrate intake.
- Eat before each match to feel comfortable and refuelled—ideally, a light snack about two hours before the start. Make sure fluids are topped up on hot days.
- Experiment with fluid and fuel replacement strategies during training sessions and practice matches to devise a suitable match plan. Long matches and hot days require extra vigilance.

These clear principles made it seem easy to devise a plan. However, as Suzi explained to the dietitian, difficulties arose because of the loose and unpredictable timetable. The day's match schedule was variable, crude and given at short notice. Unless you were drawn for the first match on a court, you could not be sure when you'd be playing. While you could predict an approximate time for the fourth match on Court 1, there was no certainty. This made it difficult to time the pre-match meal or to know what to have between two matches (a singles then a doubles match) on the same day. Suzi recounted some disastrous experiences, like the time she'd been scheduled for the third match of the afternoon and had eaten a reasonable lunch just before the start of the session. Not only had the first match lasted just 35 minutes, but the second match was forfeited after five minutes when one of the players hurt her ankle. Suddenly, Suzi found herself on the court, with a fuller stomach than she would have liked.

Another time, during a satellite tournament, Suzi had eaten her packed lunch in anticipation of her match, only to have a rain delay postpone all matches indefinitely. What should she do? Go hungry, or take a chance and eat a snack? And would the little tennis-centre kiosk stock anything that passed for high-carbohydrate, low-fat food? Apart from anything else, the worry of making the right decision interfered with her game.

Post-match eating was still a problem sometimes, even with the courtside meals available for the players. When centre-court matches stretched into the night, Suzi found herself finishing after the caterers had gone home for the day. This left only restaurants (it was often too late to find one open) or hotel room service (which had pretty unsuitable menus). And of course, with late games, sleep sometimes took priority over eating.

The dietitian suggested that two philosophies were needed to handle the situation. First was flexibility. It would be good to plan the ideal way of meeting a nutritional goal, but it would be even better to have a 'Plan B' up her sleeve in case of sudden changes in schedule. For example, the ideal match preparation would be a light meal about 2 hours or so before, followed by a warm-up hit and perhaps a top-up with extra fluids (water) before the match. Matches set to a definite schedule, such as the first match in a session, could be approached along these lines.

However, with an uncertain timetable, she should keep additional or alternative snacks on hand. Ready-to-go liquid meal supplements—for example, Powerbar Proteinplus or Sustagen Sport—would be particularly versatile in helping to fill in the gaps and handle emergencies. Being liquid and easy to digest, they could supply a nutritious, carbohydrate-based meal without the discomfort of solid food. This would be handy between two matches played close together, or as a top-up to an earlier meal when the next match was running late. They could also be a quick no-preparation snack after the game, or a boost to turn a sandwich snack into a more filling meal. With a bit of experimentation, Suzi would find many other food ideas to trouble-shoot problems like this.

Being self-reliant was the other helpful philosophy. Even at the big tournaments, where hotels and court catering are provided, many players choose to organise their own apartments so they can cook the meals they want when they want them—they can always fall back on the other food facilities when they want a break. In addition, after weeks on the circuit, it is often nice to have some home cooking rather than restaurant fare. Sometimes, it can make the difference between succumbing to homesickness/travel fatigue or not.

On the lower rungs of the circuit ladder, where the lifestyle isn't so rich and famous, being self-reliant is even more important. If players can afford to stay in a unit, perhaps sharing costs in a group, then with some organisation they can supply most of their own meals. Even in billet or hotel accommodation, players can organise some of their supplies—a travelling food kit can be a great help (see Table 22.1).

The dietitian told Suzi she was right to believe that poor nutrition could put her tennis performance below par. This happened through gradual muscle-fuel depletion and dehydration in the short term, and perhaps nutritional deficiencies and weight problems over a long tour. With better planning, not only would Suzi avoid all these physiological traps, but she could go into matches with the confidence boost of knowing she was at her best. There was every chance that she would meet an opponent, even someone with more talent than Suzi, who had not prepared so well for her nutritional needs. Suzi's commitment could well mean that opponent's loss.

CHECKLIST 22.1
A gold-medal travelling nutrition plan

Plan ahead:

- Find out what to expect at your travel destination(s) and what challenges your training or competition schedule might throw up. Good sources of information are other athletes who have been there before, and the organisers of the events you plan to compete in. Other athletes can usually give you lengthy accounts of what to do and what not to do—usually from bitter experience.
- Plan your accommodation with meals in mind. If you intend to stay in the same place for a long time, or if you have special nutritional needs that may be hard to meet by conventional arrangements (e.g. unusual meal times), then you might be best served by finding lodgings with full kitchens.
- Even facilities for minimal food preparation and storage—e.g. a fridge in your hotel room—can increase your flexibility and open up the nutritional possibilities. Another idea might be to choose an area that is close to shops or restaurants, especially if you will have limited means of transport.
- Pre-arrange meals where appropriate. If you have special needs or a complicated timetable, contact airlines, restaurants or hotels

ahead of time so they can meet your needs. This can also help to reduce waiting time and make mealtimes less confusing when travelling with a large group.

Take your own supplies:

- Take or send a supply of portable and non-perishable foods to your destination to replace important items that may be missing or to help you create well-chosen snacks that are sometimes forgotten by caterers or team managers.
- Keep in mind quarantine laws, baggage weight restrictions and other local customs that may limit the type and quantity of your supplies (see Table 22.1).

Eat and drink well en route:

- Don't succumb to 'boredom eating' just because you are confined. Instead, eat according to your real needs, taking into account the enforced rest while you are travelling.
- When moving to a new time zone, adopt eating patterns that suit your destination as soon as the trip starts. This will help your body clock to adapt.
- Recognise unseen fluid losses in air-conditioned vehicles and pressurised plane cabins and follow a suitable drinking plan that neither overhydrates nor underhydrates you.

Take care with food/water hygiene:

- Find out whether the local water supply is safe to drink. Otherwise, stick to drinks from sealed bottles, or hot drinks made from well-boiled water. Remember that ice added to drinks is often made from tap water and may be a problem.
- In high-risk environments, eat only at good hotels or well-known restaurants. Avoid food from local stalls and markets, at least until after your competition, however tempted you may be to have an 'authentic cultural experience'.
- In these environments, stick to food that has been well cooked. It is best to avoid salads or unpeeled fruit that has been in contact with local water or soil.

Adhere to your food plan:

- Choose the best of the local cuisine to meet your nutritional needs, supplementing with your own supplies where needed.
- Be assertive in asking for what you need at catering outlets—e.g. low-fat cooking styles or an extra carbohydrate choice.
- Recognise the challenges of 'all you can eat' dining. Resist the temptation to eat 'what is there' or 'what everyone else is eating' in favour of your own meal plan.

TABLE 22.1
Non-perishable food supplies for the travelling athlete

- Liquid meal supplements: In Tetra Paks if you can manage it, or in powdered versions if you need to conserve space and weight
- Breakfast cereals and powdered low-fat milk
- Dried fruit and trail mixes
- Snack packs of canned fruit
- Quick-cooking noodle and pasta varieties
- Baked beans
- Muesli bars or cereal bars
- Dried biscuits or rice cakes
- Individual packets or tubes of condiments—jam, honey, Vegemite (to prevent homesickness)
- Low-dose broad-range multivitamin mineral supplement (if you are unsure of the consistency and quality of your food intake)

Cricket

Cricket is a game of skill and tradition that touches the lives of most Australians each summer. Teams of 11 players compete against each other, with slightly different rules governing Test games (based on two complete innings for each side—four- or five-day games) and One Day International, or limited-overs matches, involving a 50-over innings for each side. The new and exciting Twenty20 format, which provides each team with an innings of 20 overs, lasts several hours.

Professional cricket competitions exist for both men and women, but it is the men's scene that dominates. A lucrative career can be made by playing in overseas leagues, such as in India or England, or by representing Australia in the various tours played between two or more countries each year, or at the World Cups. It is hard to progress through the ranks from local to district and state-level cricket to this elite level, but the players who do become household names, often in several countries. Nevertheless, most cricket in Australia is played at a social and recreational level, and there are many leagues and competitions at grades from 'F' level up.

Roughly speaking, a cricket team is broken into specialist batsmen, specialist bowlers and a wicket-keeper. Theoretically, all team members get to bat and to field, while usually only the specialists are required to bowl. The game is based on skill, and only in recent years and at a high level of play has there been talk of aerobic fitness. The Twenty20 format, which favours power hitting, may see the emergence of a new breed of strength-trained cricketers. Even so, there are many top-level players who are more aptly termed sportsmen than athletes, and whose off-field activities create as much news as their on-field exploits.

Training

Cricket is a summer sport, with the season beginning at the end of October and progressing to a final series in March. At the top level, some cricketers play all year, playing in international tours during the Northern Hemisphere summer, or travelling to England for the county cricket season. The lucrative Indian Premier League has recently provided another opening. Even if he is not playing all year round, the modern elite cricketer will continue to train, or at least to remain fit, over winter. However, the usual pattern of the old guard is to stop playing once the season is over. Unless such players get involved in another sport over winter, their fitness may have dropped off considerably by the beginning of the next season.

At first-grade level, pre-season training begins around June, most often in the form of general fitness work, and is often unsupervised or left to the individual player. As the season draws closer, organised team training takes over and the component of skills practice is increased. During the season at a top club, three team training sessions are organised each week between matches. Each lasts 2–2½ hours and involves batting and bowling practice, fielding skills and drills, and perhaps some general running or fitness work. Some individual players at the top level may be motivated to organise their own fitness program in addition to this, and may undertake extra aerobic training and perhaps a weights program. In low-grade competition there may be little or no organised training.

Competition

District cricket is played on weekends, at many grades or levels of competition. This may be in the form of two-day fixtures and/or limited-over (One Day) competitions, with the two types often happening simultaneously. Domestic competitions run concurrently over summer, with representative state teams playing against each other in each of a Twenty20 competition, a One Day (limited overs) fixture and the traditional first-class (Sheffield Shield) competitions involving four-day matches.

Summer is a busy time for international cricket in Australia. The program usually includes a Test series (five-day matches) and a tournament of One Day matches involving one or more touring teams from other cricket-playing nations. The new schedules also accommodate the Twenty20 format matches. Between matches, the cricketers may go back to their state-level competition, and may train with their state teams or district clubs. When an overseas tour is organised, the Australian team will travel together for a time, and may undergo team training sessions between matches.

The physical requirements of a cricket game vary with the format of the match and with the player's position in the team. Test games involve six hours of match play plus breaks, scheduled between 11 a.m. and 6 p.m. over the 4–5 days of competition. The limited-overs series may also involve a similar daytime schedule or a day–night timetable with the two teams each playing up to 50 overs. Twenty20 matches (20 overs each team) typically last around 2½ hours, providing a format similar in length to other team games.

Games played in mid- to late-summer are often played in great heat, and require players to stand for many hours in the sun. Those at most risk of heat stress are those who are exposed for the longest periods (e.g. the fielding team) and the fast bowlers, who may work in short, intense spells throughout the day. Batsmen who stay in for a long innings may also have to run repeatedly in the heat. The physical requirements of cricket are variable and unpredictable—between matches and between players. The duration and work–rest ratios for each type of player are dependent not only on their success on a particular day but on the success of the opposition team.

Physical characteristics

Cricketers come in all shapes and sizes—even at the top level. Only in recent years have cricket coaches demanded that body fat be kept to reasonable levels, a change paralleled by the increased fitness expected of players. Less body fat would in principle improve a player's speed, stamina and heat tolerance. Speed becomes important at a high level of play, particularly in the limited-overs matches, since skilled fielding and running between wickets are helpful for success. Several high-profile fast bowlers have received the attention of their team conditioning staff—and the media—for being over-fat and under-fit. Such criticisms are based on the belief that leaner, fitter players will have faster run-up speeds and ball delivery as well as more endurance for bowling and fielding over the day.

Wicket-keepers must be strong as well as agile—in an average day of keeping, the equivalent of 600 squats may be done. The new Twenty20 cricket game is considered a batsmen's game, favouring a power style of hitting, similar to baseball. At the time of writing, most of the changes made to accommodate this new game style relate to the technique of hitting the ball. However, we speculate that cricketers who specialise in this game might change their training and physique to more closely resemble those of baseball players.

Common nutritional issues

Body-fat levels

Even in elite cricket, there are widely publicised cases of cricket players who fight a constant battle against the bulge. One such struggle apparently led to a doping infraction, when a well-known player admitted to taking a (banned) diuretic tablet to avoid looking 'puffy' during a TV interview. The more usual disadvantages of being too fat are related to health and performance on the field.

If you think you would make your life healthier, your cricket game faster, and your captain happier by shedding some weight, then opt for a fat-loss program that is based on sensible and long-term principles. Many male (and female) cricketers find themselves wanting to lose weight but not knowing how, since nutrition and fitness haven't previously been big issues for them. The cricketing lifestyle may not help the cause either, being made up of long periods on the field with low exercise levels, and too much of the good life. Read the profile of Jason below, and Chapter 3, for ideas on healthy fat loss.

Training nutrition

Cricketers may be among the last group of sportspeople to warm to the idea of making sound nutrition part of their lifestyle. For many, the rewards may simply be improved health and vitality, and better weight control. However, for the new breed of cricket player who regards himself as an athlete and has an organised training schedule, better nutrition will also bring improvements in adaptation to training and match performance. Read Chapters 1 and 2 for an outline of the optimal diet for both health and performance.

Match-day nutrition

Until recently, match-day nutrition has often followed tradition rather than science, even at the top level. Test cricket runs on a fairly laid-back 11 a.m.-to-6 p.m. timetable. Limited-overs matches may have a daytime or a day/night schedule. Players will rise according to the needs of the day—and, in some cases, late, because of the deeds of the night before (see the comments on alcohol below). Pre-match meals are variable in quantity and quality. Some professional players who are staying in hotels may still start the day with a hearty high-fat cooked breakfast—who can resist when it's free and right there on the buffet breakfast bar? However, others are happy to keep to keep to a lighter and healthier program of cereal, fruit and dairy, toast and toppings.

Test matches are generally played with a drinks break every hour, and set breaks for lunch (40 min) and tea (20 min). A meal is usually eaten during the lunch break. Limited-overs matches have one tea break between the innings of the two teams. At the elite level, meals are catered at the ground and usually organised by a club dietitian or nutrition expert. In these circumstances, we can expect menus to include lighter hot meals—pasta and rice dishes—as well as a sandwich or salad bar that would allow players to choose for themselves. Sports foods may also be on hand to provide an alternative for people who want something more compact or just a drink. Flexibility is needed because of the different game needs of each player, the different phases of play (whether the team is batting or bowling), and individual preferences. Hopefully, the grounds at which matches are held will be able to meet the new-style catering requirements. The traditional arrangements often involved heavy, meat-focused meals.

At the other end of the scale, at many district and club cricket matches the host team provides the catering. Wives, mothers and girlfriends may be organised on a catering roster or required to 'bring a plate'. Results can be varied.

If you've read Chapter 4, you will see that modern cricket doesn't always implement state-of-the-art ideas about competition nutrition. Indeed, it might be argued that in a game of skill there is less need for such concerns. Nevertheless, cricket today requires athleticism in both the preparation and execution of a game. Even for players who don't have high fuel requirements on a particular day or session, light, carbohydrate-focused meals are more suited to hot-weather eating and more likely to preserve gut comfort.

Nutrition within a session or Twenty20 innings is another issue. Depending on the weather, the game requirements and recovery (or not) from the previous session/day, players may benefit from a proactive approach to fuel and fluid replacement.

Alcohol intake

Alcohol is, for better or worse, part of cricketing lifestyle. The traditions of the game include having a beer with the opposition team at the end of the day, or, in the case of international cricket (where being too friendly with the competition is frowned on) having a beer with your own teammates. Even during a multi-day match at the elite level, it is seen as acceptable to wine and dine or drink and dance late into the night. When the match is over, or the test series has been decided, it is almost mandatory that newspapers carry a picture of the winning team in their locker rooms celebrating heartily—often with alcohol provided by the team or series sponsor—and, as often as not, a tale of some player's misdemeanour in the hours afterwards.

Not only is alcohol intake an expected part of the game, heavy drinking is glorified and made into the stuff of legends. Cricketing aficionados can tell you how many half-centuries were made by an international cricketer on a tour of England—and also how many cans of beer he drank on the flight home, or even on the way over. In fact, from time to time we still hear of sportsmen seemingly trying to set a record for alcohol intake on a long-haul flight. According to many sources, the present record of 52 cans of full-strength beer is held by former Australian batsman David Boon, who surpassed records held by earlier cricketers. Even with player codes of conduct and team educational talks on how to drink more discreetly if not in smaller quantities, it is hard to clean up the boozy mindset of the team sports, particularly cricket.

Clearly, such drinking practices violate the principles of healthy nutrition for optimal performance. Read Chapter 1.6 and the profile in the AFL chapter for more on the role of alcohol in sport. In cricket as in other male-dominated team sports, it will take time and a change of attitude before healthier practices become widespread. It is to be hoped that the emerging group of first-class cricketers will include sensible drinking practices among their ideas of professionalism—not only looking after their own lives and sporting careers but providing a role model for thousands of young players. Checklist 18.1 provides some strategies for those who want to make changes.

Travelling on tour or abroad

Cricketers on tour live in hotels and out of suitcases, and in many cases they may be constantly on the move for months. Standing in the way of optimal nutrition are not only the usual problems associated with being a travelling athlete but the strong traditions associated with being a cricketer on tour. Remind yourself of your nutritional priorities (Chapters 1 and 2), and for specific advice on travelling nutrition read the sections in the Tennis chapter (the travelling athlete) and the Golf chapter (eating in restaurants).

Profile: Jason

Lose weight or lose match payments

There was a new order in at Jason's cricket club, and Jason was worried. He was a fast bowler, with the potential to be a very fast bowler if he could only lose some fat. The new captain-coach had called the team together at the beginning of pre-season training and explained his ideas for a new, fit team that would blast the opposition with speed and professionalism as well as skill. Each player was interviewed separately, and Jason was told to lose 9 kg or face a series of fines. A fitness program was drawn up, and Jason was given a date two weeks on, when he'd have to come in and report on his progress.

Jason had heard talk like this before. They had told him to lose weight last year, as well—the same 9 kg. But Jason had dodged his way through the season, joking to the club officials that he had developed a life of 'organised sloth'. The weight had stayed put, but his season's figures had been moderately successful, so no one had pushed things any further.

This year was different. The new captain-coach didn't look as if he would stand any nonsense, and a new fast bowler had been recruited. If Jason wanted to hold his position, he would have to make some changes. How could he lose the weight? Jason tried the Atkins diet, which suited his love of fatty foods and saw his weight drop by 3 kg almost overnight. But in the long term, how could you eat fish without the chips, or the burger without the bun? Besides, the diet made him constipated and cranky—to the point where even his mother told him to shape up or ship out. He was copping it from all ends. At his first fortnightly weigh-in with the captain-coach, Jason was fined $200 for his lack of progress. That really hurt! But then the coach explained that the money would be used to pay for a series of consultations with a sports dietitian.

Jason was surprised when the dietitian didn't immediately give him a diet sheet. She explained that rigid dietary plans were usually only successful in the short term. If Jason wanted to go to the trouble of losing weight, he might as well do it properly and lose it forever—by gradually adopting a new, healthier lifestyle. The dietitian likened this to the help he'd received from the specialist bowling coach at the club, who had carefully examined Jason's bowling style, picked out the faults and weaknesses, and helped him to remodel his delivery.

Jason told the dietitian that he lived at home but was rarely there for meals. Nevertheless, it was a potential source of food, and Jason explained that his mother had become pretty careful about her cooking since his father's heart attack four years ago. The typical intake for his day is summarised in Table 23.1.

The dietitian took careful notes, then delivered her honest assessment. Jason's diet was high in fat, and his drinking was inconsistent with a trim waistline and good performance. The uneven spread of his energy intake over the day—skipped meals and gorging late at night—also worked against him. She explained the principles of healthy training nutrition (see Chapter 1) and together they worked out an eating plan that would suit Jason's needs.

Important changes included:

- No more skipping breakfast. With fewer 'wasted' late nights, Jason would aim to get up in plenty of time for a healthy breakfast before work.
- A sandwich-based lunch to replace high-fat take-aways. This could even be toasted or grilled as long as no extra margarine was added. Jason wasn't too keen on eating fruit, but said he liked the look of the fresh fruit salads in the shop next to work.
- Some recovery snacks after training nights, to make the most of the completed session as well as preventing hunger and overstuffing at the next meal.
- Now and then, either a better chosen (low-fat) restaurant meal, or home to some of Mum's healthy cooking. Some serving sizes were given.
- A quick home-made pizza eaten on the couch instead of a greasy dial-a-pizza. The dietitian provided a recipe that even Jason could follow.
- Switching to light beer—and rationing himself to one stubbie a night. Jason was a bit reluctant, but he acknowledged that many of his mates had moved in this direction years ago because of drink-driving laws. He had used their services as designated driver without learning their self-control or repaying their effort.
- Replacing Coke with low-joule drinks.

When the plans were laid out side by side, Jason was surprised to see how much food he could now eat. The dietitian assured him that the new diet contained far fewer kilojoules, would supply more fuel on training days, and would give him more vitamins and minerals than his old diet. He tackled the new plan with gusto, and together with his fitness program and new attitude, it soon had him feeling like a new man. He surprised himself by looking forward to his bowl of cereal in the morning, though when there was time he preferred to cook up some eggs on toast. He still didn't feel like venturing too far from tried and true toppings on his homemade pizza. But one night, when the fridge was bare, he made himself baked beans on toast rather than succumb to Dial-A-Meat-Lover's. (Apparently some other famous fast bowler swore by baked beans!)

Jason's success exceeded his own expectations. Within three months, he reached what he considered his new 'fighting weight'. Being fit and motivated, his game became more aggressive and confident. Not only did he keep his place at the club, but he was recently selected to train with the state side.

Profile

The twelfth man: Carrying the drinks is an undervalued role!

Despite a long series of shake-ups from the World Series, the limited-overs format and more recently Twenty20, cricket remains a game of tradition. It evolved in the temperate climate of England, and the rules that govern its play still reflect that. They are not ideally suited to the often scorching heat of Australia—or indeed many other cricket-playing countries, from India to the West Indies and South Africa.

Not only are many cricketers required to take the field in heat exceeding 40°C, but many work hard for a number of hours in these conditions—particularly the fast bowlers. Running between wickets or fielding may also involve prolonged and heavy work during some games. The clothing worn by cricketers, including batsmen's protective gear, may add to heat stress. Clearly, sweat losses may be high in hot weather, yet the rules of cricket may interfere with adequate rehydration. Drink breaks are held each hour, with the twelfth man carrying the drinks onto the field. In very hot weather, drink breaks may be held every 40 min. Until recently, these official breaks and the luncheon and tea intervals provided the only sanctioned opportunities for fluid intake.

Chris Gore, now at the Australian Institute of Sport, investigated sweat rates, temperature control and fluid intakes in 20 first-class cricket players. Measurements were taken during a real match, and some simulated matches, in weather conditions that were designated as cool (forecast temperature 22°C), warm (forecast temperature 30°C) and hot (forecast temperature 38°C). The games were played under first-class rules, with the first session from 11 a.m. to 1 p.m., the second session from 1.40 p.m. to 3.40 p.m. and the last session from 4 p.m. to 6 p.m. Water was available according to the normal rules—before the match, every hour during the cool and warm matches, every 40 min during the hot match, and during luncheon and tea breaks. Players were able to drink as much as they desired.

The results showed that the weather significantly affected the sweat losses of players. On the cool day, the average sweat loss over the day was 540 ml per hour—470 ml per hour for the batsmen and 710 ml per hour for the bowlers. On the warm day, the average hourly sweat loss was 670 ml—600 ml for the batsmen and 690 ml for the bowlers. On the warm day, sweat rates were greater during the second and third sessions of play than during the opening session. Only bowlers were monitored on the hot day—when they recorded sweat losses of 1670 ml per hour for the first session and 1070 ml per hour for the second. There was no third session of play because these bowlers bowled out the opposition team by the tea break.

Fluid intake on the cool and warm days managed to keep pace with sweat losses. The cricket players drank about 500 ml of fluid during each hourly break on the cool day, and 600–700 ml on the warm day. Fluid intake during the luncheon break averaged about 900–1000 ml on both days, and at the tea break 400 ml and 600 ml of fluid were consumed on the cool and warm day respectively. At the end of play the players had accumulated a negligible to slight level of dehydration—averaging almost no weight change on the cool day and a deficit of 1.2 per cent of body mass on the warm day.

The hot day gave different results. Drink breaks were taken each 40 min in response to the weather, and an average of 300–600 ml of fluid was consumed on each occasion. Yet by the end of the first session of play the bowlers were significantly dehydrated, with a fluid deficit of 3.8 per cent of body mass. During the luncheon break they showered in an attempt to cool down and drank an average of 960 ml. Despite this, and despite further drink breaks during the second session, by the end of this (final) session of play the average level of dehydration was 4.3 per cent of body weight.

As in many sports, there is a maximum comfortable level of fluid intake that can be managed in a given break, regardless of the weather. In hot weather it appears that more opportunities to consume fluid are needed if total fluid intake is to match sweat losses. The level of dehydration sustained by players on the hot day would have certainly reduced their performance—and made for an uncomfortable day of cricket. Luckily, a third session was not warranted on this day!

It would have been interesting to see how the batsmen fared

in the hot-day scenario. There is a famous story from an Indian Test match in which Australian player David Hookes batted for 10 hours in temperatures of 40°C and lost 5 kg in weight (probably over 6 per cent of his body weight). These study results and anecdotes explain the recent trend for the active players on the field to have access to a drink bottle between official breaks. This can be in the form of a bottle on the boundary lines while a bowler has a spell in the field, or bottles kept with the match umpire. But apart from making the player feel more comfortable in a hot environment, how important is hydration to the outcome of a game?

In the chapters about other team games and stop-start sports, we noted that studies have linked moderate–large fluid deficits with a reduction in work output, concentration and skills—especially when a sport is played in a hot environment. There is only one study that deals specifically with cricket, carried out by researchers from RMIT University in Melbourne. It found that when sub-elite cricket players restricted their fluid intake so as to gradually build up a fluid deficit of just under 3 per cent of body weight over a session of training, they were slower at performing a shuttle run in moderate weather conditions. The fluid deficit was also associated with a reduction in the line and length of accuracy of bowling of the order of 15 per cent, although bowling speed was not affected. In contrast, bowling skills and endurance were maintained when players drank sufficient fluid over the session to keep the deficit to about 1 per cent of body weight. We might expect that the negative effects of this fluid deficit would be even more pronounced in hot conditions.

Some high-level players and their coaching staff have been dismissive of the results of this and other studies of dehydration in sport, saying that elite and experienced players are more resistant to such fatigue or more able to concentrate than lower-ranked players. We agree that individual responses to a fluid deficit vary, and that problems may not be easy to detect. However, we argue that increases in the perception of effort or need to concentrate are bound to have even small effects on performance. At the highest levels of sport, victory or loss can hinge on the margins between taking a catch or spilling the ball, judging whether it is safe to sneak a quick run or not, or hitting a fast ball or not—and that the winning edge requires optimal performance.

As in other prolonged stop-start activities, it is also likely to be worthwhile fuelling up during sessions. Therefore, active players should consider a sports drink for their fluid needs. Of course, those in sedentary roles who are likely to be able to eat regular meals or snacks during the breaks may not benefit from additional fuel (or energy intake).

Finally, it is of interest to see how well cricket players look after their hydration needs during a training session. This can be a dress rehearsal of hydration techniques for a match, as well as an opportunity to learn about individual sweat rates and the fluid deficits that might be carried from a practice day into a match. We were recently able to participate in a sweat testing session on the Australian cricket team during a 2½-hour training session (warm-up and drills, followed by bowling and batting practice in nets). The weather during the mid-morning session was hot, averaging 29°C and 50 per cent humidity. Players had access to 'drink stations', with Eskies of cold Gatorade and bottled water provided on the cricket ground and near the nets.

Urine samples collected by players that morning showed that 5 of the 12 were dehydrated from their previous day's activities. The figures from during the session suggested that the cricketers generally looked after themselves well, drinking at a rate that replaced about 72 per cent of their sweat losses. On average, the players sweated at a rate of 1200 ml per hour (3 L for the whole session), which is similar to findings from other team sports. At the individual level, however, it was a different story. There was a fourfold difference in the rates of sweat loss between players. Fluid intakes also varied, although there was a trend for the 'bigger sweaters' to drink more during the session. Four players lost more than 1.5 per cent of their body weight over the session, which might have been expected to have a detectable effect on their comfort levels if not their performance.

One player did gain a small amount of weight over the session, meaning that he drank at a rate slightly higher than his sweat losses. This player's morning urine sample had been consistent with dehydration, and he also had a lower rate of sweat loss than the others during the session. Replacing a little more fluid than he sweated out was useful in allowing him to 'make up some ground' in removing his fluid deficit. This is not to be confused with the problem of substantial overdrinking that has been reported among the slower competitors in marathons and ultra-endurance events. In these situations, athletes expose themselves to the risk of hyponatraemia (low blood-sodium levels) by drinking several litres of fluid in excess of their sweat rates and showing a substantial weight gain over the exercise session.

The players were able to make use of the information gathered at the centre to adjust their drinking practices in further training sessions and games. In particular, they noted that our testing session represented the 'best opportunities' for intake during their sport—plenty of access to fluid and plenty of reminders from their coaches to stay hydrated in the hot weather. They might need to make an effort to replicate these conditions in other circumstances or try harder when the support is less evident.

TABLE 23.1
Jason's diet—before and after

	Before	After
Breakfast	• None (late for meetings or morning training)	• Bowl of wholegrain cereal with low fat milk or 2 poached eggs on 2 slices toast • Small glass fruit juice
Lunch	• Pies/sausage rolls, flavoured milk • 1/week: counter lunch with 2–3 beers	• Salad sandwich with cheese/ham/chicken/tuna/beef • Small tub fresh fruit salad
Training 3 nights per week	• Nil or packet of chips in the car on the way home	• Small carton of low-fat flavoured milk and banana
Dinner	• Takeaways • Special likes—burgers, KFC or fish and chips • Pub meal • Special likes—veal or chicken parmigiana or T-bone and chips	• Grilled meat/fish/chicken—serve size = size of palm of hand to first finger joint, all fat trimmed. Grilled or cooked with minimum fat • On training nights: 2 bread rolls or large potato, or cup rice/pasta

	Before	After
	• Beers—tries to keep 'big nights' to 1–2/ week	OR • Pizza made on large pita bread base or fresh pizza base lean ham/ chicken breast or fresh seafood, plenty of veggies (corn, capsicum, onions, tomatoes, mushrooms) and a sprinkle of reduced-fat cheese • 1 stubbie of reduced alcohol beer or Diet Coke.
TV snacks if home	• Chips, twisties, corn chips	• 1 cup of homemade popcorn (minimum oil), Diet Coke

Golf

Golf is a sport of many levels. At one end of the spectrum are the thousands of Australians who enjoy a social round of nine or eighteen holes on weekends. At the other are some of the highest paid sportspeople in Australia and the world. Golf is basically a game of skill. A handicapping system operates to level players of differing ability, and for many recreational players the fun and motivation lie not only in playing against others but in lowering their personal handicap. Golf competition is generally played as stroke play—the winner is the individual with the lowest tally of strokes over the round or rounds. Alternatively, in match play, a team or individual accrues the most 'winning' (lowest-score) holes during a complete round. Australia's Geoff Ogilvie excels at this form.

Competitive golf is played at both amateur and professional levels. At state and national amateur titles, players often struggle to support themselves while practising and playing golf for the requisite number of hours each day. Golfers can turn professional either through an apprenticeship or by attending Player's School. Under both schemes, potential pro golfers undertake business studies as well as learning golf skills. While some professional golfers become attached to clubs and concentrate on providing golf tuition and running shops, others look to making their mark on the professional competitive circuit in Australia and overseas.

Training

Recreational golfers may practise by simply playing. Professional competition golfers, by contrast, can spend up to eight hours a day on the course, practising specific skills, playing practice rounds or playing in competitions. Even during a competition, many players will conduct a practice session at the end of the day's play.

These days, many successful professional players also include general fitness training in their competition preparation—for example, weight training or aerobic activities such as running and swimming. While this training may not directly improve golf skills, some players believe that greater fitness reduces the deterioration in skills caused by fatigue, and that improved strength may help in transferring power to the ball. Tiger Woods—a household name around the world—is reputed to train six days a week, even when on tour, with a regimen that includes weight training, distance runs, speed runs and stretching.

Competition

A round of competition golf is played over 18 holes, and tournaments are conducted either as a single round on one day, or as multi-day competitions of two or four rounds on consecutive days. In a tournament, there are usually two tee-off times—a morning group starting between 7 and 9 a.m., and an afternoon group beginning between 11 a.m. and 1 p.m. A round typically takes 3–5 hours to play, depending on the skill level of the player and the number of other players on the course. The average golf course is 7 km from first to last hole, although a player may walk 10–20 km in a game depending on the accuracy of his shots.

In Australia, professional players can travel on a circuit between club tournaments. During the pro-am season, a pro could play in ten tournaments, for a total of fifteen days of competition, each month. The events on the Australasian PGA tour are typically played from January to March and from October to December, flanking the major season overseas. The Australian Open tournament is played at the end of each year.

Australian golfers may launch themselves on the international circuit, following a range of Asian, Japanese, European, US and Sunshine

(African) tours. The four most prestigious annual tournaments in men's golf ('the majors') are the Masters (April, US), the US Open (June, US), the Open Championship (July, UK), and the PGA (August, US). The women's majors of the LPGA are the Kraft Nabisco Championships (April, US), the LPGA Championship (June, US), the US Women's Open (July US) and the Women's British Open (August, UK). The official world golf ranking is endorsed by the four major championships and the six professional tours which make up the International Federation of PGA Tours. The world's best golfers are almost continually on tour, spending only a few weeks at home each year.

Physical characteristics

Golf is a game of skill rather than physique or physical fitness, and top golfers come in many shapes and sizes. Tiger Woods and John Daly illustrate the extremes among current players in terms of their respective commitments to staying lean and fit. In general, since most players do not exercise intensely the average body-fat levels of top golfers are higher than those of aerobically trained athletes.

Common nutritional issues

Is overweight a handicap?

From time to time, 'larger-than-life' pro golfers, such as John Daly and Chris Patton, raise the question of whether high body-fat levels affect golf performance. Certainly, being significantly overweight is not ideal in terms of general health. In terms of golf skill, we might speculate that a large girth could reduce the flexibility of a player's swing; on the other hand, being heavier could increase the momentum transferred to the ball.

Theoretically, being overweight might also handicap a golfer by reducing his general fitness levels and making him more prone to physical fatigue—and thus more likely to suffer impairments of skill and concentration over the duration of a game. Since body fat works as an insulator, an overweight golfer would also be expected to tolerate heat less well. In both cases, fatigue could cause a decline in skill levels over the course of the round and the tournament.

Of course, this is all speculation: there is no scientific evidence suggesting that all overweight players will improve their golfing game by losing body fat. In fact, Craig Stadler, another heavyweight American golfer, reputedly lost body fat only to find that his swing was disrupted. To be fair, the blame might be placed as much on his emotional or psychological adjustment to the weight loss as on the physical changes.

Finally, it is likely that changes in physique that accompany an off-course training program are markers of the enhancements in strength and fitness that assist golf performance, rather than the reason for improved play. The best advice is to find body weight and body-fat levels that are healthy and comfortable for you, and to remember that a sport like golf is tolerant of a range of physical characteristics. If you do feel that your health and fitness could be improved by losing body fat, read Chapter 3 for safe and sensible advice on achieving this. By losing weight gradually with a healthy diet and exercise program, you should improve your self-confidence as well as your physical condition. Both effects could be good for your game.

Training nutrition

The principles of optimal training nutrition are essentially those of a healthy eating plan, and apply to golfers who play on weekends as well as those who spend eight hours a day on the course. As energy expenditure increases with increased training loads, so do requirements for energy and carbohydrate. Read Chapters 1 and 2 for details of the optimal training diet.

Competition and tournament nutrition

A top golfer must maintain skills and concentration over three to five hours, perhaps for days on end. Once physical fatigue sets in, deterioration in such skills can be expected. Although golfers don't exercise as strenuously as other athletes, prolonged moderate activity, accompanied by the stress of competition and often inclement weather conditions, can take a toll. Both dehydration and low blood-sugar levels may arise during competition, and each would be expected to impair golfing performance.

Sweat losses may be considerable when tournaments are played in heat and wind or even when high adrenaline levels occur in temperate conditions. The environment is often a major contributor to sweat losses, since many tournaments are played in summer, and players are on the course during the hottest parts of the day. Although many golf courses provide drink stations for players, they may be set out at infrequent intervals and may thus not be a significant source of fluid during a game. Since players usually miss a meal while playing a round, they may have no carbohydrate intake for five or six hours. Combined with exercise and nervous stress, this situation may cause a drop in blood-sugar levels in susceptible individuals, affecting brain function and skill. A recent study based on a simulated golf game found that having a caffeinated carbohydrate drink reduced perceptions of fatigue and loss of skills on the later holes. This may have been a result of the caffeine, the carbohydrate or both.

When tournaments are held over several days, there may be a carryover effect of inadequate nutrition, particularly with respect to inadequate fluid replacement. If you find yourself eating only two meals a day (before and after the day's competition), insufficient kilojoule intake can be another problem, and insufficient carbohydrate intake can add to fatigue levels. There are several easy ways to track such a situation. Does your weight drop markedly over a tournament? This is often a sign of chronic dehydration but can also signal an acute reduction in food intake. Does your first morning wee look bright yellow? Do you find yourself becoming tired and making more mistakes earlier in the round? If you answered yes to any of these questions, then you should examine your nutrition practices before and during the comp to look for avenues of improvement.

The careful golfer leaves nothing to chance, taking provisions onto the course to meet the nutritional needs that will arise in competition. There is no need to miss meals or to become dehydrated. The plan may vary with individuals and with competition settings, but you should decide for yourself how much fluid you are likely to lose through sweating and how important it is for you to keep up carbohydrate levels during a round. Experiment in practice rounds under simulated competition conditions to determine both your needs and the best ways to meet them. Chapters 1 and 2 provide some guidelines for assessing fluid and carbohydrate needs.

Carbohydrate drinks such as sports drinks, fruit juice and soft drink provide a simple way of rehydrating and refuelling simultaneously. Work out a schedule of intake that keeps you feeling comfortable over the round. Aim for frequent intake of small amounts and keep drinks cool so they are more palatable. Other sports products that may help you refuel efficiently are gels and sports bars. Everyday foods such as sandwiches, fruit or muesli bars can provide additional or alternative ways to take in carbohydrate, and unless you are extremely nervous, these are not likely to cause gastric discomfort. See Chapters 4.6 and 4.7 for more details.

Despite the stress of competition, the golfer should aim to eat well before and after the day's competition. See Chapter 4.4 for discussion about suitable pre-event meals, and be prepared to promote recovery after each round by looking out for fluid and carbohydrate needs as soon as you have finished. This might mean having a snack before you go back out onto the practice fairways. Many players enjoy the '19th hole' (see below) as a chance to unwind. However, the goals of recovery require intake of carbohydrate, protein and fluid as first priority—see Chapter 5.

Life on the circuit

When you are travelling on the golf circuit, both within the country or overseas, meeting your nutritional needs can be a challenge. Whether you are eating in restaurants or catering for yourself, it is often difficult to get what you want at the right time. And to be at your best, both in spirit and in physical form, you need to be on top of your nutrition goals. Read the Tennis chapter for advice about nutrition while travelling. It will help you survey the likely nutritional challenges at your destination and to plan ahead to meet them. Taking a food supply from home is often a good idea, and you may also be able to make some meal arrangements ahead of time. Looking after your nutritional needs in a restaurant is likely to be a skill that golfers need to master early on. Handy hints for restaurant eating are found in the Profile below.

Alcohol

A golf game traditionally finishes at the '19th hole'—the bar in the club. It is also traditional to share a round with your golf partners. Of course this does not necessarily have to mean alcohol intake, but in most cases it probably does.

Read the comments about alcohol in Chapter 1.6. While there may be no harm in having a couple of drinks, it is easy to slip into the habit of drinking more than you need. It is probably better to avoid alcohol intake during tournaments—after all, you need all the skills and concentration you can muster.

Profile

Waiter—a healthy meal, please!

Most people eat at restaurants occasionally—and for that matter, on special occasions. Under these circumstances it is usual to relax everyday dietary rules and enjoy a special meal, or even to have a total splurge. However, for athletes on the circuit, where constant travel and hotel accommodation are the norm, eating out becomes a way of life.

When restaurants are your main source of food, it is important to know how to make the food you need for good nutrition turn up on your plate. This is even more crucial when your nutritional requirements are skewed by strenuous exercise—for example, if you are training intensively or engaged in heavy competition. In the competition setting, of course, the right food intake is crucial to enable you to perform at your best.

Typically, restaurant food is more 'exotic' than home cooking and takes nutritional liberties with the cuisine of the country or region it professes to represent. Therefore, it can be higher in fat, salt and sugar, and lower in carbohydrate and fibre than the optimal training diet discussed in Chapter 1. This presents an immediate problem, since it means an athlete in heavy training may not easily achieve her daily carbohydrate requirements. Weight gain may also result because of the temptation to overeat—fat, in particular.

Of course, this is not always the fault of the restaurant or its food. Many athletes cause their own problems by forgetting their nutritional goals and their usual meal patterns. Those who are normally happy with cereal and toast for breakfast may suddenly be seduced by the eggs Benedict on the menu, and three-course hot lunches may begin to replace the customary sandwiches and fruit.

Meal timing can also be a problem. Restaurant hours may not always suit your training or competition schedule. You may finish late at night, or need to start early in the morning, and find that you are out of step with the hospitality industry. Even if you appreciate that refuelling after a strenuous session with a speedy meal that includes carbohydrates, finding those carbohydrates might be another thing. You may find a restaurant open but then be stymied by the long delay before your order is taken and the food appears in front of you.

And then there is the matter of money. Unless you are a very successful athlete, or the restaurant visit is part of the circuit hospitality, you may find yourself making food decisions on the basis of financial rather than nutritional concerns.

For general considerations about eating on the circuit, see the Tennis chapter. Meanwhile, the following hints may help you to get the most out of restaurant eating—whether it be a one-off occasion or an everyday affair. Checklist 24.1 summarises some specific guidelines for eating out, while Table 24.1 provides tips for choosing well within particular cuisines, focusing on special tactics to ensure adequate carbohydrate intake and prevent excessive kilojoule intake for those at risk of weight gain.

CHECKLIST 24.1
Eating well in a restaurant

- Set nutritional goals for a restaurant meal according to its importance in the overall scheme of your performance. If it is a special or unusual occasion, you may decide to take a more relaxed attitude. However, if this is a crucial time in training or competition, or if you are eating out every day, choose food for its nutritional contribution rather than its taste appeal alone.
- It helps to be familiar with a restaurant. If you are in an unfamiliar area, ask advice—especially from other athletes.

- When you travel to a new place, scout around to see what restaurants are available. Being armed with some knowledge lets you plan in advance where you will eat. If you wait until you are tired and desperately hungry to look for or decide on a place, you probably won't make the best choice. Also, remember that many restaurants are run as a franchise or chain—if you find a good place in one city, you may be able to use its counterparts elsewhere on your travels.
- Bear in mind that restaurants are part of the hospitality industry and by rights should be pleased to provide the service you request. Don't be afraid to ask for your special needs—whether it be the timing of a meal or the type of food you would like.
- Make the most of being well known. If you or your fellow athletes eat regularly at a restaurant, it may be prepared to make up special menus or choices for you.
- There may be times when it is important to eat straight away, to promote rapid recovery or to conserve precious sleep time. To avoid long waits in a restaurant, try phoning the restaurant ahead of time to place your order. This can be especially useful if you are in a large group.
- Choose smorgasbord restaurants if you need speedier service or more freedom of choice. However, be prepared to stay focused and avoid the distraction of quantities and types of food that are not part of your dietary plan.
- If saving money is a priority, make up your own breakfast and lunch meals from easy-to-prepare foods that you can buy or keep in your room. Make the most of dinner in a restaurant to maintain variety and make up for any nutritional shortfalls in the other meals. (Of course, depending on your schedule, you may like to make lunch the main meal of the day.)
- If body fat is an issue, use special tactics to keep your choices within your kilojoule budget:
    - Split large dishes with a friend or order a few dishes to share (and take care to eat only what you need)

- Stick to two courses—a main course and a light dessert (fruit or sorbet), or a light or vegetable soup and a small main or entrée
- Consider a skim-milk hot chocolate as a sweet alternative to dessert
- Avoid finger-food starters and garlic breads. Use the bread basket to add fuel to your meal if it is lacking in fuel choices, but don't just gobble it up because it is there and you are bored
- At a buffet, survey what is on offer, and then serve yourself. Don't have a bit of everything, and don't come back for seconds!
- Add a salad to meals to make them filling and nutritious. Avoid sun-dried and oil-marinated vegetables. Ask for a low-fat dressing, or balsamic vinegar or lemon juice and cracked pepper. At worst, ask for the dressing on the side, so you can add a small amount yourself.

TABLE 24.1
Gold-medal eating in restaurants

Restaurant	Deadliest dishes—eat at your peril!	Best low-fat options	Fuelling up with carbohydrates
Chinese Restaurants vary with the amount of oil used in cooking stir-fries	• Fried finger foods • Stir-fries with battered items	• Starters—chicken and sweet corn soup or broths • Stir-fries with beef, chicken, seafood and vegetables, added as a thin topping to plain rice. Keep to a 2 to 1 ratio of rice to topping A few words about banquets and shared eating: • Skip the fried finger foods and start with the soup • Pace yourself for a set number of bowls. Add a bed of plain rice to your bowl and top with a little of the main dishes that are suitable. Don't keep filling up or grazing from all that is on offer	• Plain rice
Mexican Unfortunately, Mexican restaurant food is usually high in fat	• Nachos—especially 'supreme' with cheese, sour cream, guacamole • Chimichanga (fried burrito)	The best choice: • Fajitas by far! Enjoy chicken/beef/seafood wrapped in soft tortilla 'bread'. Add sizzling capsicum and onion, lettuce, tomato, salsa, but go easy on the guacamole, sour cream and fried rice	• Soft tortillas—ask for a stack to go with the 'free' salsa on the table, or to accompany dips

Restaurant	Deadliest dishes—eat at your peril!	Best low-fat options	Fuelling up with carbohydrates

• corn chips and hard taco shells are fried in oil
• meals come with cheese, sour cream, beans and rice cooked in lots of oil
 	
The good part is that spicy salsas and chillies are low in fat and can dress up a meal to make it tasty (and hard to overeat)
	• Challupa (deep fried tortilla)
	• Con queso (cheese) dips
	• Relleno (deep fried capsicums)
		Not too bad strategy:
		• Order several single items to make up your own meal rather than the combination plate with lots of high fat extras
		  • Grilled/oven-baked tortillas and burritos—beef/chicken/ fish/prawn fillings
		  • Tostadas—chicken/beef/bean with lots of lettuce, tomato, a sprinkle of cheese, and a small dollop of guacamole on a single tostada base. No sour cream!
		  • Salad—ask for a low-fat dressing, or add your own topping of lemon juice and black pepper or salsa.
		  • Main meal salads (often in a tortilla basket). Beef/chicken/prawns tossed through lettuce, tomato, capsicum etc. Don't eat the fried basket!
		  • Grilled fish or chicken options are often available on larger menus
		At worst, cut back on the sour cream, cheese and guacamole added to meals
			• Ask for plain (non-fried) rice and plain beans (not refried)

Restaurant	Deadliest dishes—eat at your peril!	Best low-fat options	Fuelling up with carbohydrates
Indian	• Fried finger foods • Curries made with coconut milk and ghee very fatty • Nan, chapatti, kulcha and roti breads—these are all fried, and may range from moderate to high in fat	• Tandoori-baked meats • Tikka sauces, masala, vindaloo • Other plain stir-fries and curries without coconut milk/ghee, added as a topping to rice • Ask whether breads can be prepared with minimal oil • Shared eating—see notes on Chinese food	• Plain rice • Breads that are grilled or lightly 'dry fried'
Thai	• Fried finger food • Many dishes have coconut milk and peanut/satay sauces—these are high in fat	• Steamed finger foods—dumplings • Broth-based soups • Stirfries without coconut milk or satay, added as a topping to rice	• Plain rice • Plain noodles
Japanese Many of the items on the Japanese menu are light and low in fat	• Tempura (Battered)	Many items on the menu are low in fat • Sushi and rice rolls • Stir-fries, including teppanyaki • Noodle soups and dishes Spice up the meal with wasabi to make it tasty and hard to overeat	• Plain rice

Restaurant	Deadliest dishes—eat at your peril!	Best low-fat options	Fuelling up with carbohydrates
Italian Most creamy sauces are deadly—with oil, butter, cream and cheese	• Pasta with creamy sauces—alfredo, primavera, carbonara • Most lasagnes are topped with a white sauce and cheese. In many cases, the meat layer is also very oily. • Parmigiana (deep fried and coated with cheese and ham) • 'Frito' = fried	• Minestrone and clear soups • Pastas with a 'red sauce'—marinara, vongole (clams + marinara), arrabiata (spicy tomato) puttanesca (olives, tomato, mushrooms and basil), bolognaise, chicken + tomato • Keep to sauces with lean meat/chicken/seafood rather than salami and processed meals • Don't feel the need to eat gigantic serves—Consider entrée size serves or leave some in your bowl • Add a salad • Non-cream based risottos with plenty of veggies	Pasta or risotto with low-fat cooking style • Plain bread rather than garlic bread • Sorbet for dessert
Pizza	• Cheese stuffed crusts • Meat lovers' special • Sausage and processed meats • Garlic bread	• Thin or medium crust pizzas with ham/chicken/seafood and vegetable toppings (mushrooms, tomatoes, onion, corn, pineapple • Gourmet pizza places often have a better range of healthy toppings and let you create your own • If you are buying takeaway, consider taking it home and making up a quick salad. This way you can eat less pizza without feeling hungry	• Pizza crusts are a good source of carbohydrate. However, pan-fried thick-based and stuffed crusts are full of extra fat

Restaurant	Deadliest dishes—eat at your peril!	Best low-fat options	Fuelling up with carbohydrates
Fish 'n' chips	• Battered, deep fried fish • Skinny fries	• Grilled fish—no batter • Small serve of wedges with salsa (no sour cream) • Salad with low-fat dressing/ balsamic vinegar/ lemon juice + cracked pepper	Plain bread
Hamburger	• The 'works' • Double beef patties, cheese melts, bacon etc. • Do you want fries with that? • Meal deals • 'Upsize' or 'supersize'	• Hamburgers with a single beef patty or chicken breast and salad (skip the cheese, bacon, fried onion rings etc.) • Main meal salads	• Bread • Low-fat fruit smoothie
Sandwich bar	• Processed meats (salamis, bratwurst etc.) • Chicken and other chopped meats in a full-fat cream mayo. This often hides the crappy choice of meat as well as adding extra fat • Schnitzels	• Wraps, rolls and sandwiches are all great meals on the run • Lean meat/ham/chicken/tuna/salmon • Salad veggies (avoid sun-dried and oil-marinaded types) • Skip the butter and margarine • Low-fat dressings—light mayonnaise, salsa, spread of avocado, mustard • If full-fat mayo is the only option, keep it to a scrape • Ask for reduced-fat cheese if possible	• Bread • Low fat

ENDNOTES

Cycling

1 Lance Armstrong, *It's Not About the Bike*, Allen & Unwin, Sydney, 2000, p. 224

2 Lance Armstrong, *Every Second Counts*, Bantam Books, Sydney, 2003, p. 157

Rugby League and Union

1 AIS, *Survival from the Fittest, AIS Cookbook No. 1*, Allen & Unwin, Sydney, 1999

Football/soccer

1 The booklet can be downloaded from the FIFA website, http://www.fifa.com/aboutfifa/developing/medical/newsid=513876.html

Basketball

1 Hoffman et al. *International Journal of Sports Medicine*, 1995, 16:214–218

2 Dougherty et al. *Medicine and Science in Sports and Exercise*, 2006, 38 (9): 17650–58

3 Baker et al. *Medical Science of Sports and Exercise*, 2006, 35 (5):S177

INDEX

INDEX